Assessment & Treatment of New Addictions

Assessment & Treatment of New Addictions: Tools for Old Problems

Editors

Antoni Gual
Pablo Barrio
Laia Miquel

MDPI • Basel • Beijing • Wuhan • Barcelona • Belgrade • Manchester • Tokyo • Cluj • Tianjin

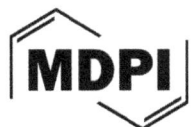

Editors
Antoni Gual
Hospital Clínic
Spain

Pablo Barrio
Hospital Clínic
Spain

Laia Miquel
Hospital Clínic
Spain

Editorial Office
MDPI
St. Alban-Anlage 66
4052 Basel, Switzerland

This is a reprint of articles from the Special Issue published online in the open access journal *Journal of Clinical Medicine* (ISSN 2077-0383) (available at: https://www.mdpi.com/journal/jcm/special_issues/Assessment_Treatment_Addictions).

For citation purposes, cite each article independently as indicated on the article page online and as indicated below:

LastName, A.A.; LastName, B.B.; LastName, C.C. Article Title. *Journal Name* **Year**, *Volume Number*, Page Range.

ISBN 978-3-03943-885-3 (Hbk)
ISBN 978-3-03943-886-0 (PDF)

© 2020 by the authors. Articles in this book are Open Access and distributed under the Creative Commons Attribution (CC BY) license, which allows users to download, copy and build upon published articles, as long as the author and publisher are properly credited, which ensures maximum dissemination and a wider impact of our publications.

The book as a whole is distributed by MDPI under the terms and conditions of the Creative Commons license CC BY-NC-ND.

Contents

About the Editors vii

Pablo Barrio, Laia Miquel and Antoni Gual
Comments from the Editors on the Special Issue "Assessment and Treatment of Addictions: New Tools for Old Problems"
Reprinted from: *J. Clin. Med.* **2019**, *8*, 1717, doi:10.3390/jcm8101717 1

Maria Garbusow, Stephan Nebe, Christian Sommer, Sören Kuitunen-Paul, Miriam Sebold, Daniel J. Schad, Eva Friedel, Ilya M. Veer, Hans-Ulrich Wittchen, Michael A. Rapp, Stephan Ripke, Henrik Walter, Quentin J. M. Huys, Florian Schlagenhauf, Michael N. Smolka and Andreas Heinz
Pavlovian-To-Instrumental Transfer and Alcohol Consumption in Young Male Social Drinkers: Behavioral, Neural and Polygenic Correlates
Reprinted from: *J. Clin. Med.* **2019**, *8*, 1188, doi:10.3390/jcm8081188 3

Alexandra Ghiţă, Olga Hernández-Serrano, Yolanda Fernández-Ruiz, Miquel Monras, Lluisa Ortega, Silvia Mondon, Lidia Teixidor, Antoni Gual, Bruno Porras-García, Marta Ferrer-García and José Gutiérrez-Maldonado
Cue-Elicited Anxiety and Alcohol Craving as Indicators of the Validity of ALCO-VR Software: A Virtual Reality Study
Reprinted from: *J. Clin. Med.* **2019**, *8*, 1153, doi:10.3390/jcm8081153 17

Ivan Herreros, Laia Miquel, Chrysanthi Blithikioti, Laura Nuño, Belen Rubio Ballester, Klaudia Grechuta, Antoni Gual, Mercè Balcells-Oliveró and Paul Verschure
Motor Adaptation Impairment in Chronic Cannabis Users Assessed by a Visuomotor Rotation Task
Reprinted from: *J. Clin. Med.* **2019**, *8*, 1049, doi:10.3390/jcm8071049 33

Pablo Barrio, Lidia Teixidor, Magalí Andreu and Antoni Gual
What Do Real Alcohol Outpatients Expect about Alcohol Transdermal Sensors?
Reprinted from: *J. Clin. Med.* **2019**, *8*, 795, doi:10.3390/jcm8060795 45

Stefano Cardullo, Luis Javier Gomez Perez, Linda Marconi, Alberto Terraneo, Luigi Gallimberti, Antonello Bonci and Graziella Madeo
Clinical Improvements in Comorbid Gambling/Cocaine Use Disorder (GD/CUD) Patients Undergoing Repetitive Transcranial Magnetic Stimulation (rTMS)
Reprinted from: *J. Clin. Med.* **2019**, *8*, 768, doi:10.3390/jcm8060768 53

Pablo Barrio, Carlos Roncero, Lluisa Ortega, Josep Guardia, Lara Yuguero and Antoni Gual
The More You Take It, the Better It Works: Six-Month Results of a Nalmefene Phase-IV Trial
Reprinted from: *J. Clin. Med.* **2019**, *8*, 471, doi:10.3390/jcm8040471 63

Hyera Ryu, Ji Yoon Lee, A Ruem Choi, Sun Ju Chung, Minkyung Park, Soo-Young Bhang, Jun-Gun Kwon, Yong-Sil Kweon and Jung-Seok Choi
Application of Diagnostic Interview for Internet Addiction (DIA) in Clinical Practice for Korean Adolescents
Reprinted from: *J. Clin. Med.* **2019**, *8*, 202, doi:10.3390/jcm8020202 71

Jia-yan Chen, Jie-pin Cao, Yun-cui Wang, Shuai-qi Li and Zeng-zhen Wang
A New Measure for Assessing the Intensity of Addiction Memory in Illicit Drug Users: The Addiction Memory Intensity Scale
Reprinted from: *J. Clin. Med.* **2018**, *7*, 467, doi:10.3390/jcm7120467 83

Zisis Bimpisidis and Åsa Wallén-Mackenzie
Neurocircuitry of Reward and Addiction: Potential Impact of Dopamine–Glutamate Co-release as Future Target in Substance Use Disorder
Reprinted from: *J. Clin. Med.* **2019**, *8*, 1887, doi:10.3390/jcm8111887 . . . . **99**

Andreas Heinz, Anne Beck, Melissa Gül Halil, Maximilian Pilhatsch, Michael N. Smolka and Shuyan Liu
Addiction as Learned Behavior Patterns
Reprinted from: *J. Clin. Med.* **2019**, *8*, 1086, doi:10.3390/jcm8081086 . . . . **133**

Albert Batalla, Hella Janssen, Shiral S. Gangadin and Matthijs G. Bossong
The Potential of Cannabidiol as a Treatment for Psychosis and Addiction: Who Benefits Most? A Systematic Review
Reprinted from: *J. Clin. Med.* **2019**, *8*, 1058, doi:10.3390/jcm8071058 . . . . **143**

About the Editors

Antoni Gual is a psychiatrist, Head of the Addictions Unit at the Neurosciences Institute, Clinic Hospital, University of Barcelona, Spain; and also acts as Alcohol Consultant at the Health Department of Catalonia. He has coordinated several EU funded projects in the field of addictions and has also been PI of several pharmacological clinical trials. He has published more than 150 articles in peer reviewed journals and edited several books. He is Vicepresident of the International Network on Brief Interventions for Alcohol Problems (INEBRIA), past-President of the European Federation of Addiction Scientific Societies (EUFAS) and past-President of the Spanish Scientific Society for the Study of Alcohol and Alcoholism.

Pablo Barrio is a Psychiatrist in the Addiction Unit at Hospital Clínic of Barcelona, Spain and an IDIBAPS researcher. He completed her Ph.D in 2017 at the University of Barcelona, focused on alcohol biomarkers and its clinical implications, which is currently one of his focus of research. He is also interested on the effects of drug use on mental health and psychiatric comorbidities. He is a member of the Spanish Network on Addictive Disorders (RTA)

Laia Miquel is a Psychiatrist in the Addiction Unit at Hospital Clínic of Barcelona, Spain and an IDIBAPS researcher. She completed her Ph.D in 2018 at the University of Barcelona. Her current work focuses on epidemiological, clinical and treatment aspects of alcohol cannabis and other substance of use. As a clinician actually involved in neuroscience research, her ultimate goal is to find novel diagnostic and therapeutic tools integrating biological and clinical measures to reduce the suffering of patients with cannabis, cocaine and alcohol use disorders. More recently, is working on psychological trauma in individuals suffering from addictive disorders. She is a member of the Spanish Network on Addictive Disorders (RTA) and the Catalan Research Workgroup on Women's Mental Health in the Catalan Society of Psichiatry and Mental Health. She is also a board member of the society Socidrogalcohol in Catalonia.

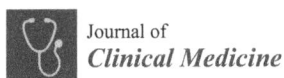

Editorial

Comments from the Editors on the Special Issue "Assessment and Treatment of Addictions: New Tools for Old Problems"

Pablo Barrio [1,2], Laia Miquel [1,2] and Antoni Gual [1,2,*]

1. Grup de Recerca en Addiccions Clínic (GRAC), Addiction Unit Hospital Clínic of Barcelona, Department of Psychiatry, 08036 Barcelona, Spain; PBARRIO@clinic.cat (P.B.); laiamiqueldemontagut@gmail.com (L.M.)
2. Institut d'Investigacions Biomèdiques August Pi i Sunyer (IDIBAPS), 08036 Barcelona, Spain
* Correspondence: agual@clinic.cat; Tel.: +34-932-271-719

Received: 15 October 2019; Accepted: 16 October 2019; Published: 17 October 2019

Abstract: New conceptual and technological solutions have been proposed to solve addictive disorders and will be presented in the future. In this Special Issue, we present some of the new assessment tools and treatment options for internet addiction, alcohol, cannabis, cocaine, and gambling disorders.

Keywords: addiction; craving; treatment; assessment instruments; digital health

Addiction represents an enormous challenge to society. Worldwide, it has been estimated that alcohol, tobacco, and illicit drugs were responsible for more than 10 million deaths [1], with a higher impact in developed countries where substance use disorders have been identified as responsible for life expectancy reversals [2]. Societal and medical responses to the problem are far from optimal, but the appearance of new technologies offers room for improvement, with lots of new initiatives launched and developed. This special issue is intended to describe and discuss how these new tools are helping to improve the assessment and treatment of such old problems (addictive disorders), covering a wide diversity of novelties that are being applied in the field.

Digital health entails the possibility to overcome existent problems around addictive disorders like stigmatization, addiction identification, treatment access, adherence and treatment efficacy by facilitating the improvement in knowledge, assessment, diagnosis, and treatment of addictive disorders. Assessment is one of the areas where new solutions have probably reached furthest. Think, for example, about transdermal sensors and ecological momentary assessment: a clear example of how new technologies can reach the core of a patient's drinking pattern. In this special issue, Barrio et al. investigate patients' attitudes towards transdermal sensors in real clinical settings. Digital technologies might be useful to assess brain damage, and they bring us closer to understanding the mechanism(s) underlying addiction. Herreros et al. present a visuomotor rotation task which might be the first step towards developing a useful tool for the detection of cerebellum dysfunction by assessing alterations in implicit learning among chronic cannabis users. New technologies have opened up the possibility of not only assessing patients "right here right now" but also of creating new realities, or should we better say virtual realities? Ghiţă et al. show us that virtual reality can enhance the assessment of alcohol-induced craving and anxiety. Technological advances in neuroimaging and genetics have allowed deepening in the understanding of some learning processes involved in substance use disorders. Garbusow et al. provide knowledge on how important processes, such as instrumental responses to relevant stimuli, are influenced by drinking patterns. In this same line, Heinz et al. conduct a review that starts with how Pavlovian and instrumental learning mechanisms interact in drug addiction and finishes with how these learning mechanisms and their respective neurobiological correlates can contribute to losing versus regaining control over drug intake.

Paradoxically enough, new technologies do also have their own risks. Take, for example, internet gaming disorder. Ryu et al. present the development of a new assessment instrument for internet addiction, the Diagnostic Interview for Internet Addiction. And keeping in mind that new psychometric instruments are also new solutions to old problems, Chen et al. investigate an interesting phenomenon in addiction: the intensity of memory addiction. They present us the development of the Addiction Memory Intensity Scale.

In the treatment area, this special issue offers an interesting combination of modalities: newly designed pharmaceutical compounds (nalmefene), naturally occurring psychoactive substances (cannabidiol), and non-pharmacological, biological therapies (rTMS). Barrio et al. report the main effectiveness analysis of a phase-IV study conducted among alcohol dependent outpatients taking nalmefene, the only approved medication for alcohol reduction aims. The use of rTMS is presented by Cardullo et al. in a sample of cocaine and gambling patients. The stimulation of the left dorsolateral prefrontal cortex yields promising results. Finally, Batalla et al. review the potential use of cannabidiol in addictive and comorbid psychotic disorders, pointing to a prominent role in the treatment of cannabis addiction.

Scientific advances and new technologies are providing new tools that let us expand our knowledge, and improve diagnosis and treatment of addictive behaviors, presenting us with opportunity for success and giving people back their health.

Conflicts of Interest: Laia Miquel has received honoraria and travel grants from Lundbeck and Neuraxpharm. Antoni Gual has received honoraria and travel grants from Lundbeck, Janssen, D&A Pharma and Servier. Pablo Barrio has received honoraria from Lundbeck.

References

1. Anderson, P.; Gual, A.; Rehm, J. Reducing the health risks derived from exposure to addictive substances. *Curr. Opin. Psychiatry* **2018**, *31*, 333–341. [CrossRef] [PubMed]
2. Rehm, J.; Anderson, P.; Fischer, B.; Gual, A.; Room, R. Policy implications of marked reversals of population life expectancy caused by substance use. *BMC Med.* **2016**, *10*, 14–42. [CrossRef] [PubMed]

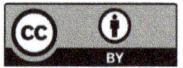

© 2019 by the authors. Licensee MDPI, Basel, Switzerland. This article is an open access article distributed under the terms and conditions of the Creative Commons Attribution (CC BY) license (http://creativecommons.org/licenses/by/4.0/).

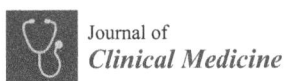

Article

Pavlovian-To-Instrumental Transfer and Alcohol Consumption in Young Male Social Drinkers: Behavioral, Neural and Polygenic Correlates

Maria Garbusow [1,*,†], Stephan Nebe [2,3,4], Christian Sommer [2], Sören Kuitunen-Paul [5,6], Miriam Sebold [1,7], Daniel J. Schad [1,7], Eva Friedel [1,8], Ilya M. Veer [1], Hans-Ulrich Wittchen [5,9], Michael A. Rapp [7], Stephan Ripke [1,10,11], Henrik Walter [1], Quentin J. M. Huys [12], Florian Schlagenhauf [1,13], Michael N. Smolka [2,3] and Andreas Heinz [1]

1. Department of Psychiatry and Psychotherapy, Charité-Universitätsmedizin Berlin, 10117 Berlin, Germany
2. Department of Psychiatry and Psychotherapy, Technische Universität Dresden, 01307 Dresden, Germany
3. Neuroimaging Center, Technische Universität Dresden, 01187 Dresden, Germany
4. Zurich Center for Neuroeconomics, Department of Economics, University of Zurich, 8006 Zurich, Switzerland
5. Institute of Clinical Psychology and Psychotherapy, Technische Universität Dresden, 01187 Dresden, Germany
6. Department of Child and Adolescent Psychiatry and Psychotherapy, Faculty of Medicine, University Hospital Carl Gustav Carus, 01307 Dresden, Germany
7. Social and Preventive Medicine, Area of Excellence Cognitive Sciences, University of Potsdam, 14469 Potsdam, Germany
8. Berlin Institute of Health (BIH), 10117 Berlin, Germany
9. Department of Psychiatry and Psychotherapy, Ludwig-Maximilians-Universität München, 80336 München, Germany
10. Analytic and Translational Genetics Unit, Massachusetts General Hospital, Boston, MA 02114, USA
11. Stanley Center for Psychiatric Research, Broad Institute of MIT and Harvard, Cambridge, MA 02142, USA
12. Division of Psychiatry and Max Planck UCL Centre for Computational Psychiatry and Ageing Research, University College London, London WC1E 6BT, UK
13. Max Planck Institute for Human Cognitive and Brain Sciences, 04103 Leipzig, Germany
* Correspondence: maria.garbusow@charite.de; Tel.: +49-30-450-517-257
† Corporate member of Freie Universität Berlin, Humboldt-Universität zu Berlin, and Berlin Institute of Health, Campus Charité Mitte.

Received: 29 June 2019; Accepted: 6 August 2019; Published: 8 August 2019

Abstract: In animals and humans, behavior can be influenced by irrelevant stimuli, a phenomenon called Pavlovian-to-instrumental transfer (PIT). In subjects with substance use disorder, PIT is even enhanced with functional activation in the nucleus accumbens (NAcc) and amygdala. While we observed enhanced behavioral and neural PIT effects in alcohol-dependent subjects, we here aimed to determine whether behavioral PIT is enhanced in young men with high-risk compared to low-risk drinking and subsequently related functional activation in an a-priori region of interest encompassing the NAcc and amygdala and related to polygenic risk for alcohol consumption. A representative sample of 18-year old men ($n = 1937$) was contacted: 445 were screened, 209 assessed: resulting in 191 valid behavioral, 139 imaging and 157 genetic datasets. None of the subjects fulfilled criteria for alcohol dependence according to the Diagnostic and Statistical Manual of Mental Disorders-IV-TextRevision (DSM-IV-TR). We measured how instrumental responding for rewards was influenced by background Pavlovian conditioned stimuli predicting action-independent rewards and losses. Behavioral PIT was enhanced in high-compared to low-risk drinkers ($b = 0.09$, $SE = 0.03$, $z = 2.7$, $p < 0.009$). Across all subjects, we observed PIT-related neural blood oxygen level-dependent (BOLD) signal in the right amygdala ($t = 3.25$, $p_{SVC} = 0.04$, $x = 26$, $y = -6$, $z = -12$), but not in NAcc. The strength of the behavioral PIT effect was positively correlated with polygenic risk for alcohol consumption ($r_s = 0.17$, $p = 0.032$). We conclude that behavioral PIT and polygenic risk for alcohol consumption might be a biomarker for a subclinical phenotype of risky alcohol consumption, even if no drug-related stimulus is present. The association between behavioral PIT effects and the amygdala might point to habitual processes related to out PIT task. In non-dependent young social drinkers, the amygdala rather than the NAcc is activated during PIT; possible different involvement in association with disease trajectory should be investigated in future studies.

Keywords: Pavlovian-to-instrumental transfer; amygdala; alcohol; polygenic risk; high risk drinkers

1. Introduction

Problematic alcohol drinking patterns like bingeing or heavy drinking during adolescence and early adulthood are associated with severe psychological, social and health problems [1]. Therefore, elucidating mechanisms that underlie high-risk drinking in young adulthood is important. Here, we assess biological factors in relation to a behavioral phenomenon that has been associated with chronic alcohol consumption theoretically [2–4] and empirically [5,6]. Specifically, we focus on behavioral effects of Pavlovian-to-instrumental transfer and at risk alcohol consumption in young male social drinkers, neural correlations and the association to polygenic risk for alcohol consumption.

Alcohol intake has been shown to be promoted by positive and negative contexts [7,8]. One mechanism implicated in the influence of contexts on ongoing behavior is Pavlovian-to-instrumental transfer (PIT). In general PIT, appetitive Pavlovian cues promote instrumental responses while aversive Pavlovian cues reduce such responses or even promote withdrawal independent of reward types [9]. In specific PIT, Pavlovian cues promote instrumental behavior associated specifically with the same outcome [10]. In animal models of addiction, drug exposure increases general and specific behavioral PIT effects [11,12] and enhanced food-related behavioral PIT was predictive for subsequent stronger cue-induced reinstatement of alcohol seeking [13]. We have recently reported increased nondrug-related behavioral PIT in detoxified alcohol-dependent patients compared to age-and gender-matched social drinkers using monetary cues [5]. In this study, we ask whether similar differences in PIT are measurable in an independent and much younger cohort of male high-versus low-risk social drinkers. Previous studies have examined alcohol-specific behavioral PIT effects in social drinkers but did not assess the association between behavioral PIT effects and individual drinking patterns [14], nor did they find an association with subclinical alcohol dependence [15,16] or neural PIT correlates using electroencephalography (EEG) [16]. In contrast to these studies, we investigate nondrug-related PIT effects in young high-versus low-risk [17] social drinkers on a behavioral and neural level using functional magnetic resonance imaging (fMRI).

On a neural level, animal studies showed that the amygdala is a core region associated with behavioral PIT [10,18–20]. Moreover, the strength of behavioral PIT is positively correlated with dopaminergic neurotransmission in the ventral striatum [21], which in turn is known to be modulated by alcohol intake [22–24]. In humans, both the nucleus accumbens (NAcc) and amygdala are activated during PIT [25–27], and amygdala activation by alcohol cues has been positively correlated with craving in alcohol-dependent patients during an alcohol-approach bias task [28]. Interestingly, PIT-related activation of the NAcc, but not the amygdala, predicted relapse after detoxification in alcohol-dependent patients [5].

Many genes can be involved in phenotypes such as alcohol use with respectively small effect sizes [29]. Therefore, we used a polygenic risk approach to investigate the genetic influence on alcohol consumption and behavioral PIT in our sample. It has been shown that higher polygenic predisposition for alcohol problems predicts earlier initial alcohol consumption and early heavy drinking patterns, as well as more alcohol-related problems in independent samples [30–32]. We therefore aimed to investigate how a polygenic risk score (PRS) for alcohol consumption derived from an independent large genome-wide association study [33] is associated with alcohol consumption and behavioral PIT in our sample.

As we previously observed stronger nondrug-related behavioral PIT in alcohol-dependent patients compared to controls as well as a stronger PIT-related NAcc activation predicting relapse [5], we wanted to assess whether there are comparable differences in nondrug-related behavioral PIT between the two groups of young male high-versus low-risk drinkers. Therefore, we examined a non-clinical sample of young males and hypothesized (1) stronger nondrug-related behavioral PIT effects in high-compared to low-risk drinkers [17]; (2) PIT-related blood oxygen level-dependent (BOLD) activity in an a-priori region of interest (ROI) encompassing amygdala and NAcc; and (3) a positive association between alcohol-related polygenic risk [33] and both the strength of nondrug-related behavioral PIT and alcohol consumption in our sample.

2. Materials and Methods

2.1. Participants and Procedure

1974 males were randomly drawn from local registration offices in two sites (Berlin & Dresden, Germany [34]) shortly after their 18th birthday representing their local legal adult age. We screened 445 respondents via telephone. Exclusion criteria were left-handedness, history of major neurological or psychiatric disorders (except for nicotine dependence and alcohol abuse), current alcohol abstinence and MRI-specific contraindications. In total, 209 subjects were included and tested. After quality control, 191 behavioral, 139 imaging and 157 genetic datasets could be analyzed (see Figure 1). Subjects were descriptively comparable to similar cohorts drawn from the German general population (see Supplementary Table S1).

All participants were assessed with the Composite International Diagnostic Interview (CIDI) [35,36] according to the Diagnostic and Statistical Manual of Mental Disorders (DSM-IV-TR) [37] and completed a neuropsychological test battery. On a second appointment (mean = 8.5 (SD = 16.2) days later), participants performed a task battery during a functional magnetic resonance imaging (fMRI) scan. The experimental procedure comprised a two-step Markov decision making task [38,39] and the PIT task with nondrug-and drug-related contexts [40]. Blood samples for genetic analyses were taken at first (Berlin) or second (Dresden, after MRI scan) appointment. The study procedures (clinical trials identifier: NCT01744834) adhered to the Declaration of Helsinki and were approved by local ethics committees of Charité Universitätsmedizin Berlin (EA/1/157/11) and Technische Universität Dresden (EK 227062011). All participants gave written informed consent prior to participation.

2.2. Experimental Design

The PIT task consisted of four parts:

Instrumental training. Participants collected shells by repeated button presses receiving probabilistic feedback (see Figure 2A). To control for instrumental performance, participants trained until they reached a criterion of 80% correct choices over 16 trials (for a minimum of 60 or a maximum of 120 trials).

Pavlovian conditioning. Trials began with presenting for 3 s a compound stimulus consisting of fractal-like pictures and pure tones (conditioned stimulus, CS); followed by a 3 s delay, and finally an unconditioned stimulus (US: picture of a coin) for 3 s (see Figure 2B). Participants were instructed to memorize the pairings. All participants completed 80 trials.

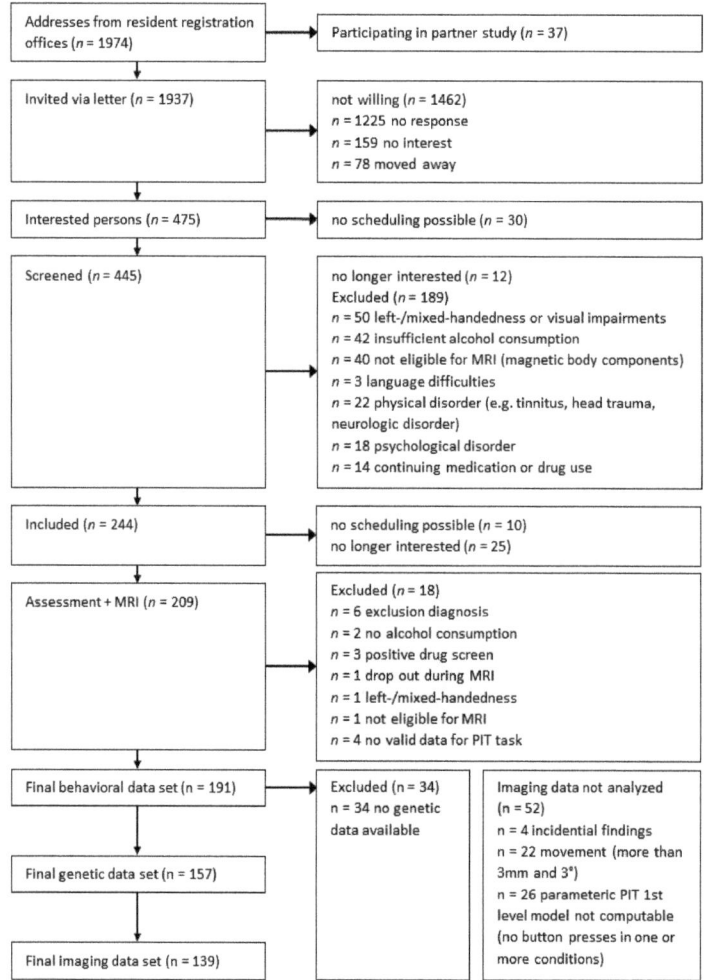

Figure 1. Recruiting and exclusion procedure leading to the final behavioral, genetic and imaging datasets. MRI: magnetic resonance imaging; PIT: Pavlovian-to-instrumental transfer.

Pavlovian-to-instrumental transfer. Participants performed the instrumental task now with CS tiling the background (see Figure 2C). Note that the instrumental task was independent of the value of the background stimulus. No outcomes were presented, but participants were instructed that their choices still counted towards the final monetary outcome. The pairings of CS in background und shell in foreground were counterbalanced with each combination showing three times, resulting in 90 trials.

Forced choice task. Finally, participants chose one of two CSs (Figure 2D). All possible CS pairings were presented three times in randomized order.

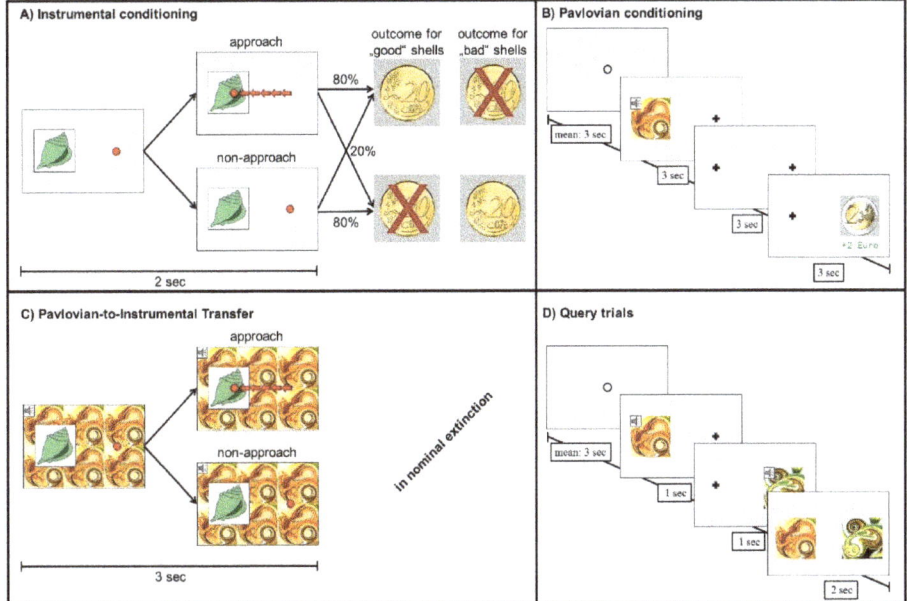

Figure 2. Pavlovian-to-instrumental Transfer (PIT) task. (**A**): Instrumental training: collecting a 'good' shell was rewarded in 80% while not collecting a 'good' shell punished in 80%. The opposite reinforcement contingencies applied to 'bad' shells. Red arrows indicate the five or more button presses required to approach and collect the presented shell. By trial and error, subjects learned to collect or not to collect three out of six shells. (**B**): Pavlovian conditioning: subjects passively viewed a conditioned stimulus (CS), which was deterministically followed by an unconditioned stimulus (US). As CS, a compound of a tone and five fractal-like visual stimulus was used. USs were pictures of a coin (−2€, −1€, 0€, +1€, +2€). (**C**): Transfer: subjects were asked for the instrumental response, while the background was tiled with the CS. Trials with drink-related background stimuli are not displayed. (**D**): Query trials: Subjects were asked to choose the better (i.e., that was associated with the highest reward or lowest punishment during Pavlovian conditioning) between sequentially presented CSs.

2.3. Self-Reported Questionnaires

We used self-reported measures for sample description measuring alcohol dependence severity (ADS) [41], alcohol craving (Obsessive Compulsive Drinking Scale, OCDS) [42] and nicotine dependence severity (Fagerström Test for Nicotine Dependence, FTND) [43].

2.4. Measures of Alcohol Consumption

In accordance with previous analyses of nondrug-related PIT group differences between alcohol-dependent patients and matched social drinkers [5], we used the World Health Organization (WHO) definition for risk of acute alcohol-related problems [17] based on average ethanol consumption on a drinking occasion within the last year. Accordingly, subjects qualified as low-risk drinkers (≤60 g of alcohol on a single occasion) or high-risk drinkers (>60 g), respectively. To further characterize participants' drinking behavior and how this relates to polygenic risk, we calculated a sum score of drinking variables (henceforth referred to as drink score) from the z-scaled CIDI items with higher values indicating higher or more risky alcohol consumption [44] (see supplementary materials for calculations "measures of alcohol consumption").

2.5. MRI Data Acquisition

Functional imaging was performed on a Siemens Trio 3 Tesla MRI scanner with an Echo Planar Imaging (EPI) sequences (repetition time, 2410 ms; echo time, 25 ms; flip angle, 80°; field of view, 192 × 192 mm^2; voxel size, 3 × 3 × 2 mm^3, 1 mm gap; 480 volumes) comprising 42 slices acquired in descending order and rotated approximately −25° to the bicommissural plane. For coregistration and normalization during pre-processing, a three-dimensional magnetization-prepared rapid gradient echo image was acquired (repetition time, 1900 ms; echo time, 2.52 ms; flip angle, 9°; field of view, 256 × 256 mm^2; 192 sagittal slices; voxel size, 1 × 1 × 1 mm^3). A field map was recorded to account for individual homogeneity differences of the magnetic field.

The PIT task was programmed using Matlab with the Psychophysics Toolbox Version 3 (PTB-3) extension [45]. Responses during PIT were made using a current-design MRI-compatible response box with the right index finger.

2.6. Polygenic Risk Score

To genotype our sample, DNA was extracted semi-automatically with a Chemagen Magnetic Separation Module (Perkin Elmer) from whole blood drawn in EDTA tubes before fMRI assessment. All samples were genotyped with the Illumina Infinium Psych Array Bead Chip [46]. Content for the PsychArray includes 265,000 proven tag SNPs found on the HumanCoreBeadChip, 245,000 markers from the Human Exome Bead Chip and 50,000 additional markers.

For calculating the polygenic risk score (PRS), we used a standard approach [47]. Our training data set derived from a large genome-wide association study (GWAS) investigating the genetic basis of alcohol consumption in $n > 105,000$ healthy social drinkers [33]. To calculate a polygenic risk score for each individual in our independent sample we summed up the number of alleles for each single nucleotide polymorphism (SNP) weighted by the effect size (association between each SNP and alcohol consumption) drawn from GWAS from the training data set. The score was computed at different p-value thresholds ($p = 1$, $p = 0.5$, $p = 0.2$, $p = 0.1$, $p = 0.05$, $p = 0.01$) representing the composite additive effect of all SNPs ($p = 1$, $n = 100,000$ SNPs) or the number of SNPs above the respective threshold. This gives the SNPs with higher significance automatically more weight than SNPs with lower significance.

2.7. Statistical Analysis

Data were analyzed in Matlab 2011a [48] and the R System for Statistical Computing Version 3.3.3 [49]. Functional magnetic resonance imaging (fMRI) data were analyzed using Statistical Parametric Mapping (SPM 12) software package [50]. All analyses refer to the transfer part of the PIT task (Figure 2C).

2.8. Behavioral Analysis

We conducted a generalized linear mixed-effects model implemented in the lme4 package (version 1.1-12). In order to assess the individual contribution of Pavlovian values on behavior, we built a Poisson distributed model where the number of button presses in each trial was predicted by the value of the background CS (−2, −1, 0, +1, +2; linear effect) and the instrumental condition (collect/not collect; coded as +0.5/−0.5). The within-subject factors (intercept, main effect of CS value, instrumental condition, and their interaction) were taken as random effects across subjects. Instrumental stimuli (shells) and Pavlovian CSs were taken as separate crossed random effects with varying intercepts in order to control for potential item effects. We included group (high-versus low-risk drinkers; coded as +0.5/−0.5) as between-subject factor to this model, performing two-tailed statistical tests on the a-priori hypothesis that behavioral PIT effects are stronger in high-compared to low-risk drinkers. Furthermore, we extracted individual regression slopes from the original generalized linear mixed-effects model as a measure of individual strength of behavioral PIT for further testing the association between the strength of the behavioral PIT effect and polygenic risk for alcohol consumption.

2.9. Imaging Analysis

Preprocessing. For preprocessing information see supplementary materials.

First-level analysis. The influence of Pavlovian stimulus values on instrumental responses (PIT effect) was measured by constructing a linear contrast, which weighted the parametric modulator of each condition (i.e., trial-by-trial number of button presses) by their associated Pavlovian values (−2, −1, 0, +1, +2) [5], i.e., the neural PIT effect was modeled by number of button presses times value of background stimulus (onset: appearance of shell in foreground). To account for variance caused by motor responses, button presses for all trials together were modeled with a regressor of no interest. Regressors were then convolved with the canonical hemodynamic response function. The six realignment parameters and their first derivatives were included as regressors of no interest. For a measure of the neural PIT effect a linear contrast was constructed, which weighted the parametric modulators for each condition by the related Pavlovian background value. The neural CS value effect was measured with a similar linear contrast on the CS event regressors.

Second-level analysis. Linear contrast images for neural PIT and neural CS contrasts were taken to the second level. To test for the neural PIT effect, we conducted a one-sample t-test. Study site was included as covariate. Using the wake Forest University (WFU) Pick Atlas software [51], we computed one ROI for a small volume correction (SVC) approach including both the bilateral NAcc and bilateral amygdala to avoid multiple testing. Next, we extracted individual mean beta values of the observed neural PIT effect to test the association of neural and individual behavioral PIT effect. We expected a positive association, yet conducted a two-tailed test.

2.10. Polygenic Analyses

We computed a PRS (see methods above), to verify genetic risk for alcohol consumption computed at threshold $p = 1$, thus including all genetic signal. To present the full picture, we also report results at other p-levels. Spearman's correlation coefficient was used to compute the respective association between PRS and (i) the continuous composite drink score, and (ii) behavioral PIT slope extracted from the glmer model described above. We expected a positive association between these measures and tested two-tailed. While the first analysis (i) provides evidence of whether the PRS is associated with drinking in our sample (replications see [30,31]), the second analysis (ii) explores a direct association between PRS and behavioral PIT (p-values for descriptive reasons only).

3. Results

3.1. Sample Characteristics by Drinking Group

Supplementary Table S2 summarizes sample characteristics comparing high-risk drinkers ($n = 94$) to low-risk drinkers ($n = 97$) according to WHO stratification [17]. Pure alcohol consumed in life in kg, ADS and OCDS are for clinical description of severity of alcohol use problems. According to that, high-risk drinkers reported higher lifetime alcohol intake, stronger craving in the past seven days and more problems associated with alcohol dependence. Groups did not differ significantly in terms of smoking severity, age, socio economic status and verbal intelligence.

3.2. Behavioral Results

Behavioral PIT effects were significantly stronger in high-compared to low-risk drinkers (for PIT effect in whole sample see supplementary material Figure S1). Specifically, the regression analyses showed an interaction effect between Pavlovian background and group on instrumental response rate ($b = 0.09$, $SE = 0.03$, $z = 2.7$, $p < 0.009$, $n = 191$, two-tailed; see Figure 3 and Supplementary Table S3) in the way that with higher value of the background stimulus the instrumental response rate increases. Crucially, this was not due to smoking severity (see Supplementary Table S4), or differences in instrumental performance ($p = 0.54$, see Supplementary Table S3).

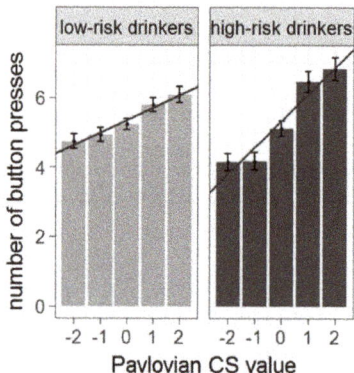

Figure 3. Behavioral PIT effect in low-versus high-risk drinkers ($n = 191$). Number of button presses for each Pavlovian background condition. The behavioral PIT effect is stronger in high-risk drinkers (as indicated by a steeper group regression slope).

3.3. Imaging Results

The ROI analysis (encompassing bilateral amygdalae and NAcc) for the whole sample revealed a significant PIT-related activation in the right amygdala ($t_{(137)} = 3.25$, $p_{SVC} = 0.04$, $x = 26$, $y = -6$, $z = -12$, $k = 29$, $n = 139$, see Figure 4A), which could not be explained by a pure CS effect (see Supplementary Figure S2). Extracted mean beta-values within the right amygdala showed a positive association with the behavioral PIT effect ($b = 0.07$, $SE = 0.014$, $z = 4.7$, $p < 0.001$, two-tailed, $n = 139$). High-versus low-risk drinkers according to the WHO did not differ significantly in neural activation during PIT. Within our single ROI, there was no significant activation in the NAcc. For exploratory whole brain analyses at $p_{uncorr} < 0.001$ and $k = 10$ see Supplementary Table S5.

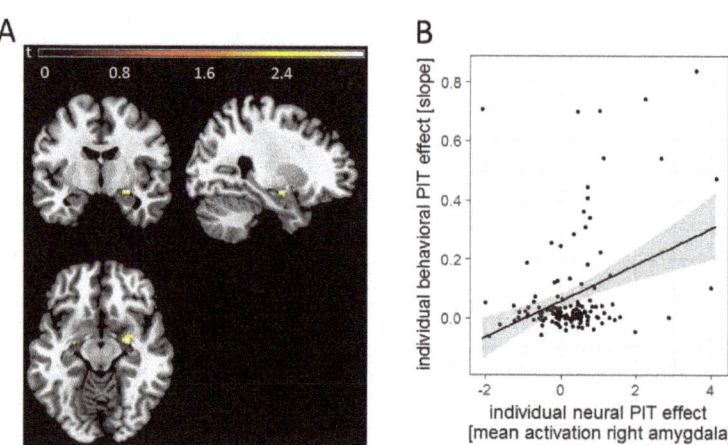

Figure 4. (**A**). Neural PIT effect in the right amygdala for the whole group ($n = 139$). For illustrational purposes, this effect was masked for the bilateral amygdala (region of interest (ROI) derived from wake Forest University (WFU) Pick Atlas). (**B**). The PIT-related activation in the right amygdala positively correlated with the behavioral PIT effect.

3.4. Polygenic Risk in Association with Behavioral PIT

We found a significant positive correlation between the PRS and the composite drink score in our sample ($r_s = 0.17$, $p = 0.032$, $n = 157$, two-tailed see Figure 5A). Figure 5B illustrates this association between polygenic risk and drink score in our sample using PRS computed at different thresholds ranging from $p = 0.01$ to $p = 1$. Furthermore, there was a significant positive correlation between the strength of the behavioral PIT effect and the PRS ($r_s = 0.17$, $p = 0.032$, $n = 157$, two-tailed, see Figure 5C). Figure 5D illustrates this association between polygenic risk and behavioral PIT using PRS computed at different thresholds ranging from $p = 0.01$ to $p = 1$. For a multi-level approach using multi-modal information (behavioral PIT, neural PIT effect and PRS), see Supplementary Table S6.

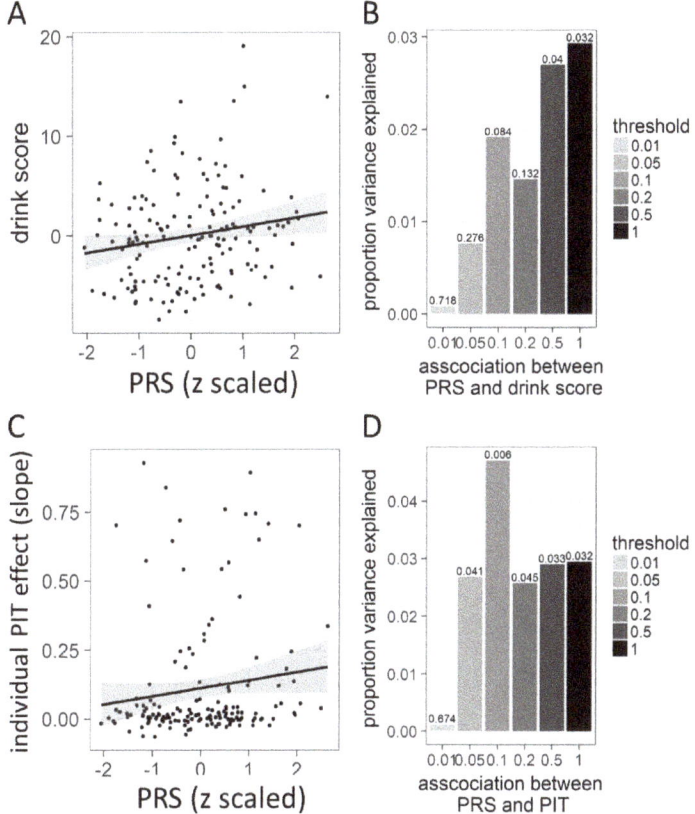

Figure 5. Polygenic risk score (PRS) for alcohol consumption in association with alcohol intake and PIT in our sample ($n = 157$). (**A**): Association between PRS and alcohol intake as measured by the drink score in our sample. (**B**): Explained variance of the association between PRS and drink score as indicated by r_s^2 for each threshold. Values at each bar represent the p-values, tested two-tailed. (**C**): Association between PRS and behavioral PIT effect slope. (**D**): Explained variance of the association between PRS and behavioral PIT slope as indicated by r_s^2 for each threshold. Values at each bar represent the *p*-values, tested two-tailed.

4. Discussion

We aimed to investigate the nondrug-related behavioral PIT effect in a cohort of young male high-versus low-risk [17] drinkers and the neural correlate of this PIT effect. We further explored the association of behavioral PIT with polygenic risk for alcohol consumption. Our main finding of enhanced behavioral PIT in high-risk drinkers suggests that strong effects of Pavlovian cues on instrumental behavior could be a core behavioral signature of risky alcohol consumption. We further observed PIT-related amygdala activation and a positive association between the strength of the behavioral PIT effect and polygenic risk related to alcohol consumption. A similarly assessed behavioral PIT effect was previously enhanced in alcohol-dependent patients compared to matched controls [5]. However, whether this is a vulnerability marker for developing alcohol use disorder or a consequence of substance exposure requests investigation in future longitudinal studies.

On a neurobiological level, we observed PIT-related activation in the right amygdala, which is in line with animal [52] and human studies [25,26,53], supporting previous reports of a key role for the amygdala in PIT [10]. Lesions of the basolateral amygdala abolished the selective excitatory effects of reward-related Pavlovian stimuli, while lesions of the central amygdala abolish general motivational effects of such cues [10]. A human study by Prevost et al. [26] confirmed the dissociation within the amygdala and general and specific PIT. Although our task has repeatedly identified Pavlovian modulation of instrumental responses [5,6,9], we cannot distinguish between general and specific PIT effects, as the reward used for Pavlovian and instrumental conditioning was both monetary, preventing conclusions about the specificity of the Pavlovian influence on instrumental behavior. Moreover, the amygdala was involved in cue-elicited habitual rather than goal-directed reward seeking in healthy humans [54]. Thus, our results on PIT effects in the amygdala might point to habitual processes that are related to enhanced PIT effects in our task.

Interestingly, PIT-related NAcc activity was related to poor treatment outcome in alcohol-dependent patients [5] supporting the known role of chronic alcohol intake on striatal dopaminergic neurotransmission [55], while in this sample of young at-risk drinkers, we could not observe PIT-related NAcc activity. This may suggest that the neurobiology by which CSs come to guide behavior is different in at risk alcohol consumption versus alcohol-dependent patients. The amygdala may be involved in cue-induced modulation of instrumental behavior among young adults and the NAcc might be associated with the nondrug-related PIT effect in alcohol dependence only. These biological differences may be associated with the shift from impulsive to habitual drug intake during the development of substance use disorders [3,56–58]. Further studies should assess whether these PIT activation differences are correlated with loss of control over alcohol intake.

Moreover, we observed alcohol-related polygenic risk to be associated with higher alcohol consumption in our sample. This effect is in line with numerous studies that emphasize a polygenic risk for risky alcohol consumption [30,31]. In addition, our study reveals that this polygenic risk is also related to a possible underlying mechanism associated with risky alcohol consumption, namely PIT. Thus, the strength of contextual stimuli in influencing ongoing instrumental behavior might be modulated by an underlying genotype for alcohol consumption, strengthening PIT to be a relevant mechanism to understand alcohol intake.

In terms of clinical implications, Ostafin et al. [59] showed that prevention programs boosting the explicit motivation to reduce alcohol consumption are only effective in hazardous drinkers with low automatic approach tendencies towards alcohol, and can even result in increased alcohol consumption if they fail to address implicit motivational processes [60]. Our data suggest that high-risk drinkers may be more susceptible to cue-triggered processes; this group may particularly profit from interventions focusing on implicit motivational processes to reduce hazardous alcohol consumption [61].

Limitations of our study include potential selection bias during recruitment: due to ethical guidelines, we were required to state in the invitation letter that we wish to recruit for a study on alcohol consumption. Subjects with high alcohol consumption might have been more reluctant to participate. Moreover, we excluded alcohol-dependent subjects, as we aimed to investigate PIT in social drinkers only. These two reasons might explain why most of our sample reported low life-time alcohol consumption (kg pure alcohol), a comparably small number of dependence problems as measured by the ADS as well as little numbers of DSM-IV-TR alcohol abuse diagnoses. Moreover, we focused on high risk for acute alcohol-related problems as defined by the WHO. Therefore, our data cannot make conclusions about chronic alcohol problems. In line with DSM 5, a dimensional approach to AUD has been applied, which needs to also identify risky variants at the lower end which might convert into high risk drinkers. Here, the reported study design is cross-sectional, which limits conclusions about how PIT effects change over the course of alcohol consumption and it limits mechanistic statements and explanations. Moreover, we included male subjects exclusively, thus limiting the generalization to female alcohol consumers. However, female drinking has been reported to be manifested in a different way that lack some of the very public and overt ways that male drinking presents [62]. We only assessed males to avoid loss of power due to potential gender differences; findings need to be replicated for women. Furthermore, as expected, especially the genetic effects sizes are rather small, which limits the predictive power on an individual level. Finally, we cannot draw conclusions about other substance-related disorders, as we focused our analyses on alcohol only.

In summary, we observed enhanced behavioral PIT effects in young high-risk drinkers, which were associated with functional activation in the right amygdala and correlated with an alcohol-related polygenic risk. Together with previous findings on behavioral PIT effects in alcohol-dependent patients [5], these data suggest that stronger behavioral PIT effects are a trait marker for high-risk alcohol use. How this is related to the risk of developing alcohol dependence should be further explored in longitudinal studies. Although the behavioral effects reported here were similar to the previously reported effects in patients, the neural correlates involved the amygdala rather than the NAcc [5], suggesting a differential involvement of these structures at different time points in the disease trajectory. Given the well-documented effects of alcohol on striatal dopaminergic neurotransmission [55], future studies should explore alcohol effects on striatal versus amygdala function and their malleability in longitudinal settings.

Supplementary Materials: The following are available online at http://www.mdpi.com/2077-0383/8/8/1188/s1, Figure S1: PIT effect in the whole sample (n = 191). Number of button presses are displayed relative to the zero (0€) condition. Grey line reflects the group regression slope, Figure S2: Pure CS effect during the PIT task. This effect was significant for the whole imaging group of n = 139 subjects in the right NAcc only (p_{SVC} = 0.041). Table S1: Comparing our study cohort to a reference population, Table S2: Sample characteristics for the two groups of low-and high-risk drinkers, Table S3: Regression coefficients indicating the influence of Pavlovian background conditions (−2€, −1€, 0€, +1€, +2€), instrumental conditions (collect versus not-collect) and drinking group, Table S4: Regression coefficients indicating the influence of Pavlovian background conditions (−2€, −1€, 0€, +1€, +2€), instrumental conditions (collect versus not-collect) and drinking group controlled for smoking severity, Table S5: Exploratory whole brain analysis of PIT-related activations, Table S6: Generalized linear mixed-effects model for predicting number of button presses as a function of instrumental task (collect versus not collect) and Pavlovian background stimulus value (−2€, −1€, 0€, +1€, +2€). Moreover, this analysis includes additional predictors, namely alcohol risk group, neural PIT effect and polygenic risk (n = 115).

Author Contributions: Conceptualization, M.G., E.F., I.M.V., H.-U.W., M.A.R., S.R., H.W., Q.J.M.H., F.S., M.N.S. and A.H.; Data curation, M.G., S.N., C.S., S.K.-P., M.S. and I.M.V.; Formal analysis, M.G., D.J.S. and F.S.; Funding acquisition, H.-U.W., M.A.R., Q.J.M.H., M.N.S. and A.H.; Investigation, M.G., S.N., S.K.-P. and M.S.; Methodology, M.G., S.K.-P., D.J.S., I.M.V., H.-U.W., M.A.R., S.R., Q.J.M.H. and F.S.; Project administration, M.G., S.N., S.K.-P. and E.F.; Resources, H.-U.W., M.A.R., H.W., M.N.S. and A.H.; Software, Q.J.M.H.; Supervision, H.-U.W., M.A.R., H.W., F.S., M.N.S. and A.H.; Validation, S.R., Q.J.M.H., F.S. and A.H.; Visualization, M.G.; Writing—original draft, M.G. and A.H.; Writing—review & editing, M.G., S.N., C.S., S.K.-P., M.S., D.J.S., E.F., I.M.V., H.-U.W., M.A.R., S.R., H.W., Q.J.M.H., F.S., M.N.S. and A.H.

Funding: This work was supported by the German Research Foundation (Deutsche Forschungsgemeinschaft, DFG, FOR 1617 grants FR 3572/1-1, HE 2597/13-1, HE 2597/13-2, HE 2597/15-1, HE 2597/15-2, RA 1047/2-1, SCHL 1969/2-2/4-1, SM 80/7-1, SM 80/7-2, WA 1539/7-1, WI 709/10-1, WI 709/10-2, as well as DFG grants SFB 940/1 and SFB 940/2). Eva Friedel is a participant in the BIH Charité Clinician Scientist Program funded by the Charité—Universitätsmedizin and the Berlin Institute of Health.

Acknowledgments: MR-imaging for this study was performed at the Berlin Center for Advanced Neuroimaging (BCAN) and Neuroimaging Centre (NIC) at TU Dresden. We acknowledge support from the German Research Foundation (DFG) and the Open Access Publication Fund of Charité—Universitätsmedizin Berlin.

Conflicts of Interest: The authors declare no conflict of interest.

References

1. Maggs, J.L.; Schulenberg, J.E. Initiation and course of alcohol consumption among adolescents and young adults. In *Recent Developments in Alcoholism: An Official Publication of the American Medical Society on Alcoholism, the Research Society on Alcoholism, and the National Council on Alcoholism*; National Institute on Alcohol Abuse and Alcoholism: Bethesda, MD, USA, 2005; Volume 17, pp. 29–47.

2. Robbins, T.W.; Everitt, B.J. Drug addiction: Bad habits add up. *Nature* **1999**, *398*, 567–570. [CrossRef] [PubMed]
3. Everitt, B.J.; Robbins, T.W. Neural systems of reinforcement for drug addiction: From actions to habits to compulsion. *Nat. Neurosci.* **2005**, *8*, 1481–1489. [CrossRef] [PubMed]
4. Everitt, B.J.; Robbins, T.W. Drug addiction: Updating actions to habits to compulsions ten years on. *Annu. Rev. Psychol.* **2016**, *67*, 23–50. [CrossRef] [PubMed]
5. Garbusow, M.; Schad, D.J.; Sebold, M.; Friedel, E.; Bernhardt, N.; Koch, S.P.; Steinacher, B.; Kathmann, N.; Geurts, D.E.; Sommer, C.; et al. Pavlovian-to-instrumental transfer effects in the nucleus accumbens relate to relapse in alcohol dependence. *Addict. Biol.* **2016**, *21*, 719–731. [CrossRef] [PubMed]
6. Sommer, C.; Garbusow, M.; Jünger, E.; Pooseh, S.; Bernhardt, N.; Birkenstock, J.; Schad, D.J.; Jabs, B.; Glockler, T.; Huys, Q.M.; et al. Strong seduction: Impulsivity and the impact of contextual cues on instrumental behavior in alcohol dependence. *Transl. Psychiatry* **2017**, *7*, e1183. [CrossRef] [PubMed]
7. Victorio-Estrada, A.; Mucha, R.F. The inventory of drinking situations (ids) in current drinkers with different degrees of alcohol problems. *Addict. Behav.* **1997**, *22*, 557–565. [CrossRef]
8. Heinz, A.J.; Beck, A.; Meyer-Lindenberg, A.; Sterzer, P.; Heinz, A. Cognitive and neurobiological mechanisms of alcohol-related aggression. *Nat. Rev. Neurosci.* **2011**, *12*, 400–413. [CrossRef] [PubMed]
9. Huys, Q.J.; Cools, R.; Golzer, M.; Friedel, E.; Heinz, A.; Dolan, R.J.; Dayan, P. Disentangling the roles of approach, activation and valence in instrumental and pavlovian responding. *PLoS Comput. Biol.* **2011**, *7*, e1002028. [CrossRef] [PubMed]
10. Corbit, L.H.; Balleine, B.W. Double dissociation of basolateral and central amygdala lesions on the general and outcome-specific forms of pavlovian-instrumental transfer. *J. Neurosci. Off. J. Soc. Neurosci.* **2005**, *25*, 962–970. [CrossRef] [PubMed]
11. LeBlanc, K.H.; Maidment, N.T.; Ostlund, S.B. Repeated cocaine exposure facilitates the expression of incentive motivation and induces habitual control in rats. *PLoS ONE* **2013**, *8*, e61355. [CrossRef] [PubMed]
12. Corbit, L.H.; Janak, P.H. Ethanol-associated cues produce general pavlovian-instrumental transfer. *Alcohol. Clin. Exp. Res.* **2007**, *31*, 766–774. [CrossRef] [PubMed]
13. Barker, J.M.; Torregrossa, M.M.; Taylor, J.R. Low prefrontal psa-ncam confers risk for alcoholism-related behavior. *Nat. Neurosci.* **2012**, *15*, 1356–1358. [CrossRef] [PubMed]
14. Hogarth, L.; Retzler, C.; Munafo, M.R.; Tran, D.M.; Troisi, J.R., 2nd; Rose, A.K.; Jones, A.; Field, M. Extinction of cue-evoked drug-seeking relies on degrading hierarchical instrumental expectancies. *Behav. Res. Ther.* **2014**, *59*, 61–70. [CrossRef] [PubMed]
15. Hardy, L.; Mitchell, C.; Seabrooke, T.; Hogarth, L. Drug cue reactivity involves hierarchical instrumental learning: Evidence from a biconditional pavlovian to instrumental transfer task. *Psychopharmacology* **2017**, *234*, 1977–1984. [CrossRef] [PubMed]
16. Martinovic, J.; Jones, A.; Christiansen, P.; Rose, A.K.; Hogarth, L.; Field, M. Electrophysiological responses to alcohol cues are not associated with pavlovian-to-instrumental transfer in social drinkers. *PLoS ONE* **2014**, *9*, e94605. [CrossRef] [PubMed]
17. World Health Organization; Department of Mental Health and Substance DependenceNoncommunicable Diseases. *International Guide for MONITORING Alcohol Consumption and Related Harm. Technical Document who/msd/msb/00.4*; World Health Organisation: Geneva, Switzerland, 2000.
18. Campese, V.D.; Kim, J.; Lazaro-Munoz, G.; Pena, L.; LeDoux, J.E.; Cain, C.K. Lesions of lateral or central amygdala abolish aversive pavlovian-to-instrumental transfer in rats. *Front. Behav. Neurosci.* **2014**, *8*, 161. [CrossRef] [PubMed]
19. Holland, P.C.; Hsu, M. Role of amygdala central nucleus in the potentiation of consuming and instrumental lever-pressing for sucrose by cues for the presentation or interruption of sucrose delivery in rats. *Behav. Neurosci.* **2014**, *128*, 71–82. [CrossRef]
20. McCue, M.G.; LeDoux, J.E.; Cain, C.K. Medial amygdala lesions selectively block aversive pavlovian-instrumental transfer in rats. *Front. Behav. Neurosci.* **2014**, *8*, 329. [CrossRef]
21. Wassum, K.M.; Ostlund, S.B.; Loewinger, G.C.; Maidment, N.T. Phasic mesolimbic dopamine release tracks reward seeking during expression of pavlovian-to-instrumental transfer. *Biol. Psychiatry* **2013**, *73*, 747–755. [CrossRef]
22. Di Chiara, G.; Bassareo, V. Reward system and addiction: What dopamine does and doesn't do. *Curr. Opin. Pharmacol.* **2007**, *7*, 69–76. [CrossRef]

23. Deserno, L.; Beck, A.; Huys, Q.J.; Lorenz, R.C.; Buchert, R.; Buchholz, H.G.; Plotkin, M.; Kumakara, Y.; Cumming, P.; Heinze, H.J.; et al. Chronic alcohol intake abolishes the relationship between dopamine synthesis capacity and learning signals in the ventral striatum. *Eur. J. Neurosci.* **2015**, *41*, 477–486. [CrossRef] [PubMed]
24. Volkow, N.D.; Wang, G.J.; Fowler, J.S.; Logan, J.; Hitzemann, R.; Ding, Y.S.; Pappas, N.; Shea, C.; Piscani, K. Decreases in dopamine receptors but not in dopamine transporters in alcoholics. *Alcohol. Clin. Exp. Res.* **1996**, *20*, 1594–1598. [CrossRef]
25. Talmi, D.; Seymour, B.; Dayan, P.; Dolan, R.J. Human pavlovian-instrumental transfer. *J. Neurosci. Off. J. Soc. Neurosci.* **2008**, *28*, 360–368. [CrossRef] [PubMed]
26. Prevost, C.; Liljeholm, M.; Tyszka, J.M.; O'Doherty, J.P. Neural correlates of specific and general pavlovian-to-instrumental transfer within human amygdalar subregions: A high-resolution fmri study. *J. Neurosci. Off. J. Soc. Neurosci.* **2012**, *32*, 8383–8390. [CrossRef] [PubMed]
27. Geurts, D.E.; Huys, Q.J.; den Ouden, H.E.; Cools, R. Aversive pavlovian control of instrumental behavior in humans. *J. Cogn. Neurosci.* **2013**, *25*, 1428–1441. [CrossRef] [PubMed]
28. Wiers, C.E.; Stelzel, C.; Park, S.Q.; Gawron, C.K.; Ludwig, V.U.; Gutwinski, S.; Heinz, A.; Lindenmeyer, J.; Wiers, R.W.; Walter, H.; et al. Neural correlates of alcohol-approach bias in alcohol addiction: The spirit is willing but the flesh is weak for spirits. *Neuropsychopharmacology* **2014**, *39*, 688–697. [CrossRef] [PubMed]
29. Manolio, T.A.; Collins, F.S.; Cox, N.J.; Goldstein, D.B.; Hindorff, L.A.; Hunter, D.J.; McCarthy, M.I.; Ramos, E.M.; Cardon, L.R.; Chakravarti, A.; et al. Finding the missing heritability of complex diseases. *Nature* **2009**, *461*, 747–753. [CrossRef]
30. Taylor, M.; Simpkin, A.J.; Haycock, P.C.; Dudbridge, F.; Zuccolo, L. Exploration of a polygenic risk score for alcohol consumption: A longitudinal analysis from the alspac cohort. *PLoS ONE* **2016**, *11*, e0167360. [CrossRef]
31. Kapoor, M.; Chou, Y.L.; Edenberg, H.J.; Foroud, T.; Martin, N.G.; Madden, P.A.; Wang, J.C.; Bertelsen, S.; Wetherill, L.; Brooks, A.; et al. Genome-wide polygenic scores for age at onset of alcohol dependence and association with alcohol-related measures. *Transl. Psychiatry* **2016**, *6*, e761. [CrossRef]
32. Li, J.J.; Cho, S.B.; Salvatore, J.E.; Edenberg, H.J.; Agrawal, A.; Chorlian, D.B.; Porjesz, B.; Hesselbrock, V.; Dick, D.M. The impact of peer substance use and polygenic risk on trajectories of heavy episodic drinking across adolescence and emerging adulthood. *Alcohol. Clin. Exp. Res.* **2017**, *41*, 65–75. [CrossRef]
33. Schumann, G.; Liu, C.; O'Reilly, P.; Gao, H.; Song, P.; Xu, B.; Ruggeri, B.; Amin, N.; Jia, T.; Preis, S.; et al. Klb is associated with alcohol drinking, and its gene product beta-klotho is necessary for fgf21 regulation of alcohol preference. *Proc. Natl. Acad. Sci. USA* **2016**, *113*, 14372–14377. [CrossRef] [PubMed]
34. Livingston, M.; Room, R. Variations by age and sex in alcohol-related problematic behaviour per drinking volume and heavier drinking occasion. *Drug Alcohol Depend.* **2009**, *101*, 169–175. [CrossRef] [PubMed]
35. Jacobi, F.; Mack, S.; Gerschler, A.; Scholl, L.; Hofler, M.; Siegert, J.; Burkner, A.; Preiss, S.; Spitzer, K.; Busch, M.; et al. The design and methods of the mental health module in the german health interview and examination survey for adults (degs1-mh). *Int. J. Methods Psychiatr. Res.* **2013**, *22*, 83–99. [CrossRef] [PubMed]
36. Wittchen, H.-U.; Pfister, H. *Dia-x-Interviews: Manual für Screening-Verfahren und Interview; Interviewheft Längsschnittuntersuchung (Dia-x-Lifetime); Ergänzungsheft (Dia-x-Lifetime); Interviewheft Querschnittuntersuchung (Dia-x-12 Monate); Ergänzungsheft (dia-x Monate); Pc-Programm zur Durchführung des Interviews (Längs- und Querschnittuntersuchung); Auswertungsprogramm*; Swets & Zeitlinger: Frankfurt, Germany, 1997.
37. Saß, H.; Wittchen, H.-U.; Zaudig, M.H.I. *Diagnostisches und Statistisches Manual Psychischer Störungen—Textrevision—Dsm-iv-tr*; Hogrefe: Göttingen, Germany, 2003.
38. Sebold, M.; Nebe, S.; Garbusow, M.; Guggenmos, M.; Schad, D.J.; Beck, A.; Kuitunen-Paul, S.; Sommer, C.; Frank, R.; Neu, P.; et al. When habits are dangerous: Alcohol expectancies and habitual decision making predict relapse in alcohol dependence. *Biol. Psychiatry* **2017**, *82*, 847–856. [CrossRef] [PubMed]
39. Daw, N.D.; Gershman, S.J.; Seymour, B.; Dayan, P.; Dolan, R.J. Model-based influences on humans' choices and striatal prediction errors. *Neuron* **2011**, *69*, 1204–1215. [CrossRef] [PubMed]
40. Garbusow, M.; Schad, D.J.; Sommer, C.; Jünger, E.; Sebold, M.; Friedel, E.; Wendt, J.; Kathmann, N.; Schlagenhauf, F.; Zimmermann, U.S.; et al. Pavlovian-to-instrumental transfer in alcohol dependence: A pilot study. *Neuropsychobiology* **2014**, *70*, 111–121. [CrossRef] [PubMed]
41. Skinner, H.A.; Horn, J.L. *Alcohol Dependence Scale (ads): Users Guide*; Addiction Research Foundation: Toronto, ON, Canada, 1984.

42. Mann, K.; Ackermann, K. Die ocds-g: Psychometrische kennwerte der deutschen version der obsessive compulsive drinking scale. *Sucht* **2000**, *46*, 90–100. [CrossRef]
43. Heatherton, T.F.; Kozlowski, L.T.; Frecker, R.C.; Fagerstrom, K.O. The fagerstrom test for nicotine dependence: A revision of the fagerstrom tolerance questionnaire. *Br. J. Addict.* **1991**, *86*, 1119–1127. [CrossRef]
44. Nebe, S.; Kroemer, N.B.; Schad, D.J.; Bernhardt, N.; Sebold, M.; Muller, D.K.; Scholl, L.; Kuitunen-Paul, S.; Heinz, A.; Rapp, M.A.; et al. No association of goal-directed and habitual control with alcohol consumption in young adults. *Addict. Biol.* **2017**, *23*, 379–393. [CrossRef]
45. Brainard, D.H. The psychophysics toolbox. *Spat. Vis.* **1997**, *10*, 433–436. [CrossRef]
46. Infinium PsychArray-24 Kit | Psychiatric Predisposition Microarray. Available online: https://www.illumina.com/products/by-type/microarray-kits/infinium-psycharray.html (accessed on 25 June 2019).
47. Purcell, S.M.; Wray, N.R.; Stone, J.L.; Visscher, P.M.; O'Donovan, M.C.; Sullivan, P.F.; Sklar, P. Common polygenic variation contributes to risk of schizophrenia and bipolar disorder. *Nature* **2009**, *460*, 748–752. [PubMed]
48. *Matlab*, version 7.12.0; The MathWorks Inc.: Natick, MA, USA, 2011.
49. R Development Core Team. *R: A Language and Environment for Statistical Computing*; R Foundation for Statistical Computing: Vienna, Austria, 2013.
50. Statistical Parametric Mapping. Available online: http://www.fil.ion.ucl.ac.uk/spm (accessed on 7 August 2019).
51. Pick Atlas Software. Available online: http://www.fmri.wfubmc.edu/download.htm (accessed on 7 August 2019).
52. Wassum, K.M.; Izquierdo, A. The basolateral amygdala in reward learning and addiction. *Neurosci. Biobehav. Rev.* **2015**, *57*, 271–283. [CrossRef]
53. Mendelsohn, A.; Pine, A.; Schiller, D. Between thoughts and actions: Motivationally salient cues invigorate mental action in the human brain. *Neuron* **2014**, *81*, 207–217. [CrossRef] [PubMed]
54. Van Steenbergen, H.; Watson, P.; Wiers, R.W.; Hommel, B.; de Wit, S. Dissociable corticostriatal circuits underlie goal-directed vs. Cue-elicited habitual food seeking after satiation: Evidence from a multimodal mri study. *Eur. J. Neurosci.* **2017**, *46*, 1815–1827. [CrossRef] [PubMed]
55. Boileau, I.; Assaad, J.M.; Pihl, R.O.; Benkelfat, C.; Leyton, M.; Diksic, M.; Tremblay, R.E.; Dagher, A. Alcohol promotes dopamine release in the human nucleus accumbens. *Synapse* **2003**, *49*, 226–231. [CrossRef]
56. Belin, D.; Mar, A.C.; Dalley, J.W.; Robbins, T.W.; Everitt, B.J. High impulsivity predicts the switch to compulsive cocaine-taking. *Science* **2008**, *320*, 1352. [CrossRef]
57. Robbins, T.W.; Gillan, C.M.; Smith, D.G.; de Wit, S.; Ersche, K.D. Neurocognitive endophenotypes of impulsivity and compulsivity: Towards dimensional psychiatry. *Trends Cogn. Sci.* **2012**, *16*, 81–91. [CrossRef]
58. Robinson, T.E.; Berridge, K.C. The neural basis of drug craving: An incentive-sensitization theory of addiction. *Brain Res. Brain Res. Rev.* **1993**, *18*, 247–291. [CrossRef]
59. Ostafin, B.D.; Palfai, T.P. When wanting to change is not enough: Automatic appetitive processes moderate the effects of a brief alcohol intervention in hazardous-drinking college students. *Addict. Sci. Clin. Pract.* **2012**, *7*, 25. [CrossRef]
60. Wiers, R.W.; Bartholow, B.D.; van den Wildenberg, E.; Thush, C.; Engels, R.C.; Sher, K.J.; Grenard, J.; Ames, S.L.; Stacy, A.W. Automatic and controlled processes and the development of addictive behaviors in adolescents: A review and a model. *Pharmacol. Biochem. Behav.* **2007**, *86*, 263–283. [CrossRef]
61. Wiers, R.W.; Eberl, C.; Rinck, M.; Becker, E.S.; Lindenmeyer, J. Retraining automatic action tendencies changes alcoholic patients' approach bias for alcohol and improves treatment outcome. *Psychol. Sci.* **2011**, *22*, 490–497. [CrossRef] [PubMed]
62. Erol, A.; Karpyak, V.M. Sex and gender-related differences in alcohol use and its consequences: Contemporary knowledge and future research considerations. *Drug Alcohol Depend.* **2015**, *156*, 1–13. [CrossRef] [PubMed]

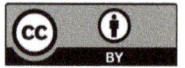 © 2019 by the authors. Licensee MDPI, Basel, Switzerland. This article is an open access article distributed under the terms and conditions of the Creative Commons Attribution (CC BY) license (http://creativecommons.org/licenses/by/4.0/).

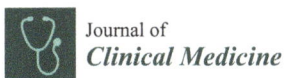

Article

Cue-Elicited Anxiety and Alcohol Craving as Indicators of the Validity of ALCO-VR Software: A Virtual Reality Study

Alexandra Ghiță [1], Olga Hernández-Serrano [2], Yolanda Fernández-Ruiz [1], Miquel Monras [3], Lluisa Ortega [3], Silvia Mondon [3], Lidia Teixidor [3], Antoni Gual [3], Bruno Porras-García [1], Marta Ferrer-García [1] and José Gutiérrez-Maldonado [1,*]

1. Department of Clinical Psychology and Psychobiology, University of Barcelona, Passeig de la Vall d' Hebron 171, 08035 Barcelona, Spain
2. Department of Physical Therapy, EUSES University of Girona, 17190 Salt, Spain
3. Addictive Behaviors Unit, Hospital Clinic of Barcelona, 08036 Barcelona, Spain
* Correspondence: jgutierrezm@ub.edu; Tel.: +34-933-125-124

Received: 17 July 2019; Accepted: 30 July 2019; Published: 2 August 2019

Abstract: Background: This study is part of a larger project aiming to develop a virtual reality (VR) software to be implemented as a clinical tool for patients diagnosed with alcohol use disorder (AUD). The study is based on previous research in which we identified factors that elicit craving for alcohol in a sample of AUD patients, and which led to the development of a virtual reality software to be used in cue exposure treatments of alcohol use disorder (ALCO-VR). The main objective of this study was to test the effectiveness of ALCO-VR to elicit cue-induced craving and anxiety responses among social drinkers (SD) and AUD patients. Our secondary objective was to explore which responses (cue-induced craving or anxiety) can best differentiate between AUD patients and the SD group. Method: Twenty-seven individuals (13 AUD patients and 14 SD) participated in this study after giving written informed consent. Their anxiety and alcohol craving levels were measured by different instruments at different stages of the procedure. The VR equipment consisted of Oculus Rift technology, and the software consisted of the ALCO-VR platform. Results: Our data indicate that the ALCO-VR software can elicit responses of anxiety and alcohol craving, especially in the group of AUD patients. The cue-induced anxiety response differentiated AUD patients and the SD group better than the cue-induced craving response. Conclusions: The general interest in applying new technologies to the assessment and treatment of mental health disorders has led to the development of immersive real-life simulations based on the advantages of VR technology. Our study concluded that the ALCO-VR software can elicit anxiety and craving responses and that cue-induced anxiety responses can distinguish between AUD and SD groups better than cue-induced craving. The data on craving and anxiety were assessed consistently by different instruments. In addition, we consider that ALCO-VR is able to ecologically assess cue-induced anxiety and alcohol craving levels during exposure to VR alcohol-related environments.

Keywords: ALCO-VR; virtual reality; cue-exposure; alcohol use disorder; alcohol craving; anxiety; social drinkers

1. Introduction

Alcohol misuse is considered to be a serious condition with important negative consequences at a personal and societal level [1–4]. Numerous studies have emphasized that excessive alcohol use may establish a solid basis for general heavy drinking patterns, binge-drinking episodes, and further development of alcohol use disorder (AUD) in adulthood [5–8]. In AUD, a substantial number of patients respond to treatment by accomplishing individual goals such as controlled drinking or total abstinence [9]. However, many individuals struggle with maintaining long-term abstinence; despite treatment, they experience relapses, especially in the first three months [10,11]. AUD is a complex disorder and many factors contribute to its development and maintenance. The current study focuses on the interplay between anxiety and alcohol craving as factors interfering in long-term abstinence.

Anxiety, ranging from momentary distress to a psychopathological diagnosis, is common in the majority of patients with AUD, and is considered a facilitating factor in the onset of alcohol consumption [12]. Anxiety is involved not only in the pre-phase of drinking behaviors, but is also a predominant symptom experienced during alcohol withdrawal in patients with AUD [13]. A growing and solid body of research has focused on understanding the phenomena underlying anxiety disorders and AUD, since individuals with dual diagnoses are more vulnerable in terms of recovery and maintaining abstinence [14–16]. A network modeling analysis revealed that anxiety-related states such as social anxiety and stress are directly engaged in craving elicitation in patients diagnosed with AUD [14]; thus, a strong causal relationship was established between anxiety and craving for alcohol, which further precipitates drinking behaviors and, implicitly, relapse. This new model explains the critical involvement of this causative relationship between anxiety and alcohol craving in patients diagnosed with AUD.

Alcohol craving, described in the literature as a "pathological appetite", is an unbearable desire to use alcohol [17] and has a crucial role in alcohol misuse behaviors [18]. Explained by the classical conditioning theory [19], alcohol craving is acquired through repetitive drinking behaviors accompanied by positive emotional valence [20]. Over the past two decades, laboratory research [21,22] and clinical research [23–25] have emphasized the strong relationship between proximity of alcohol-related stimuli that trigger alcohol craving. This context dependency theory indicates that alcohol-related stimuli gain incentive salience over time [26,27] and therefore, cues and contexts related to alcohol consumption emerge as high-risk stimuli for individuals who misuse alcohol [28]. A common method for exploring alcohol craving responses is based on the cue-exposure paradigm, which involves in vivo alcohol cue presentation, or exposure to photographic alcohol-related stimuli in non-realistic experimental or clinical settings [29]. Over the past years, an increasing interest in new technologies like virtual reality (VR) has led to the development of more ecologically valid methods to explore alcohol craving [30]. VR may add effectiveness to the classical cue-exposure paradigm by including multiple inputs like visual, auditory, olfactory or tactile stimuli, thus creating an immersive experience based on naturalistic daily-life contexts [31]. This three-dimensional (3D) system allows a high degree of interaction, which further increases the individual's level of momentary presence within the VR environment [32]. These are fundamental variables for developing ecological momentary assessment (EMA) instruments, particularly for its use in clinical settings, as most assessment instruments in clinical psychology rely on self-reported scales [33,34]. In drug cue reactivity, VR has been included in many protocols, primarily studying craving for alcohol [35,36], tobacco [37–39], methamphetamine [40] or cocaine [41]. In AUD, VR has also been implemented in the treatment of patients with the final aim of reducing craving levels and, implicitly, of preventing further relapses. A comprehensive review of the existing studies indicated that all studies focused on the applications of VR as a therapy tool showed consistent results in terms of craving reduction, thus favoring the inclusion of this technology in the treatment of substance use disorders [30].

The present study is based on the results of a previous study, in which we identified triggering factors for alcohol craving, aiming to develop significant VR alcohol-related environments. Our main objective was to validate the ALCO-VR platform (a virtual reality software to be used in cue exposure treatments of alcohol use disorder) and to test its effectiveness in terms of the elicitation of cue-induced alcohol craving and anxiety responses in a sample of social drinkers (SD) and patients diagnosed with AUD. A secondary objective of our study was to explore which cue-elicited response (alcohol craving or anxiety) differentiates better between AUD patients and SD. We expected to obtain significant differences between the neutral VR condition and the VR alcohol-related environments regarding cue-induced anxiety and alcohol craving responses in the two groups, AUD patients and SD. Similarly, we expected to find statistically significant differences between AUD and SD groups in terms of their alcohol craving and anxiety responses. Based on an earlier study in bulimia nervosa [42], we expected cue-induced anxiety responses to differentiate between AUD patients and SD better than cue-induced alcohol craving responses.

2. Method

2.1. Participants

Twenty-seven individuals participated in this study, 13 patients from the Addictive Behaviors Unit, Hospital Clinic of Barcelona and 14 SD, students at the University of Barcelona. Ethical approval was obtained from the Ethics Committees at the University of Barcelona and Hospital Clinic of Barcelona. All patients and students participated in this study after providing written informed consent. The clinical sample consisted of 13 outpatients, 8 men and 5 women (M_{age} = 48, SD = 4.8), diagnosed with AUD according to the *Diagnostic and Statistical Manual of Mental Disorders* (5th ed.) [43]. Patients presented comorbid diagnoses of borderline personality disorder, anxiety, and attention deficit hyperactivity disorder (ADHD). Their pharmacotherapy included anxiolytic, antidepressant, disulfiram, and antipsychotic medication. Seven patients reported occasional tobacco, cannabis, and cocaine use in the month prior to the experiment, but none reported alcohol consumption in the last month as they were under treatment for AUD at Hospital Clinic of Barcelona. The mean abstinence period was 68 days, ranging from one month to one year. Self-reports of substance use and abstinence data were supported by results of urine analyses performed in all patients. The inclusion criteria were having an AUD diagnosis and receiving outpatient treatment for AUD. Individuals with comorbid disorders like personality disorders or anxiety disorders and occasional use of illicit drugs (e.g., cannabis or cocaine) or tobacco were included, but those with severe comorbid psychopathology (e.g., psychosis or dementia), severe cognitive impairment that might interfere with the task completion, or anti-craving medication (e.g., naltrexone) were excluded. Pregnant women were also excluded.

The control group consisted of 14 SD, 2 men and 12 women (M_{age} = 23, SD = 5.6), all students at the University of Barcelona. Among this group, there were self-reports of one diagnosis of depression and one diagnosis of ADHD. One student reported using anxiolytic medication, and one student antidepressant medication. Tobacco and cannabis use were self-reported by six students in the last month prior to the experiment. SD also reported their monthly consumed standard drink units (SDU). A Spanish SDU is a single consumption of 10 g of ethanol (the standard quantity of wine or beer and half the standard quantity of liquor) [44]. Students consumed approximately 9 SDU (M = 9.2, SD = 9.9) per month, ranging from 3 to 24 SDU/month. Abstinence data (M_{days} = 15, SD = 18) in this group were based on self-reports from the students. The inclusion criterion was a social drinking pattern (i.e., individuals who use alcohol on a social basis and are not identified as having a problematic pattern of alcohol use). As in the clinical group, comorbid disorders (personality disorders or anxiety) and occasional use of illicit drugs (e.g., cannabis or cocaine) or tobacco were not considered exclusion criteria. However, any participants with severe comorbid psychopathology or severe cognitive impairment were excluded.

2.2. Measures

Alcohol consumption was assessed with the Alcohol Use Disorder Identification Test (AUDIT) [45]. The Spanish version of AUDIT [46] is a 10-item scale assessing alcohol misuse and severity of alcohol-related problems. Responses are scored from 0 to 4 with a maximum score of 40.

Alcohol craving was assessed with the Multidimensional Alcohol Craving Scale (MACS) [47]. The MACS is a Spanish self-reported scale aiming to assess the "intensity of alcohol craving experienced by the participant in the previous week". Scores on each item range from 1 ("Strongly disagree") to 5 ("Strongly agree"). There are three MACS outcome scores: "desire to drink," "behavioral disinhibition," and the total score, which were each graded as nonexistent, mild, moderate or intense. Moreover, a modified version of MACS (MACS-VR) was introduced in the experimental procedure to explore alcohol craving immediately after VR exposure to alcohol-related contexts and cues. The items, scores, and outcomes of the MACS-VR remained the same as in the original MACS, although the instructions were now to assess the "intensity of alcohol craving experienced during VR exposure".

Anxiety was explored with the Spanish version of the State-Trait Anxiety Inventory (STAI) [48]. The STAI is a self-reported questionnaire with two subscales assessing how a person feels at the moment (STAI-state, state anxiety) and how a person feels in general (STAI-trait, trait anxiety). Each subscale consists of 20 items, and scores of each item range from 0 ("Not at all") to 3 ("Very much so"). Higher scores on each subscale indicate higher levels of trait and/or state anxiety.

Alcohol craving and anxiety experienced during VR exposure were explored with visual analogue scales (VAS). These scales are widely used as instruments to measure craving (VAS-C) and anxiety (VAS-A) during VR exposure [35]. The VAS-C is a self-reported virtual craving scale, with scores ranging from 0 to 100, where 0 is interpreted as "no craving" and 100 indicates "intense craving". Similarly, VAS-A is a self-reported scale aiming to explore anxiety levels, with scores ranging from 0 to 100, where 0 is interpreted as "no anxiety" and 100 as "intense anxiety". VAS-C and VAS-A are ecological scales used during exposure to VR environments.

2.3. Instruments

2.3.1. Hardware

The VR equipment consisted of Oculus Rift head-mounted display (HMD), 1080 × 1200 resolution per eye, a 90 Hz refresh rate, and 110° field of view, sensors, touch controllers, and a computer compatible with the VR technology (INTEL(R) Core(TM) i7-2600 CPU, 16.0 GB RAM, Operating System 64 bits, processor ×64, graphic card NVIDIA GeForce GTX 1080 Ti).

2.3.2. "ALCO-VR" Software

"ALCO-VR" software was developed based on the results of a previous study [49], in which we identified factors that contribute to the elicitation of alcohol craving in a sample of patients diagnosed with AUD. Based on that study, the ALCO-VR software was created, consisting of four VR alcohol-related environments: a restaurant, a bar, a pub, and at-home environments (Figure 1). These VR environments were created considering multiple variables, as in our previous research, such as social interactions (including avatars in the environments), different alcohol-related cues (a menu of 22 alcoholic drinks), or different times of day (daytime or nighttime). Hence, there were two environments during daylight (bar and restaurant) and two environments during nighttime (pub and at-home), one environment with no social interaction (the at-home environment) and three with social interaction (bar, pub, restaurant). All environments were created to simulate real-life scenarios based on patients' experiences. The ALCO-VR platform consisted of two parts, assessment and therapy. The assessment part was the focus of the current study and the ALCO-VR created a hierarchy of exposure from the lowest rated environment with the lowest rated alcoholic drink to the highest rated environment and the highest rated alcoholic drink. On the VAS-A and VAS-C, users were asked to rate how much cue-induced anxiety and craving they considered the environments and alcoholic drinks triggered on a scale from 0 to 100. The assessment part of the ALCO-VR centered on the first five rated alcoholic beverages, the favorite drinks of each participant, which were presented in each VR environment. In addition, the software consisted of a neutral environment (a room with a white background and a glass of water), where the participants could familiarize themselves with the VR technology. A high interaction level between the user and the VR platform was considered fundamental and individuals could approach their alcoholic beverages, hold them and observe them from all angles with Oculus Touch controllers.

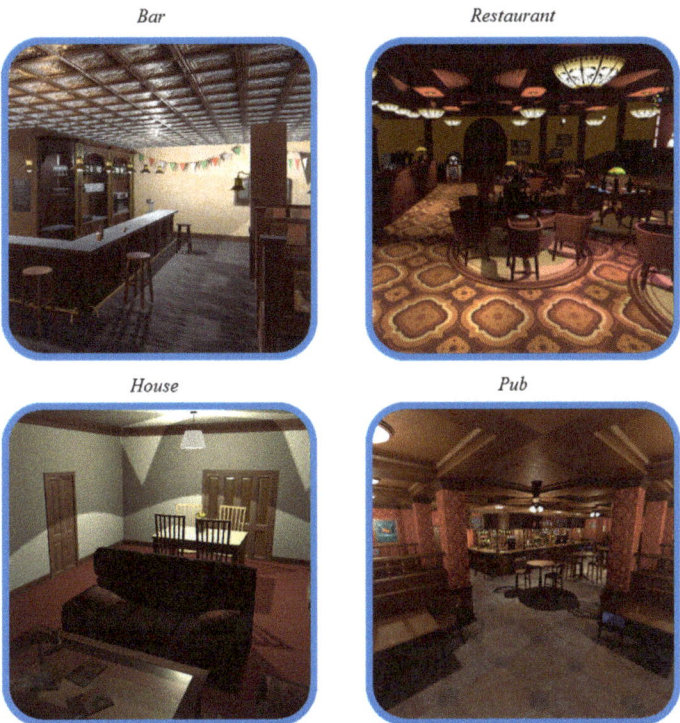

Figure 1. Pictures of the VR environments.

2.4. Procedure

Participants from the control group (SD group) were recruited through social media platforms at the University of Barcelona. Patients from the clinical group (AUD group) were informed about the study during one of their appointments with their psychiatrists or clinical psychologists at the Addictive Behaviors Unit at the Hospital Clinic of Barcelona. Once they had agreed to participate, they were referred to the researcher in charge of the study. Participants were asked to sign the informed consent document after a short explanatory introduction regarding the technology used. Subsequently, clinical data were collected from the patients such as dual diagnoses, medication, abstinence data, alcohol consumption, and other substance use (illicit or licit) during the month prior to the experiment. These data were confirmed by their clinical psychologist. Participants were then asked to complete the AUDIT, STAI (the trait part), and MACS. Upon completion of these self-reported scales, the researcher instructed participants how to use the touch controllers, and they were given water to drink in order to not interfere with alcohol consumption patterns. The ALCO-VR software started by assessing how much craving and anxiety was triggered by 2D images of each VR environment (pub, at home, restaurant, and bar) and each alcoholic drink on a VAS from 0 to 100. Based on these responses, the individualized exposure hierarchy consisted of the interplay between the first five chosen alcoholic beverages, and the four contexts, gradually increasing from the lowest rated drink and the lowest rated VR environment to the highest rated alcoholic beverage and highest rated environment. When this initial part of the procedure was completed, the Oculus Rift HMD was attached to the participant's head. This represented the start of the 3D virtual experience and each participant was exposed to the VR environments following his/her hierarchy. The first instruction was to approach the beverage and observe it from all angles for approximately 20 s, but without attempting to virtually drink from it. The VR exposure started with a neutral environment, exposure to a glass of water in a white room, aiming to familiarize participants with the VR technology. This environment served as a neutral condition in the analyses and as training for the participants. The hierarchy created by the ALCO-VR platform consisted of exposure to each alcoholic drink, which appeared in each environment. Hence, participants self-reported their cue-induced alcohol craving and anxiety levels on the VAS-C and VAS-A throughout exposure to the ALCO-VR software (4 environments × 5 drinks = 20 ratings × 2 (craving and anxiety) = 40 ratings). Olfactory stimuli were introduced during the exposure procedure and corresponded to each drink. Previously prepared alcoholic beverages were transferred onto cotton pads and placed on the table, close to the participant each time a new alcoholic drink appeared during the exposure procedure. Overall, the exposure lasted for approximately 10–15 min. After the experiment, participants were asked to complete the MACS-VR, and STAI (the state part). In addition, they were also asked to rate several variables of the ALCO-VR platform on a scale from 0 to 10, with 0 considered "very low" and 10 was considered "excellent"; these variables were user-friendliness, overall quality of the software, realism of the environments, and realism of the alcoholic beverages. Finally, for the AUD group, a debriefing session was carried out at the end of the procedure with the aim of reducing momentary craving and anxiety levels and to minimize any further possible alcohol use. Each session lasted for approximately one hour. The cross-sectional sessions were delivered by an experienced clinician-scientist at VR-Psy Lab, University of Barcelona.

2.5. Statistical Analysis

As the assumption of normality of data was not satisfied according to the Shapiro–Wilks test p-value of ≤0.05, non-parametric tests were applied in this study. First, Friedman tests were run separately for each group to compare participants' levels of craving and anxiety experienced during VR exposure to the neutral environment and to the four alcohol-related environments. Post-hoc Wilcoxon signed-rank tests were used to determine specific significant differences in craving and anxiety between the conditions in both groups. In addition, Mann–Whitney U tests were applied to explore differences between the AUD group and SD in terms of anxiety and alcohol craving levels experienced during exposure to the VR alcohol-related environments. Spearman correlations were conducted to explore the relationship between self-reported craving and anxiety responses on VAS-C/VAS-A and the results of AUDIT, STAI, and MACS. Finally, due to the gender and age imbalance, we performed analysis of covariance (ANCOVA) after converting our data into rank scores. All statistical analyses were carried out using IBM SPSS version 24.

3. Results

Table 1 indicates the data of the self-reported questionnaires in terms of alcohol misuse (AUDIT), trait-anxiety (STAI, trait part), alcohol craving during the last week prior to the experiment (MACS), state anxiety (STAI, state part), and momentary cue-induced alcohol craving immediately after exposure to the ALCO-VR software (MACS-VR).

Table 1. Data of the self-reported scales.

Scales	Alcohol Use Disorder (AUD) Patients M (SD)	Social Drinkers M (SD)
Alcohol Use Disorder Identification Test (AUDIT)	23.77 (13)	4.5 (2.2)
State-Trait Anxiety Inventory (STAI) (trait part)	34.85 (12)	19 (13)
Multidimensional Alcohol Craving Scale (MACS)	29.23 (9.3)	20 (4.1)
STAI (state part)	18.77 (12.4)	15.64 (14.41)
MACS-VR	36 (12.17)	26.64 (10.9)

Data of the Self-Reported Questionnaires

Significant differences were found in self-reported levels of anxiety and alcohol craving across exposure to the VR environments. The Friedman test indicated statistically significant differences in self-reported anxiety levels reported on the VAS-A across the VR environments in both AUD patients (χ^2 (4) = 11.26, p = 0.02) and the SD group (χ^2 (4) = 15.78, p = 0.003). In the AUD group, post-hoc Wilcoxon rank test confirmed that there were significant differences in cue-induced anxiety reported on the VAS-A between the neutral and at-home environments (Z = −2.621, p = 0.009), between neutral and bar environments (Z = −2.447, p = 0.01), between neutral and restaurant scenarios (Z = −2.762, p = 0.006) and between neutral and pub environments (Z = −2.691, p = 0.007). No statistically significant differences were found between the four VR alcohol-related environments on self-reported anxiety on the VAS-A (p > 0.05). Figure 2 confirms that self-reported levels of anxiety were higher during exposure to the VR alcohol-related environments than during exposure to the neutral environment. However, in the SD group, we found the opposite pattern. Although there were statistically significant differences between neutral and at-home environments (Z = −2.707, p = 0.007), between neutral and bar environments (Z = −2.621, p = 0.009), between neutral and restaurant environments (Z = −2.589, p = 0.01), and between neutral and pub environments (Z = −2.135, p = 0.03), the scores of self-reported anxiety were higher in the neutral environment than in the four VR alcohol-related environments, as Figure 2 shows.

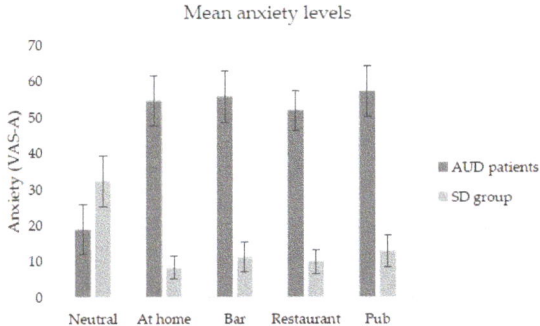

Figure 2. Self-reported mean levels of anxiety (A) on visual analogue scales (VAS)-A.

Regarding self-reports of alcohol craving on the VAS-C, the Friedman test revealed a statistically significant difference across the VR environments in the AUD patients' group (χ^2 (4) = 22.83 p = 0.000), but not in the SD group (p > 0.05). In the AUD group, post-hoc analyses with Wilcoxon rank test showed significant differences in self-reported alcohol craving on the VAS-C between the neutral and at-home environments (Z = −3.041, p = 0.002), between neutral and bar environments (Z = −3.180, p = 0.001), between neutral and restaurant environments (Z = −3.110, p = 0.002), and between neutral and pub environments (Z = −3.110, p = 0.002). As can be seen in Figure 3, no statistically significant differences in alcohol craving reports on the VAS-C were found across the four VR alcohol-related environments. Both Figures 2 and 3 indicate significantly higher scores in the AUD group than in the SD group regarding self-reported anxiety and alcohol craving levels on the VAS-A and VAS-C, respectively. As there were more significant differences in terms of anxiety levels compared to craving levels, we consider that cue-induced anxiety responses can better differentiate between SD and AUD patients than self-reported craving responses.

The results of the Mann–Whitney U test indicated a statistically significant difference between AUD and SD groups when comparing the mean anxiety and alcohol craving responses in each VR alcohol-related environment (p < 0.05). As can be seen in Table 2, self-reported anxiety and alcohol craving levels were higher in the AUD group than in the SD group across all VR alcohol-related environments. There were no statistically significant differences between AUD and SD groups regarding their anxiety and alcohol craving responses in the neutral environment (p > 0.05).

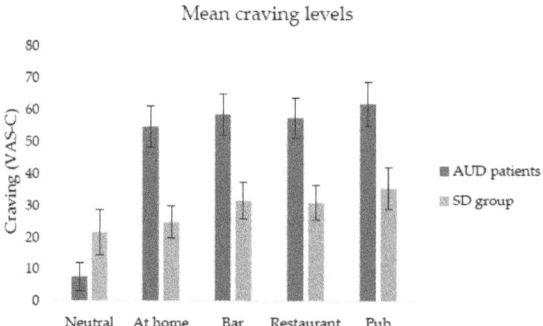

Figure 3. Self-reported mean levels of alcohol craving (C) on VAS-C.

Table 2. Differences in anxiety and alcohol craving self-reports on VAS-A and VAS-C.

	AUD Patients (N = 13)			Social Drinkers (N = 14)			
	Mean (SD)	Median	IQR [a]	Mean (SD)	Median	IQR	Z [b]
			Neutral env [c]				
Anxiety	18.85 (24.54)	5.00	40	32.21 (26.45)	34.00	50	−1.347
Craving	7.69 (16.05)	0.00	7	21.64 (26.38)	11.00	32	−1.726
			At home				
Anxiety	54.54 (24.97)	54.00	36	8.21 (11.82)	.50	15	−4.064 ***
Craving	54.77 (22.86)	62.00	33	24.93 (18.71)	19.00	33	−3.180 ***
			Bar				
Anxiety	55.69 (25.70)	52.00	43	11.21 (15.55)	2.50	22	−3.980 ***
Craving	58.62 (23.11)	61.00	44	31.64 (21.57)	32.00	42	−2.719 *
			Restaurant				
Anxiety	51.77 (20.17)	53.00	41	9.93 (12.17)	5.50	17	−4.162 ***
Craving	57.54 (22.74)	59.00	44	30.93 (20.58)	34.50	39	−2.671 *
			Pub				
Anxiety	57.15 (25.32)	54.00	46	12.86 (16.61)	5.00	27	−3.896 ***
Craving	61.85 (24.46)	64.00	50	35.64 (24.48)	39.00	46	−2.258 *

[a] IQR, interquartile range; [b] Mann–Whitney U test. Bonferroni adjustment for multiple testing; *** $p < 0.001$; * $p < 0.05$; [c] env, environment.

In addition, in the AUD group, there was a strong, positive correlation between alcohol dependence severity as shown by AUDIT and total craving reported on the VAS-C ($r_s = 0.783$, $p = 0.002$) and total anxiety reported on the VAS-A ($r_s = 0.650$, $p = 0.016$). In addition, there was a significant relationship between trait-anxiety as assessed by the STAI (the trait part of the questionnaire) and the total alcohol craving score reported on the VAS-C ($r_s = 0.667$, $p = 0.013$). A positive correlation was also found between cue-induced craving as explored by the MACS-VR and total alcohol craving responses reported on the VAS-C ($r_s = 0.581$, $p = 0.03$). No other correlations were found in anxiety and craving levels assessed by different instruments ($p > 0.05$). Regarding the SD group, the only correlations were found between cue-induced craving as assessed by MACS-VR and mean total craving reported on the VAS-C ($r_s = 0.629$, $p = 0.016$) and mean total anxiety reported on the VAS-A ($r_s = 0.707$, $p = 0.005$).

Addressing the age and gender imbalance in our study, ANCOVA analyses were run to determine the effect regarding gender and age on total mean levels of anxiety and alcohol craving in SD and AUD patients. After converting the scores to ranks, we performed ANCOVA analyses on the rank scores. After adjustment for gender, there was a statistically significant group difference regarding their total mean anxiety levels reported on VAS-A $F(1, 24) = 39.313$, $p < 0.001$, partial $\eta^2 = 0.621$. Post-hoc analysis was performed with a Bonferroni adjustment. Anxiety levels were significantly greater in AUD patients (M = 54.8, SE = 6.33) than the SD group (M = 10.5, SE = 3.47), a mean difference of 13.7, 95% confidence interval (CI) (9.23, 18.3), $p < 0.001$. Similarly, after adjusting for gender, there was a statistically significant group difference regarding total mean craving levels reported on VAS-C $F(1, 24) = 10.075$, $p < 0.005$, partial $\eta^2 = 0.296$. Post-hoc Bonferroni analysis revealed that AUD patients (M = 58.2, SE = 6.05) reported significantly greater craving levels than the SD group (M = 30.79, SE = 5.4) (mean difference of 9.63, 95% CI (3.37, 15.90), $p < 0.005$).

In addition, after adjusting for age, there were statistically significant differences between SD and AUD groups in terms of their cue-induced responses. There was a statistically significant difference between the two groups regarding their total mean anxiety levels $F(1, 24) = 12.317$, $p < 0.005$, partial $\eta^2 = 0.339$. Anxiety levels were significantly greater in AUD patients (M = 48.23, SE = 6.33) compared to the SD group (M = 23, SE = 3.4) (mean difference of 17.65, 95% CI (7.27, 28.04), $p < 0.005$). Finally, there was no statistically significant difference between groups in terms of total mean craving regardless of age $F(1, 24) = 3.764$, $p > 0.05$, partial $\eta^2 = 0.136$. These results can be appreciated in Figures 4 and 5.

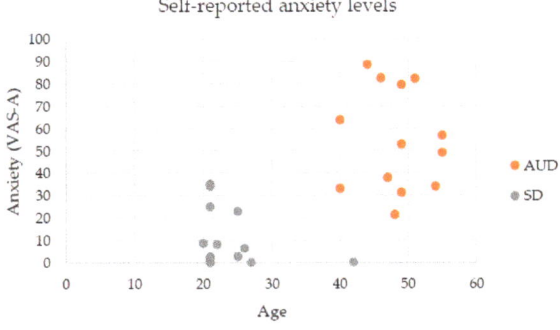

Figure 4. Self-reports of total mean anxiety in AUD and social drinkers (SD) groups.

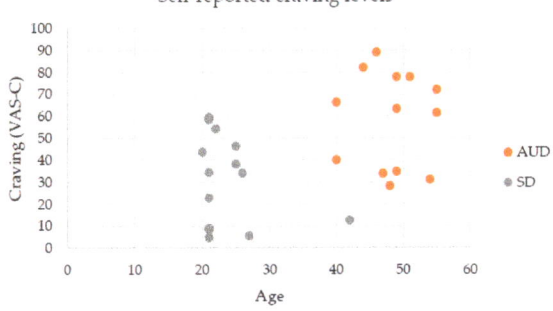

Figure 5. Self-reports of total mean craving in AUD and SD groups.

Finally, the participants rated the ALCO-VR software according to the following variables: user-friendliness ($M_{AUD} = 9.15$, SD = 0.89; $M_{SD} = 8.93$, SD = 0.91), overall quality of the software ($M_{AUD} = 8.23$, SD = 1.58; $M_{SD} = 8$, SD = 1.3), realism of the environments ($M_{AUD} = 7.77$, SD = 1.53; $M_{SD} = 7.8$, SD = 1.5), and realism of the alcoholic beverages ($M_{AUD} = 7.38$, SD = 1.93; $M_{SD} = 7.21$, SD = 1.31).

4. Discussion

The current study was centered on testing the effectiveness of ALCO-VR software to induce anxiety and craving responses. Its secondary objective was to assess which craving or anxiety responses could best differentiate between the AUD and SD groups. The VR alcohol-related environments induced significantly greater anxiety levels than the neutral environment in our clinical group, but not in our control group. On the contrary, the VR alcohol-related environments induced greater craving levels than the neutral environment in both clinical and control groups. More significant alcohol craving responses were found among AUD patients.

Our results are consistent with previous research [35] and confirm the effectiveness of the ALCO-VR platform for inducing anxiety and craving responses. Patients diagnosed with AUD displayed high levels of anxiety during exposure to alcohol-related contexts compared to our control group. Furthermore, craving responses in the AUD group were even higher than in the SD group during exposure to the VR alcohol-related environments than during exposure to the neutral environment. This response pattern is supported by previous research showing greater levels of craving within alcohol-related VR environments [36,50]. In substance use disorders, VR smoking-related environments elicited higher craving levels in nicotine-dependent undergraduate students than in the control condition [51]. In a virtual reality-methamphetamine (VR-METH) cue-exposure paradigm, methamphetamine users experienced higher craving levels than in the neutral condition [40]. Additionally, in behavioral addictions, a significant internet gaming VR environment induced higher craving levels in patients diagnosed with internet gaming disorder than in a control group [52]. Similarly, in gambling disorder, frequent gamblers experienced higher craving induced by the VR environment than non-frequent gamblers [53].

Furthermore, although there were no statistically significant differences across the VR environments in our SD group, we observed a gradual increase in alcohol craving during exposure to the VR alcohol-related environments compared to the neutral scenario. We interpret this result as being representative of a group of young social drinkers, whose drinking patterns involve social interaction and peer pressure, especially in bars and pubs. The result also confirms the contextual specificity of craving for alcohol [49,54].

It is worth mentioning that both SD and AUD patients did not self-report high levels of anxiety and there were no statistically significant differences between groups at baseline measurement. For instance, 20 or 30 self-reported anxiety levels on a VAS from 0 to 100 during the VR neutral environment did not represent significant levels of anxiety. The fact that the SD group had slightly lower anxiety levels in VR alcohol-related environments indicated that these participants did not associate alcohol-related stimuli with the aversive consequences of drinking patterns. However, in our examination of the effectiveness of the ALCO-VR, we found significant differences between AUD and SD groups in anxiety and craving responses across all VR alcohol-related environments. Interestingly, in terms of cue-induced anxiety and craving responses, AUD patients reported similar levels of craving and anxiety during exposure to the VR alcohol-related environments. However, SD cue-induced anxiety responses were lower than their craving responses. SD had a different response tendency from the clinical group regarding anxiety levels. Cue-induced anxiety responses better differentiated the AUD patients and the SD group than craving. It should be noted that craving is elicited by stimuli in both groups, but it may not be associated with anxiety in SD, while, due to the ambivalence of patients in treatment (want to drink and want to remain abstinent) the same cravings may lead to high levels of anxiety.

Addressing age and gender imbalance in this study, our results confirm that AUD patients self-reported greater anxiety and alcohol craving levels compared to participants from the SD group. Similar results were found in a previous study in patients diagnosed with bulimia nervosa (BN), in which anxiety responses discriminated best between BN patients and healthy participants [42]. Although BN and AUD are apparently different disorders, we consider these similar results as an indicator that BN and AUD share common causal and maintenance mechanisms [55].

Apart from the craving and anxiety responses self-reported on the VAS-C and VAS-A respectively, our participants completed the following instruments: AUDIT, MACS, STAI, and MACS-VR. The results showed significantly higher scores in all the instruments in the clinical group than in the control group. The strong correlation between the results of these questionnaires and the scores reported on the VAS-C and the VAS-A confirms the validity of the ALCO-VR software for measuring cue-induced alcohol craving and anxiety, and so we consider that ALCO-VR software may be a useful EMA tool to assess craving and anxiety levels. Interestingly, the MACS-VR instrument exploring alcohol craving immediately after ALCO-VR exposure indicated higher levels of cue-induced alcohol craving than the MACS instrument exploring alcohol craving in the week prior to the experiment. This confirms that the ALCO-VR software can elicit momentary alcohol craving not only in AUD patients, but in SD as well. Therefore, we argue that the ALCO-VR software is a valid instrument for exploring cue-induced anxiety and alcohol craving responses and can differentiate between groups of AUD patients and SD.

The current study is part of a larger project aiming to develop a VR therapy tool based on the cue-exposure paradigm to alcohol-related cues and contexts in patients with severe AUD and with several failed attempts to cease alcohol use. First, we conducted a pilot study testing a VR software based on alcohol-related cues and environments; the results indicated that the software distinguished between heavy drinkers (HD) and light drinkers (LD) in terms of behavioral parameters. LD displayed a preference for non-alcoholic drinks, whereas most heavy drinking individuals preferred alcoholic beverages [56]. In view of these results, we attempted to develop a new VR platform designed to treat patients diagnosed with AUD who were considered "resistant-to-treatment-as-usual" (TAU). A common procedure for identifying specific triggers for alcohol craving is to conduct exhaustive interviews with relevant populations, in our case, with patients with AUD. Therefore, we conducted a second study in which we developed an ad-hoc questionnaire to determine significant factors such as cues and contexts that elicit craving in AUD patients with the aim of creating naturalistic real-life environments [49]. We developed the ALCO-VR software based on the results of the previous study. In addition, the current study is the preceding step to test the efficacy of the cue-exposure therapy (CET) approach using the VR technology in AUD patients.

As substance use disorders and eating disorders resemble addictive behavior mechanisms [57], our study was based on a previous study centered on patients diagnosed with BN, which was conducted at VR-Psy Lab from the University of Barcelona. The aim of the study was to test the efficacy of a VR-cue exposure therapy (VR-CET) for patients diagnosed with BN. The study showed positive results in terms of abstinence rates, anxiety, and craving levels in patients with BN in the VR-CET group compared to the control group. The first step was to perform exhaustive interviews with BN patients to determine triggering factors for binge eating behaviors [58]. Based on the results of that study, VR environments were created and tested in BN patients to examine the elicitation of food craving [42]. These two studies were essential to develop a VR-CET for BN patients. The efficacy of the VR-based therapy software was tested in a multi-site clinical trial and it was found to achieve better outcomes than cognitive-behavioral therapy (CBT) both at the post-treatment assessment [59] and at six-month follow-up [55]. Several limitations should be noted with regard to our study. First, our control group consisted mostly of young women from the Faculty of Psychology, where the majority of students are female. Second, our clinical and control samples were limited. For future studies, we propose that larger samples should be used and that the effectiveness of the ALCO-VR software to differentiate between patients with long-term versus short-term abstinence period in terms of alcohol craving and anxiety should be tested. In addition, to address the gender and age imbalance between our groups, we will consider these limitations for upcoming studies of the same project.

5. Conclusions

The current study demonstrated the validity of the ALCO-VR software to induce alcohol craving and anxiety responses, particularly in patients diagnosed with AUD. The ALCO-VR can perform the ecological assessment of momentary cue-induced alcohol craving and anxiety levels, and can differentiate between individuals with AUD and those that are SD.

Considering the promising results of this study, the next step would be to test the therapeutic use of the software in patients diagnosed with AUD. The ALCO-VR is currently being implemented in a multi-site clinical trial testing its efficacy as a cue-exposure therapy tool for patients diagnosed with AUD, who are considered resistant to TAU. The ultimate goal of the project is to reduce relapse rates upon completion of treatment, since relapse remains one of the greatest challenges in AUD treatment and follow-up.

Author Contributions: Conceptualization, J.G.-M., M.F.-G. and A.G. (Alexandra Ghiţă); methodology, J.G.-M., M.F.-G. and A.G. (Alexandra Ghiţă); software, J.G.-M., M.F.-G., A.G. (Alexandra Ghiţă) and B.P.-G.; validation, A.G. (Alexandra Ghiţă), O.H.-S., Y.F.-R., B.P.-G., M.M., L.O., S.M., L.T. and A.G. (Antoni Gual); formal analysis, A.G. (Alexandra Ghiţă); investigation, A.G. (Alexandra Ghiţă), O.H.-S., Y.F.-R., B.P.-G., M.M., L.O., S.M., L.T. and A.G. (Antoni Gual); resources, J.G.-M.; data curation, A.G. (Alexandra Ghiţă); writing—original draft preparation, A.G. (Alexandra Ghiţă); writing—review and editing, A.G. (Alexandra Ghiţă), J.G.-M., O.H.-S., M.F.-G., B.P.-G., M.M., A.G. (Antoni Gual); supervision, J.G.-M.; project administration, J.G.-M.; funding acquisition, J.G.-M.

Funding: This research was funded by the Spanish Ministry of Health, Social Services and Equality, Delegation of the Government for the National Plan on Drugs (FEDER/UE/Project 2016I078: "ALCO-VR: Virtual Reality-based protocol for the treatment of patients diagnosed with severe alcohol use disorder"). The study also received support from AGAUR, Generalitat de Catalunya, 2017SGR1693.

Acknowledgments: This study was supported by the Spanish Ministry of Health, Social Services and Equality, Delegation of the Government for the National Plan on Drugs (FEDER/UE/Project 2016I078: "ALCO-VR: Virtual Reality-based protocol for the treatment of patients diagnosed with severe alcohol use disorder"). The study also received support from AGAUR, Generalitat de Catalunya, 2017SGR1693.

Conflicts of Interest: The authors declare no conflict of interest.

References

1. Thursz, M.; Kamath, P.S.; Mathurin, P.; Szabo, G.; Shah, V.H. Alcohol-related liver disease: Areas of consensus, unmet needs and opportunities for further study. *J. Hepatol.* **2019**, *65*, 2271–2283. [CrossRef] [PubMed]
2. Connor, J.P.; Haber, P.S.; Hall, W.D. Alcohol use disorders. *Lancet* **2016**, *387*, 988–998. [CrossRef]
3. Rehm, J.; Anderson, P.; Barry, J.; Dimitrov, P.; Elekes, Z.; Feijão, F.; Frick, U.; Gual, A.; Gmel, G.; Kraus, L.; et al. Prevalence of and potential influencing factors for alcohol dependence in Europe. *Eur. Addict. Res.* **2015**, *21*, 6–18. [CrossRef] [PubMed]
4. Shield, K.D.; Parry, C.; Rehm, J. Chronic diseases and conditions related to alcohol use. *Alcohol. Res. Curr. Rev.* **2014**, *35*, 155–173.
5. Prince, M.A.; Read, J.P.; Colder, C.R. Trajectories of college alcohol involvement and their associations with later alcohol use disorder symptoms. *Prev. Sci.* **2019**, *20*, 741–752. [CrossRef] [PubMed]
6. King, A.C.; Hasin, D.; O'Connor, S.J.; McNamara, P.J.; Cao, D. A prospective 5-year re-examination of alcohol response in heavy drinkers progressing in alcohol use disorder. *Biol. Psychiatry* **2016**, *79*, 489–498. [CrossRef] [PubMed]
7. Schulte, M.T.; Ramo, D.; Brown, S.A. Gender differences in factors influencing alcohol use and drinking progression among adolescents. *Clin. Psychol. Rev.* **2009**, *296*, 535–547. [CrossRef]
8. Dawson, D.A.; Goldstein, R.B.; Chou, S.P.; June-Ruan, W.; Grant, B.F. Age at first drink and the first incidence of adult-onset DSM-IV alcohol use disorders. *Alcohol. Clin. Exp. Res.* **2008**, *32*, 2149–2160. [CrossRef]
9. Coriale, G.; Fiorentino, D.; Rosa, F.; Solombrino, S.; Scalese, B.; Ciccarelli, R.; Attilia, F.; Vitali, M.; Musetti, A.; Fiore, M.; et al. Treatment of alcohol use disorder from a psychological point of view. *Riv. Psichiatr.* **2018**, *53*, 141–148.
10. Andersson, H.W.; Wenaas, M.; Nordfjærn, T. Relapse after inpatient substance use treatment: A prospective cohort study among users of illicit substances. *Addict. Behav.* **2019**, *90*, 222–228. [CrossRef]
11. Sinha, R.; Fox, H.C.; Hong, K.; Hansen, J.; Tuit, K.; Kreek, M.J. Effects of adrenal sensitivity, stress- and cue-induced craving, and anxiety on subsequent alcohol relapse and treatment outcomes. *Arch. Gen. Psychiatry* **2011**, *68*, 942–952. [CrossRef]
12. Blanco, C.; Flórez-Salamanca, L.; Secades-Villa, R.; Wang, S.; Hasin, D.S. Predictors of initiation of nicotine, alcohol, cannabis, and cocaine use: Results of the National Epidemiologic Survey on Alcohol and Related Conditions (NESARC). *Am. J. Addict.* **2018**, *27*, 477–484. [CrossRef]
13. Gilpin, N.W.; Herman, M.A.; Roberto, M. The central amygdala as an integrative hub for anxiety and alcohol use disorders. *Biol. Psychiatry* **2015**, *77*, 859–869. [CrossRef]
14. Anker, J.J.; Kummerfeld, E.; Rix, A.; Burwell, S.J.; Kushner, M.G. Causal Network Modeling of the determinants of drinking behavior in comorbid alcohol use and anxiety disorder. *Alcohol. Clin. Exp. Res.* **2018**, *43*, 91–97. [CrossRef]
15. Miloyan, B.; Van Doorn, G. Longitudinal association between social anxiety disorder and incident alcohol use disorder: Results from two national samples of US adults. *Soc. Psychiatry Psychiatr. Epidemiol.* **2019**, *54*, 469–475. [CrossRef]

16. Wolitzky-Taylor, K.; Niles, A.N.; Ries, R.; Krull, J.L.; Rawson, R.; Roy-Byrne, P.; Craske, M. Who needs more than standard care? Treatment moderators in a randomized clinical trial comparing addiction treatment alone to addiction treatment plus anxiety disorder treatment for comorbid anxiety and substance use disorders. *Behav. Res. Ther.* **2018**, *107*, 1–9. [CrossRef]
17. Drummond, D.C. Theories of drugs craving, ancient and modern. *Addiction* **2001**, *96*, 33–46. [CrossRef]
18. Van Lier, H.G.; Pieterse, M.E.; Schraagen, J.M.C.; Postel, M.G.; Vollenbroek-Hutten, M.M.R.; de Haan, H.A.; Noordzij, M.L. Identifying viable theoretical frameworks with essential parameters for real-time and real world alcohol craving research: A systematic review of craving models. *Addict. Res. Theory* **2018**, *26*, 35–51. [CrossRef]
19. Pavlov, I.P. Conditioned reflexes: An investigation of the physiological activity of the cerebral cortex. *Ann. Neurosci.* **1927**, *17*, 136–141. [CrossRef]
20. Pina, M.M.; Williams, R.A. Alcohol cues, craving, and relapse: Insights from animal models. In *Recent Advances in Drug Addiction Research and Clinical Applications*; IntechOpen: London, UK, 2016; pp. 47–79.
21. Wrase, J.; Schlagenhauf, F.; Kienast, T.; Wustenberg, T.; Bermpohl, F.; Kahnt, T.; Beck, A.; Strohle, A.; Juckel, G.; Knutson, B.; et al. Dysfunction of reward processing correlates with alcohol craving in detoxified alcoholics. *Neuroimage* **2007**, *35*, 787–794. [CrossRef]
22. Kim, D.J.; Jeong, J.; Kim, K.S.; Chae, J.H.; Jin, S.H.; Ahn, K.J.; Myrick, H.; Yoon, S.J.; Kim, H.R.; Kim, S.Y. Complexity changes of the EEG induced by alcohol cue exposure in alcoholics and social drinkers. *Alcohol. Clin. Exp. Res.* **2003**, *27*, 1955–1961. [CrossRef]
23. Witteman, J.; Post, H.; Tarvainen, M.; De Bruijn, A.; De Elizabeth, S.F.P.; Ramaekers, J.G.; Wiers, R.W. Cue reactivity and its relation to craving and relapse in alcohol dependence: A combined laboratory and field study. *Psychopharmacology* **2015**, *232*, 3685–3696. [CrossRef]
24. Sinha, R.; Fox, H.C.; Hong, K.A.; Bergquist, K.; Bhagwagar, Z.; Siedlarz, K.M. Enhanced negative emotion and alcohol craving, and altered physiological responses following stress and cue exposure in alcohol dependent individuals. *Neuropsychopharmacology* **2009**, *34*, 1198–1208. [CrossRef]
25. Bottlender, M.; Soyka, M. Impact of craving on alcohol relapse during, and 12 months following, outpatient treatment. *Alcohol Alcohol.* **2004**, *39*, 357–361. [CrossRef]
26. Valyear, M.D.; Villaruel, F.R.; Chaudhri, N. Alcohol-seeking and relapse: A focus on incentive salience and contextual conditioning. *Behav. Process.* **2017**, *141*, 26–32. [CrossRef]
27. Olney, J.J.; Warlow, S.M.; Naffziger, E.E.; Berridge, K.C. Current perspectives on incentive salience and applications to clinical disorders. *Curr. Opin. Behav. Sci.* **2018**, *22*, 59–69. [CrossRef]
28. Stasiewicz, P.R.; Brandon, T.H.; Bradizza, C.M. Effects of extinction context and retrieval cues on renewal of alcohol-cue reactivity among alcohol-dependent outpatients. *Psychol. Addict. Behav.* **2007**, *21*, 244–253. [CrossRef]
29. Conklin, C.A.; Tiffany, S.T. Applying extinction research and theory to cue-exposure addiction treatments. *Addiction* **2002**, *97*, 155–167. [CrossRef]
30. Ghiţă, A.; Gutiérrez-Maldonado, J. Applications of virtual reality in individuals with alcohol misuse: A systematic review. *Addict. Behav.* **2018**, *81*, 1–11. [CrossRef]
31. Riva, G. Virtual reality: An experiential tool for clinical psychology. *Br. J. Guid. Couns.* **2009**, *37*, 335–343. [CrossRef]
32. Ferrer-García, M.; García-Rodríguez, O.; Gutiérrez-Maldonado, J.; Pericot-Valverde, I.; Secades-Villa, R. Efficacy of Virtual Reality in triggering the craving to smoke: Its relation to level of presence and nicotine dependence. *Annu. Rev. Cyberther. Telemed.* **2010**, *8*, 99–106.
33. Serre, F.; Fatseas, M.; Swendsen, J.; Auriacombe, M. Ecological momentary assessment in the investigation of craving and substance use in daily life: A systematic review. *Drug Alcohol. Dep.* **2015**, *148*, 1–20. [CrossRef]
34. Shiffman, S.; Stone, A.A.; Hufford, M.R. Ecological momentary assessment. *Annu. Rev. Clin. Psychol.* **2008**, *4*, 1–32. [CrossRef]
35. Bordnick, P.S.; Traylor, A.; Copp, H.L.; Graap, K.M.; Carter, B.; Ferrer, M.; Waton, A.P. Assessing reactivity to virtual reality alcohol based cues. *Addict. Behav.* **2008**, *33*, 743–756. [CrossRef]
36. Cho, S.; Ku, J.; Park, J.; Han, K.; Lee, H.; Choi, Y.K.; Jung, Y.-C.; Namkoong, K.; Kim, J.-J.; Kim, I.Y.; et al. Development and Verification of an Alcohol Craving–Induction Tool Using Virtual Reality: Craving Characteristics in Social Pressure Situation. *CyberPsychol. Behav.* **2008**, *11*, 302–309. [CrossRef]

37. Pericot-Valverde, I.; Secades-Villa, R.; Gutierrez-Maldonado, J.; Garcia-Rodriguez, O. Effects of systematic cue exposure through virtual reality on cigarette craving. *Nicotine Tob. Res.* **2014**, *16*, 1470–1477. [CrossRef]
38. Acker, J.; MacKillop, J. Behavioral economic analysis of cue-elicited craving for tobacco: A Virtual Reality study. *Nicotine Tob. Res.* **2013**, *15*, 1409–1416. [CrossRef]
39. Bordnick, P.S.; Graap, K.M.; Copp, H.L.; Brooks, J.; Ferrer, M. Virtual Reality cue reactivity assessment in cigarette smokers. *Cyberpsychol. Behav.* **2005**, *8*, 487–492. [CrossRef]
40. Culbertson, C.; Nicolas, S.; Zaharovits, I.; London, E.D.; Garza, R.; Brody, A.L.; Newton, T.F. Methamphetamine craving induced in an online virtual reality environment. *Pharmacol. Biochem. Behav.* **2010**, *96*, 454–460. [CrossRef]
41. Saladin, M.E.; Brady, K.T.; Graap, K.; Rothbaum, B.O. A preliminary report on the use of virtual reality technology to elicit craving and cue reactivity in cocaine dependent individuals. *Addict. Behav.* **2006**, *31*, 1881–1894. [CrossRef]
42. Pla-Sanjuanelo, J.; Ferrer-García, M.; Vilalta-Abella, F.; Riva, G.; Dakanalis, A.; Ribas-Sabaté, J.; Andreu-Gracia, A.; Fernandez-Aranda, F.; Sanchez-Diaz, I.; Escandón-Nagel, N.; et al. Testing virtual reality-based cue-exposure software: Which cue-elicited responses best discriminate between patients with eating disorders and healthy controls? *Eat. Weight Disord.* **2019**, *24*, 757–769. [CrossRef]
43. American Psychiatric Association. *Diagnostic and Statistical Manual of Mental Disorders*; American Psychiatric Publishing: Arlington, VA, USA, 2013.
44. Llopis Llácer, J.J.; Gual Solé, A.; Rodríguez-Martos Dauer, A. Registro del consumo de bebidas alcohólicas mediante la unidad de bebida estándar. Diferencias geográficas. *Adicciones* **2000**, *12*, 11–20. [CrossRef]
45. Saunders, J.B.; Aasland, O.G.; Babor, T.F.; De La Fuente, J.R.; Grant, M. Development of the Alcohol Use Disorders Identification Test (AUDIT): WHO Collaborative Project on Early Detection of Persons with Harmful Alcohol Consumption-II. *Addiction* **1993**, *88*, 791–804. [CrossRef]
46. Contel Guillamón, M.; Gual Solé, A.; Colom Farran, J. Test para la identificación de trastornos por uso de alcohol (AUDIT): Traducción y validación del AUDIT al catalán y castellano. *Adicciones* **1999**, *11*, 337–347. [CrossRef]
47. Guardia Serecigni, J.; Segura García, L.; Gonzalvo Cirac, B.; Trujols Albet, J.; Tejero Pociello, A.; Suárez González, A.; Martí Gil, A. Estudio de validación de la Escala Multidimensional de Craving de Alcohol. *Med. Clin.* **2004**, *123*, 211–216. [CrossRef]
48. Spielberger, C.D.; Gonzalez-Reigosa, F.; Martinez-Urrutia, A.; Natalicio, L.F.S.; Natalicio, D.S. Development of the Spanish Edition of the State-Trait Anxiety Inventory. *Interam. J. Psychol.* **1971**, *5*, 145–158.
49. Ghiță, A.; Teixidor, L.; Monras, M.; Ortega, L.; Mondon, S.; Gual, A.; Paredes, S.M.; Villares-Urgell, L.; Porras-Garcia, B.; Ferrer-Garcia, M.; et al. Identifying triggers of alcohol craving to develop effective virtual environments for cue exposure therapy. *Front. Psychol.* **2019**, *10*, 74. [CrossRef]
50. Lee, J.S.; Namkoong, K.; Ku, J.; Cho, S.; Park, J.Y.; Choi, Y.K.; Kim, J.J.; Kim, I.Y.; Kim, S.I.; Jung, Y.C. Social pressure-induced craving in patients with alcohol dependence: Application of virtual reality to coping skill training. *Psychiatry Investig.* **2008**, *5*, 239–243. [CrossRef]
51. Gamito, P.; Oliveira, J.; Baptista, A.; Morais, D.; Lopes, P.; Rosa, P.; Santos, N.; Brito, R. Eliciting nicotine craving with virtual smoking cues. *Cyberpsychol. Behav. Soc. Netw.* **2014**, *17*, 556–561. [CrossRef]
52. Shin, Y.B.; Kim, J.J.; Kim, M.K.; Kyeong, S.; Jung, Y.H.; Eom, H.; Kim, E. Development of an effective virtual environment in eliciting craving in adolescents and young adults with internet gaming disorder. *PLoS ONE* **2018**, *13*, e0195677. [CrossRef]
53. Bouchard, S.; Robillard, G.; Giroux, I.; Jacques, C.; Loranger, C.; St-Pierre, M.; Chrétien, M.; Goulet, A. Using virtual reality in the treatment of gambling disorder: The development of a new tool for cognitive behavior therapy. *Front. Psychiatry* **2017**, *8*, 27. [CrossRef] [PubMed]
54. Ryan, J.J.; Kreiner, D.S.; Chapman, M.D.; Stark-Wroblewski, K. Virtual reality cues for binge drinking in college students. *CyberPsychol. Behav.* **2010**, *13*, 159–162. [CrossRef] [PubMed]
55. Ferrer-García, M.; Pla-Sanjuanelo, J.; Dakanalis, A.; Vilalta-Abella, F.; Riva, G.; Fernandez-Aranda, F.; Forcano, L.; Riesco, N.; Sánchez, I.; Clerici, M.; et al. A randomized trial of Virtual Reality-based cue exposure second-level therapy and cognitive-behavior second-level therapy for bulimia nervosa and binge-eating disorder: Outcome at six-month follow-up. *Cyberpsychol. Behav. Soc. Netw.* **2018**, *22*, 60–68. [CrossRef] [PubMed]

56. Ghiță, A.; Ferrer-Garcia, M.; Gutiérrez-Maldonado, J. Behavioral, craving, and anxiety responses among light and heavy drinking college students in alcohol-related virtual environments. *Annu. Rev. Cyberther. Telemed.* **2017**, *15*, 135–140.
57. Bordnick, P.S.; Carter, B.L.; Traylor, A.C. What virtual reality research in addictions can tell us about the future of obesity assessment and treatment. *J. Diabetes Sci. Technol.* **2011**, *5*, 265–271. [CrossRef] [PubMed]
58. Pla-Sanjuanelo, J.; Ferrer-García, M.; Gutiérrez-Maldonado, J.; Riva, G.; Andreu-Gracia, A.; Dakanalis, A.; Fernandez-Aranda, F.; Forcano, L.; Ribas-Sabaté, J.; Riesco, N.; et al. Identifying specific cues and contexts related to bingeing behavior for the development of effective virtual environments. *Appetite* **2015**, *87*, 81–89. [CrossRef] [PubMed]
59. Ferrer-García, M.; Gutiérrez-Maldonado, J.; Pla-Sanjuanelo, J.; Vilalta-Abella, F.; Riva, G.; Clerici, M.; Ribas-Sabate, J.; Andreu-Garcia, A.; Fernandez-Aranda, F.; Forcano, L.; et al. A randomised controlled comparison of second-level treatment approaches for treatment-resistant adults with bulimia nervosa and binge eating disorder: Assessing the benefits of virtual reality cue exposure therapy. *Eur. Eat. Disord. Rev.* **2017**, *25*, 479–490. [CrossRef]

© 2019 by the authors. Licensee MDPI, Basel, Switzerland. This article is an open access article distributed under the terms and conditions of the Creative Commons Attribution (CC BY) license (http://creativecommons.org/licenses/by/4.0/).

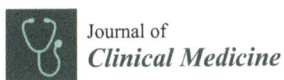

Article

Motor Adaptation Impairment in Chronic Cannabis Users Assessed by a Visuomotor Rotation Task

Ivan Herreros [1,†], Laia Miquel [2,3,*,†], Chrysanthi Blithikioti [2,3], Laura Nuño [2], Belen Rubio Ballester [4], Klaudia Grechuta [4], Antoni Gual [2,3], Mercè Balcells-Oliveró [2,‡] and Paul Verschure [4,5,‡]

1. SPECS Lab, Universitat Pompeu Fabra, 08002 Barcelona, Spain
2. GRAC, Grup de Recerca en Addiccions Clínic, Villarroel, 170 08036 Barcelona, Spain
3. IDIBAPS, Institut d'Investigacions Biomèdiques August Pi i Sunyer, Villarroel, 170 08036 Barcelona, Spain
4. IBEC, Institute for Biomedical Engineering of Catalonia, Universitat Politècnica de Catalunya, 08028 Barcelona, Spain
5. ICREA, Institució Catalana de Recerca i Estudis Avançats, Passeig Lluís Companys, 08010 Barcelona, Spain
* Correspondence: MIQUEL@clinic.cat; Tel.: +34-93-227-17-19; Fax: +34-93-227-54-54
† These authors contributed equally as the first authorship.
‡ These authors contributed equally as the last authorship.

Received: 31 May 2019; Accepted: 16 July 2019; Published: 18 July 2019

Abstract: Background—The cerebellum has been recently suggested as an important player in the addiction brain circuit. Cannabis is one of the most used drugs worldwide, and its long-term effects on the central nervous system are not fully understood. No valid clinical evaluations of cannabis impact on the brain are available today. The cerebellum is expected to be one of the brain structures that are highly affected by prolonged exposure to cannabis, due to its high density in endocannabinoid receptors. We aim to use a motor adaptation paradigm to indirectly assess cerebellar function in chronic cannabis users (CCUs). Methods—We used a visuomotor rotation (VMR) task that probes a putatively-cerebellar implicit motor adaptation process together with the learning and execution of an explicit aiming rule. We conducted a case-control study, recruiting 18 CCUs and 18 age-matched healthy controls. Our main measure was the angular aiming error. Results—Our results show that CCUs have impaired implicit motor adaptation, as they showed a smaller rate of adaptation compared with healthy controls (drift rate: 19.3 +/− 6.8° vs. 27.4 +/− 11.6°; t(26) = −2.1, $p = 0.048$, Cohen's $d = −0.8$, 95% CI = (−1.7, −0.15)). Conclusions—We suggest that a visuomotor rotation task might be the first step towards developing a useful tool for the detection of alterations in implicit learning among cannabis users.

Keywords: cerebellum; cannabis; implicit motor learning; motor adaptation; visuomotor rotation

1. Introduction

Cannabis is the most consumed illicit drug of abuse worldwide, ranking right after alcohol and tobacco [1,2]. The effects of the principal active component of cannabis, Delta9-tetrahydrocannabinol (THC), on the brain are still not well characterized. The cerebellum has several motor and cognitive functions [3] and has been suggested as a crucial structure for the addiction brain network [4]. It is well known that the cerebellum has a very high density of Cannabinoid receptor type 1 (CB1) receptors; however, little is known about its functional deficits due to chronic cannabis use. Motor adaptation is a cerebellum-dependent motor function that can be assessed with a visuomotor rotation (VMR) task and it might be altered in chronic cannabis users. Until now, there are no diagnostic tools that allow us to rate possible cerebellar impairments. We suggest that the VMR task could become a tool to assess cerebellar alterations due to chronic cannabis use (CCU).

Given the current trend towards the tolerance/legalization of its medical and recreational uses [5,6], it is crucial to clarify how long-term cannabis consumption affects brain function and performance. Numerous studies have evaluated the behavioral effects of acute and non-acute cannabis use [7], showing effects of cannabis not only on cognitive processes such as attention and memory [8–10], but also on psychomotor tasks, where reaction times and the ability to inhibit motor actions are impaired [11,12]. In addition, acute cannabis consumption increases the risk of driving accidents two- to three-fold [13]. However, there is still no correlation between the known molecular effects of cannabis and changes in overt behavior. This hampers our ability to assess cannabis-induced levels of dysfunction and the associated risks of chronic use and cannabis addiction.

Progress in understanding the consequences of cannabis requires linking its effects on the biological substrate with deficits in performance. THC [14] acts in the central nervous system through the CB1 receptor [15,16]. CB1 receptors are located in presynaptic terminals and have a regulatory effect on synaptic transmission [17,18]. The distribution and density of CB1 receptors in the brain may indicate which brain areas are more affected by the prolonged use of cannabis. Even though CB1 receptors are expressed all over the brain [19,20] (e.g., hippocampus, amygdala, striatum), their concentration is especially high in the molecular layer of the cerebellum [19]. In particular, cannabis consumption has been shown to down-regulate the CB1 receptors in the cerebellar molecular layer [21], affecting cerebellar plasticity mechanisms [22]. Indeed, chronic use of cannabis affects cerebellar-dependent behaviors both in animals and humans—specifically eye-blink conditioning, which is one of the basic paradigms for studying cerebellar associative learning [23]. CB1 knock-out mice and mice exposed to CB1 antagonists display a decreased acquisition of cerebellar-dependent eye-blink responses [24]. In humans, this result has been replicated in non-acute chronic cannabis users tested after 24 h of abstinence [25]. However, it is still not clear how deficits in eye-blink conditioning translate to easily administered diagnostic tests and instrumental activities of daily life.

Motor adaptation is a cerebellar-dependent function that has not been studied in chronic cannabis users (CCUs). Through adaptation, the motor control system readjusts to changes in the dynamics of their musculoskeletal system and body configuration [26,27]. Motor adaptation occurs in automatically when a difference between the predicted trajectory and the observed movement exists. Motor adaptation is frequently studied with visuomotor rotation paradigms [28], where a specific perturbation creates a mismatch between the motor action and the observed outcome. Healthy individuals will gradually compensate for this mismatch and adjust to sizeable perturbations, without awareness of the process (implicit motor learning). One way to speed up adaptation is by introducing a strategy that enables participants to explicitly adjust their aiming direction to hit a given target, as Mazzoni and Krakauer did (MK task) [29]. By inserting a rule, healthy participants manage to immediately cancel aiming errors (explicit motor learning) but at the expense of setting the predicted trajectory and the actual trajectory in conflict. In other words, with practice, participants make increasingly larger errors (implicit motor learning occurs). In general, cerebellar pathologies induce reduced adaptation [30,31]. Specifically, in the MK task, cerebellar-ataxic patients, despite using an explicit strategy [32], performed "better" (with less systematic error), as implicit adaptation is impaired.

Given the above observations, we sought to assess the impact of chronic cannabis use (CCU) in motor adaptation using a VMR paradigm. We hypothesize that THC, acting as an exogenous agonist of the cannabinoid receptors, will diminish cerebellar plasticity. For this reason, we look for a measurable impact on motor adaptation—a cerebellar-dependent process that facilitates maintaining accurate control of motor behavior [27]—that can be studied with the VMR task [29,32]. We expect that, alike to cerebellar ataxic patients, chronic cannabis consumers will have reduced implicit motor adaptation and thus will perform more accurately than healthy controls on the VMR task.

2. Experimental Section

2.1. Design

We conducted a case-control study. The study protocol is registered in clinicaltrials.gov, ID: NCT02816034. The study was approved by the Ethics Committee of Hospital Clínic de Barcelona (decision number HCB/2016/0018).

2.2. Participants

Study participants were between 18 and 50 years old. We included in the experimental group individuals following Diagnostic and Statistical Manual of Mental Disorders (DSM–V) criteria for Cannabis Use Disorder that screened positive for cannabis in the urine analysis performed the same day of their assessment. For the experimental and control groups, we recruited right-handed participants, without another active substance-use disorder (except of tobacco use disorder), with normal or corrected-to-normal vision. Participants with a cognitive impairment, such as mental retardation, or with psychotic disorders were excluded. Cannabis users were recruited among the patients of the Addiction Unit of a tertiary Hospital and their acquaintances. The sample included 17 CCUs and 18 healthy age-matched controls. All the participants signed an informed consent form before the initiation of the experiment. Participants were compensated for their effort with a voucher equivalent to a lunch ticket.

2.3. Procedures

A clinical interview was performed by a psychiatrist and a psychologist with mental health and addiction expertise. Socio-demographic data, including gender and age, were collecteddduring the clinical interviews. DSM-V criteria were used to diagnose patients with Cannabis Use Disorder. Furthermore, we gathered information about the frequency and quantity of cannabis consumed during the last week and the last 6 months using an ad hoc questionnaire. We used the first question of the Cannabis Use Disorder Identification Test (CUDIT) [33] to determine the frequency of cannabis use. In order to quantify cannabis use we used the Standard Joint Unit (1 SJU = 1 joint = 7 mg THC) [34]. The Scale for the Assessment and Rating of Ataxia (SARA) [35] was administered to assess ataxia. The SARA is a semi-quantitative scale, which has 8 items and assesses motor changes in gait, stance, sitting, speech disturbances, finger chase, nose-finger chase, fast alternating hand movements and heel–shin slide.

Participants sat in front of a desk (Figure 1A,B) and were asked to control a cursor that was displayed on a screen, using an optical pen. Its position was recorded using a high-resolution digitizing tablet (Intuos3, Wacom, Saitama, Japan) at a sampling rate of 100 Hz. During the task, every trial required moving the stylus with the right hand over the digitization tablet from an initial central position. Visual feedback was projected on a surface placed in front of the subject. This surface occluded the subject's view of the movements of their arm. The projection displayed eight circles over the surface, arranged in a circle (Figure 1C,D). For each trial, a target marked with a bulls-eye appeared inside one of these eight circles. Participants were instructed to perform a center–out reaching movement from the initial position towards the target with the pen. Participants moved as fast as possible to reach the target, which in turn turned red Then they then returned the pen to the start position. Depending on the phase of the experiment, the correct target was either the bulls-eye or the clockwise adjacent marker.

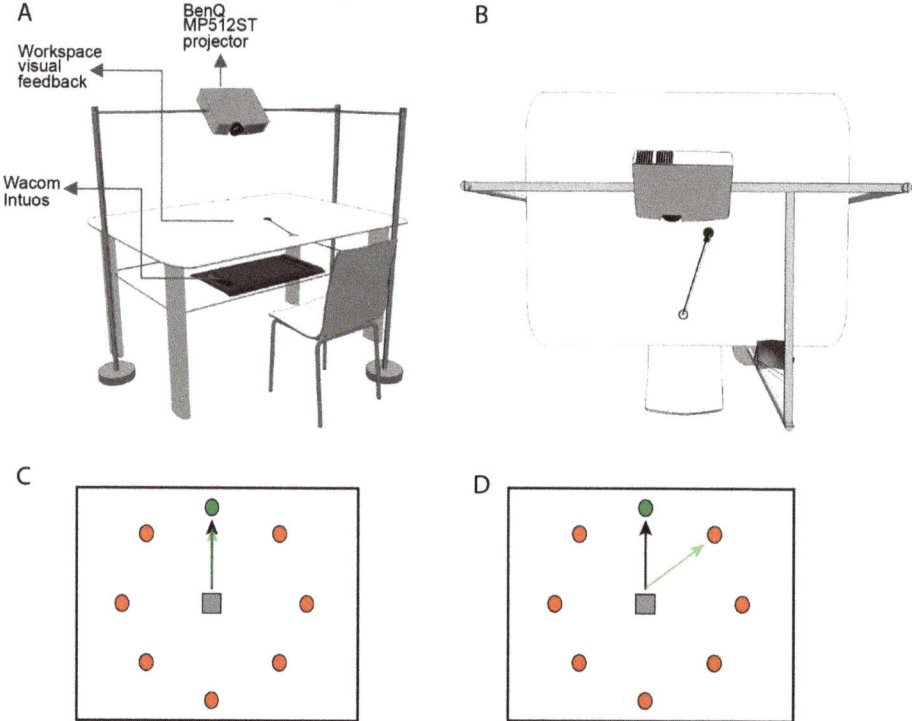

Figure 1. Perspective (**A**) and top view (**B**) of the experimental setup. Subjects were seated approximately 25 cm in front of a table with both hands occluded to vision. Movement trajectories were recorded through a digitizing tablet (Intuos Pro, Wacom, Saitama) located at waist height at the lower part of the table. We used a projector (BenQ MP512ST, Texas Instruments, Taoyuan, Taiwan), mounted 55 cm above the table, to display the behavioral tasks. The size of the projection was 46 × 61 cm; data were sampled and stimuli displayed at 100 Hz. Prior to the experiment, we adjusted the seat in order to ensure that the distance between the center of the projection and the eyes of each participant was approximately 40 cm. (**C**) Visuomotor task. A centered home position (gray square) and eight circles (red) are projected over the surface, arranged in a circle. For each trial, a target appeared inside one of these eight circles (green circle). (**D**) During the Rotation and Rotation Strategy phases, the visual feedback (black arrow) of actual center–out reaching movements (green arrow) deviate by 45 degrees in a counter-clockwise direction.

The experimental protocol constisted of 7 phases and a total amount of 242 movements. These movements were grouped in 30 blocks of 8 trials and 1 of only 2trials. We replicated the protocol performed in cerebellar ataxic patients [32]. The protocol started with two baseline adaptation phases (B1 and B2) separated by a cognitive control phase (practice strategy, PS). Each baseline phase consisted of 24 movements (three blocks) where the participants moved towards the indicated target, and the visually projected cursor reproduced the participants' movement trajectory. In the PS phase, participants were asked to aim to the marker adjacent to the target in the clock-wise direction (that is, the marker appearing at 45 degrees to the clock-wise direction). After these three phases, a visual rotation was introduced without warning during two trials. In these trials, the mapping of the movement-to-visual coordinates was altered such that the position of the displayed cursor was rotated 45 degrees counter-clockwise relative to the starting position. In order to force fast reaching movements, trials were repeated when movements were not completed within a time limit of 1.5 seconds after target appearance.

After these two trials, participants started the main experimental phase, i.e., the rotation plus strategy (RS) phase, where they were instructed to overcome the rotation by applying the strategy learned in the PS phase. The RS phase lasted 80 trials (10 blocks), that is, ten movements towards each target in random order. The last phase of the experiment started with a no-feedback washout (NF) phase, where participants were instructed not to apply the rotation strategy anymore, while they performed a series of 8 reaching movements, in the absence of visual feedback. Finally, in an 80 trials long washout phase (W), visual feedback was reinstalled in the absence of any rotation. The whole task lasted approximately 20 min.

2.4. Analysis

We measured performance in terms of the angular error—the angular difference between the executed movement and target directionsThis measure can be very noisy on a trial by trial basis, mostly because participants sometimes lapse and they apply the aiming rule incorrectly. For this reason we used the median angular error per block of 8 trials, noting that within a block all eight target positions were presented once.

One patient and one control were removed from the final sample because of laterality problems and were not included in the analyses. An additional patient was discarded because her behavior was a clear outlier (3 SD) from the mean performance score and was not included in the analyses. Additionally, to avoid acute cannabis use effects on performance, we removed from the analysis all participants that had consumed cannabis within the 6 hours prior to performing the task ($n = 4$), as this interval has been used as a criterion for cannabis' acute effects [36].

If not stated otherwise, sample estimates are reported as mean +/− standard deviation, and qualitative data are described as percentages. Chi-square test and t-tests were done to compare groups depending on the type of data. Bonferroni correction was performed for multiple comparisons and Cohen coefficient for effect size.

3. Results

CCUs ($n = 11$, 4 women) had a mean age of 28.7 +/− 8.6 years old, which was age-matched by the control group (CG) ($n = 17$, 8 women; 30.7 +/− 7.1 years old). CCUs were diagnosed with a severe cannabis use disorder (≥ 6 criteria) and 75% were marijuana smokers. One subject was diagnosed with an attention deficit hyperactivity disorder in childhood but did not fulfill DSM-V criteria at the time of inclusion in the study. Experimental subjects showed significant differences in educational level compared to controls. For more details on clinical and sociodemographic characteristics, see Table 1.

Table 1. Sociodemographic and clinical characteristics of the experimental (chronic cannabis users) and control groups.

	Experimental ($n = 11$)				Control ($n = 17$)				χ^2/t/fisher	p-Value
	n	%	Mean	SD	n	%	Mean	SD		
Men	7	63.6			9	52.9			0.3	0.6
Age			28.3	8.1			30.7	7.1	−0.8	0.41
Academic Level									13.7	<0.001
High school	8	72.7			1	5.9				
University	3	27.3			16	94.1				
Civil Status									0.05	0.8
Single	8	72.7			13	76.5				
Married	3	27.3			4	23.5				
Age at first cannabis consumption			16.6	3			15	2		

Table 1. *Cont.*

	Experimental (n = 11)				Control (n = 17)				χ^2/t/fisher	p-Value
	n	%	Mean	SD	n	%	Mean	SD		
Age at regular cannabis use			19	2.1						
Regular cigarette smokers (yes)	4	36.4			1	6.3			0.134	0.07
Frequency of Cannabis use last 6 months										
4 to 6 times per week	2	18.2								
Daily	9	75.0								
SJU/day last 6 months			3.7	3.7						
Frequency of Cannabis use last week										
Never	2	18.2								
2 to 3 times per week	1	69.1								
4 to 6 times per week	2	18.2								
Daily	6	54.5								
SJU/day last week			2	2.2						
Standard drink units per week			6.7	8.3			2.9	3.9	1.6	0.1
SARA			0				0			

SD: Standard Deviation; SJU: Standard Joint Unit (1 SJU = 7 mg THC); SDU: Standard Drink Unit (1 SDU = 10 gr of pure alcohol). SARA: Scale for the Assessment and Rating of Ataxia. Bonferroni correction = p-value = 0.006.

The evolution of the angular error during the VMR task was our main behavioral outcome (Figure 2A). Cannabis users as well as controls demonstrated an average evolution of the angular error consistent with the expected interference between the use of an explicit strategy and an implicit adaptation process, as reported for healthy subjects in relevant studies [28,37]. Both groups experienced an increase in error (a drift towards positive angular errors) as trials accumulated in the RS phase. To assess implicit motor adaptation, we used both the maximum aiming error (degrees in cursor space) during the RS phase, or the *peak drift* [31], together with the *drift rate*, measured as the slope of the adaptation curve in the RS phase (in degrees per trial). To reduce the noise that was introduced by outlying trials, both measures were computed based on block scores, obtained as the median error for the eight trials in each block. Drift rate was significantly smaller for CCUs compared to controls (0.1 +/− 0.1°/trial vs. 0.2 +/− 0.1°/trial; $t(26) = -2.2$, $p = 0.037$, Cohen's $d = -0.9$, 95% CI = (−1.8, −0.1)) and so was peak drift (19.3 +/− 6.7° vs. 27.4 +/− 11.6°; $t(26) = -2.1$, $p = 0.048$, Cohen's $d = -0.8$, 95% CI = −1.7, −0.1), confirming the experimental hypothesis that chronic cannabis consumption can reduce motor adaptation. However, even though CCUs tended to display larger after-effects than controls, which were measured as the remnant error during the no-feedback washout phase (9.1 +/− 8.7° vs. 13.5 +/− 4.5°; $t(26) = -1.8$; $p = 0.09$), the difference did not reach significance. Notably, adaptation occurred very rapidly at the onset of the RS phase in comparison to the literature [38], which suggests that the use of continuous feedback might have provoked a fast explicit adaptation process in addition to implicit adaptation.

The difference in performance was not due to an intrinsic difference between CCUs and controls in unperturbed aiming, as both groups scored similarly in both baseline periods (−2.3 +/− 3.4° vs. −2.1 +/− 2.5°; $t(26) = -0.1$, $p = 0.89$ and −1.4 +/− 1.8° vs. −1.4 +/− 2.1°; $t(26) = -0.1$, $p = 0.95$ in B1 and B2, respectively). Differences were also minor in execution at either the onset or the offset of the PS phase (block 4: −6.4 +/− 5.8° vs. −5.0 +/− 5.2°; $t(26) = -0.7$, $p = 0.51$ and block 6: −4.0 +/− 5.7° vs. −2.1 +/− 3.1°; $t(26) = -1.1$, $p = 0.26$). No significant differences were found between CCUs and the CG in VMR task performance in terms of timings.

Finally, even though the experimental and control groups did not differ significantly in terms of alcohol and tobacco consumption, one could not a-priori discard their involvement in the reduced adaptation observed in this study, as they both are psycho-active substances. To clarify this, we performed an ordinary least-squares analysis, where we added the levels of tobacco and alcohol consumption as possible confounds in addition to the group variable. Given the reduced sample size, the contrast between CCUs vs. controls only at the trend level ($p = 0.10$), but this was in striking contrast with the almost null influence observed both for tobacco ($p = 0.75$) and alcohol ($p = 0.99$).

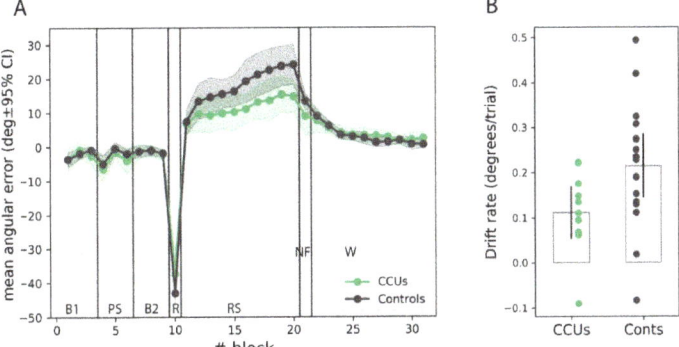

Figure 2. Motor adaptation in chronic cannabis users (CCUs) and control participants (Conts). (**A**): Evolution of the average error. Vertical lines separate different phases of the experiment, indicated by the labels: B1, first baseline period; PS: practice strategy; B2: second baseline period; R: rotation; RS: rotation plus strategy; NF: no feedback washout; W: regular washout. (**B**): Rate of error increase in the RS phase. Shaded areas and error bars indicate the 95% confidence interval of the mean.

4. Discussion

This is the first study that analyzes the effects of chronic cannabis consumption on a visuomotor rotation task to assess the processes involved in motor adaptation. CCUs displayed impaired adaptation, manifested as lower aiming errors in the VMR task than controls.

Our results are consistent with our hypothesis that chronic cannabis use has an impact on cerebellar-dependent functions and, more specifically, on motor adaptation. The visuomotor adaptation paradigm has been used as a marker of cerebellar damage in ataxic patients, who show impaired implicit learning, putatively, due to disrupted forward internal models [32]. More specifically, cerebellar ataxic patients accumulate fewer aiming errors during the rotation and strategy (RS) phase, indicating a decreased motor adaptation [32]. It is interesting to note that the effect size of the original study with ataxic patients is very sizeable (Cohen's d = −2.627), while the effect size on CCUs is moderate (Cohen's d= −0.8). This is not surprising, as the clinical manifestation of cerebellar dysfunction of ataxia is severe, while cannabis-induced cerebellar alterations do not lead to a clinical phenotype (all the participants assessed scored zero on the SARA scale). However, we suggest that our results are clinically meaningful for two reasons: First of all, in several brain disorders, early alterations in the patient's brain are present even decades before the first clinical symptoms appear [39,40]. Our paper shows an altered performance of CCUs in a visuomotor adaptation task, indicating subtle cerebellar alterations in the users' brains. These results were obtained after excluding experimental participants under the acute effects of cannabis (on the suggestion of an anonymous reviewer). Interestingly, even though this reduced the sample size (from $n = 33$ to $n = 28$), statistical significance, and therefore the underlying effect size, increased (from d = −0.7 to −0.8). Our finding suggests that CCUs adapt less when they are not under the acute effects of cannabis. This deficit might be explained by the hypothesis of CB1 receptor down-regulation due to cannabis use [21]. More specifically, it has been shown that repeated cannabis exposure causes endocytosis of the endocannabinoid receptors, resulting in reduced activity of those receptors in the absence of their exogenous agonist. If this hypothesis explains our results, it would be plausible that acute cannabis use in CCUs may indeed hide an underlying impairment in cerebellar-dependent motor adaptation. Although our results show very subtle alterations compared to ataxic patients, these might be the first signs of a future clinically significant impairment that will only manifest with continuous heavy use [41]. Future longitudinal studies will clarify whether these early cerebellar alterations prelude long-term clinical symptoms. Secondly, it is noteworthy that even though, CCUs show no measurable motor deficits clinically, they share a certain degree of alterations in motor adaptation with cerebellar ataxic patients. Future research will show the reliability of the task as a potential tool for assessing brain alterations, as well as whether the latter are present exclusively in cannabis users or they are part of addiction-induced brain alterations.

Globally, these results indicate that VMR tasks might be a simple, non-invasive and novel way to start exploring a basic cerebellar function in CCUs. The cerebellum is crucial for motor adaptation, among other functions. As implicit learning is an essentialskill for everyday functioning, our findings are the first step towards understanding more complex cerebellar deficits. Our results are in line with the increasingly recognized role of the cerebellum in higher cognitive functions and emotional processes, and a recent review that points out a cerebellar involvement in cannabis addiction [42]. Future research should examine whether there are changes in the performance of users after cessation of use, as well as if this task can capture cerebellar alterations in individuals dependent on other substances, such as tobacco, alcohol, amphetamines, etc.

This study has limitations that have to be taken into consideration when interpreting the results. First of all, the small sample size might have compromised the power of the study, so further studies should increase the sample size and also explicitly indicate in the protocol that participants are required to refrain from cannabis use for at least 6 hours prior to the study. Regardless of the small sample size, the moderate effect size might be due to the fact that CCUs do not show any clinically significant motor deficits (SARA score equals to 0), unlike ataxic patients. Secondly, significant differences were found between groups in terms of educational level. While we propose that educational level should not be an important confounder, due to the implicit nature of the task, tobacco and alcohol use might have had an effect on performance. Indeed, even though an ordinary least-squares analysis showed inexistent correlation with performance in the present study, one should take into account for future studies that reduced adaptationmight arise due to the synergistic effects of all substances, and not exclusively of cannabis. Thirdly, even if the small differences that we found in motor adaptation are representative of cerebellar alterations in CCUs, no causation can be inferred, as the brain differences might have been preceded cannabis use. Future longitudinal studies should clarify this matter. Finally, in previous studies where participants only received end-point position feedback, the systematic aiming error accumulated slowly during the 80 trials of the RS phase. However, we opted for providing participants with continuous feedback, evaluating the angular orientation using the initial part of the trajectory. The increased level of feedback has introduced discrepancies with the literature. First, as intended, it may have accelerated (implicit) adaptation, consistently with Taylor et al. [38], where a different VMR task was used. Indeed, the drift rate in our control group (0.2°/trial) is twice as fast as in Taylor et al. [32] (circa 0.1°/trial). Secondly, it has produced a shift in the maximum peak drift, which here reached 27.2° for the control group whereas in previous experiments it remained near 10° [29,32]. This increased peak drift might be due to fast explicit processes [38], as suggested by the high level of adaptation already manifested in the first block of the RS phase. However, we expect to have minimized the influence of the explicit learning in our main result by reporting the drift rate, which was computed taking into account the median performance for each one of the ten blocks of eight trials of the RS phase. In other words, our measure of drift rate is not affected by the high level of adaptation which had already been reached at the first block of the RS phase. Besides, even though we report a tendency in the after-effects that is consistent with our hypothesis of decreased implicit adaptation in CCUs, the difference only reached trend-level significance ($p < 0.09$). Hence, the replication of these results with a bigger sample size may be needed to confirm that the difference in performance reported here is due to putatively-cerebellar implicit motor learning. Indeed, a possibility to avoid involving explicit processes would be using newer VMR paradigms more precisely targeted at measuring implicit learning [43].

5. Conclusions

Taken altogether, CCUs showed a moderately decreased motor adaptation compared to controls, assessed with the VMR task. This tool is easy to implement and might be able to detect subtle changes in brain function before clinical symptoms of damage occur. Future research will clarify whether the VMR task can emerge as a potential assessment tool of brain dysfunction secondary to chronic cannabis consumption.

Author Contributions: Conceptualization, I.H., L.M., M.B.-O., P.V.; Methodology, I.H., L.M.; Data analysis, I.H.; L.M. Investigation, I.H., L.M., C.B., L.N., K.G., B.R.B.; Writing—Original Draft Preparation, I.H., L.M.; Writing—Review & Editing, All authors; Supervision, M.B.-O., P.V., A.G.

Funding: This work was supported by MINECO "Retos Investigacion I+d+i", Plan Nacional project, SANAR (Gobierno de España)—under agreement TIN2013-44200-REC, FPI grant nr. BES-2014-068791, and by the European Research Council under grant agreement 341196 (CDAC).

Acknowledgments: The authors wish to thank all subjects participating in this study. CERCA Programme/ Generalitat de Catalunya.

Conflicts of Interest: LM has received honoraria from Lundbeck, outside of the work for this project. AG has received honoraria and travel grants from Lundbeck, Janssen, D&A Pharma and Servier, all outside the work for this project. The other authors declare that they have no competing interests.

References

1. UNODC. World Drug Report. 2016. Available online: https://www.unodc.org/wdr2016/ (accessed on 16 July 2019).
2. Al-Imam, A. The Most Popular Chemical Categories of NPS in Four Leading Countries of the Developed World: An Integrative Analysis of Trends Databases, Surface Web, and the Deep Web. *Glob. J. Health Sci.* **2017**, *9*, 40. [CrossRef]
3. Koziol, L.F.; Budding, D.; Andreasen, N.; Darrigo, S.; Bulgheroni, S.; Imamizu, H.; Ito, M.; Manto, M.; Marvel, C.; Parker, K.; et al. Consensus Paper: The Cerebellum's Role in Movement and Cognition. *Cerebellum* **2014**, *13*, 151–177. [CrossRef] [PubMed]
4. Miquel, M.; Vazquez-Sanroman, D.; Carbo-Gas, M.; Gil-Miravet, I.; Sanchis-Segura, C.; Carulli, D.; Manzo, J.; Coria-Avila, G.A. Have we been ignoring the elephant in the room? Seven arguments for considering the cerebellum as part of addiction circuitry. *Neurosci. Biol. Rev.* **2016**, *60*, 1–11. [CrossRef] [PubMed]
5. Hasin, D.S.; Sarvet, A.L.; Cerdá, M.; Keyes, K.M.; Stohl, M.; Galea, S.; Wall, M.M. US Adult Illicit Cannabis Use, Cannabis Use Disorder, and Medical Marijuana Laws1991–1992 to 2012–2013. *JAMA Psychiatry* **2017**, *74*, 579–588. [CrossRef] [PubMed]
6. Hall, W.; Weier, M. Assessing the Public Health Impacts of Legalizing Recreational Cannabis Use in the USA. *Clin. Pharmacol. Ther.* **2015**, *97*, 607–615. [CrossRef] [PubMed]
7. Volkow, N.D.; Swanson, J.M.; Evins, A.E.; DeLisi, L.E.; Meier, M.H.; Gonzalez, R.; Bloomfield, M.A.P.; Curran, H.V.; Baler, R. Effects of cannabis use on human behavior, including cognition, motivation, and psychosis: A review. *JAMA Psychiatry* **2016**, *73*, 292–297. [CrossRef] [PubMed]
8. Crane, N.A.; Schuster, R.M.; Fusar-Poli, P.; Gonzalez, R. Effects of cannabis on neurocognitive functioning: Recent advances, neurodevelopmental influences, and sex differences. *Neuropsychol. Rev.* **2013**, *23*, 117–137. [CrossRef]
9. Ramaekers, J.; Kauert, G.; Theunissen, E.; Toennes, S.; Moeller, M. Neurocognitive performance during acute THC intoxication in heavy and occasional cannabis users. *J. Psychopharmacol.* **2009**, *23*, 266–277. [CrossRef]
10. Meier, M.H.; Caspi, A.; Ambler, A.; Harrington, H.; Houts, R.; Keefe, R.S.E.; McDonald, K.; Ward, A.; Poulton, R.; Moffitt, T.E. Persistent cannabis users show neuropsychological decline from childhood to midlife. *Proc. Natl. Acad. Sci. USA* **2012**, *109*, E2657–E2664. [CrossRef]
11. Prashad, S.; Filbey, F.M. Cognitive motor deficits in cannabis users. *Curr. Opin. Behav. Sci.* **2017**, *13*, 1–7. [CrossRef]
12. Ramaekers, J.G.; Kauert, G.; van Ruitenbeek, P.; Theunissen, E.L.; Schneider, E.; Moeller, M.R. High-Potency Marijuana Impairs Executive Function and Inhibitory Motor Control. *Neuropsychopharmacology* **2006**, *31*, 2296–2303. [CrossRef] [PubMed]

13. Hall, W. What has research over the past two decades revealed about the adverse health effects of recreational cannabis use? *Addiction* **2015**, *110*, 19–35. [CrossRef] [PubMed]
14. Gaoni, Y.; Mechoulam, R. Isolation, structure, and partial synthesis of an active constituent of hashish. *J. Am. Chem. Soc.* **1964**, *86*, 1646–1647. [CrossRef]
15. Matsuda, L.; Lolait, S.; Brownstein, M.; Young, A.; Bonner, T. Structure of a cannabinoid receptor and functional expression of the cloned cDNA. *Nature* **1990**, *346*, 561–564. [CrossRef] [PubMed]
16. Devane, W.A.; Dysarz, F.A.; Johnson, M.R.; Melvin, L.S.; Howlett, A.C. Determination and characterization of a cannabinoid receptor in rat brain. *Mol. Pharmacol.* **1988**, *34*, 605–613. [PubMed]
17. Kano, M.; Ohno-Shosaku, T.; Hashimotodani, Y.; Uchigashima, M.; Watanabe, M. Endocannabinoid-mediated control of synaptic transmission. *Physiol. Rev.* **2009**, *89*, 309–380. [CrossRef] [PubMed]
18. Cadogan, A.K.; Alexander, S.P.; Boyd, E.A.; Kendall, D.A. Influence of cannabinoids on electrically evoked dopamine release and cyclic AMP generation in the rat striatum. *J. Neurochem.* **1997**, *69*, 1131–1137. [CrossRef] [PubMed]
19. Tsou, K.; Brown, S.; Sañudo-Peña, M.; Mackie, K.; Walker, J. Immunohistochemical distribution of cannabinoid CB1 receptors in the rat central nervous system. *Neuroscience* **1998**, *83*, 393–411. [CrossRef]
20. Egertova, M.; Elphick, M.R. Localisation of cannabinoid receptors in the rat brain using antibodies to the intracellular C-terminal tail of CB1. *J. Comp. Neurol.* **2000**, *422*, 159–171. [CrossRef]
21. Cutando, L.; Busquets-Garcia, A.; Puighermanal, E.; Gomis-González, M.; Delgado-García, J.M.; Gruart, A.; Maldonado, R.; Ozaita, A. Microglial activation underlies cerebellar deficits produced by repeated cannabis exposure. *J. Clin. Investig.* **2013**, *123*, 2816–2831. [CrossRef]
22. Safo, P.K.; Regehr, W.G. Endocannabinoids control the induction of cerebellar LTD. *Neuron* **2005**, *48*, 647–659. [CrossRef] [PubMed]
23. Hesslow, G.; Yeo, C.H. The functional anatomy of skeletal conditioning. In *A Neuroscientist's Guide to Classical Conditioning*; Springer: Berlin, Germany, 2002; pp. 86–146.
24. Kishimoto, Y. Endogenous Cannabinoid Signaling through the CB1 Receptor Is Essential for Cerebellum-Dependent Discrete Motor Learning. *J. Neurosci.* **2006**, *26*, 8829–8837. [CrossRef] [PubMed]
25. Skosnik, P.D.; Edwards, C.R.; O'Donnell, B.F.; Steffen, A.; Steinmetz, J.E.; Hetrick, W.P. Cannabis use disrupts eyeblink conditioning: Evidence for cannabinoid modulation of cerebellar-dependent learning. *Neuropsychopharmacology* **2008**, *33*, 1432–1440. [CrossRef] [PubMed]
26. Shadmehr, R.; Smith, M.A.; Krakauer, J.W. Error correction, sensory prediction, and adaptation in motor control. *Annu. Rev. Neurosci.* **2010**, *33*, 89–108. [CrossRef] [PubMed]
27. Herreros, I.; Verschure, P.F.M.J. Nucleo-olivary inhibition balances the interaction between the reactive and adaptive layers in motor control. *Neural Netw.* **2013**, *47*, 64–71. [CrossRef] [PubMed]
28. Krakauer, J.W.; Pine, Z.M.; Ghilardi, M.F.; Ghez, C. Learning of visuomotor transformations for vectorial planning of reaching trajectories. *J. Neurosci.* **2000**, *20*, 8916–8924. [CrossRef] [PubMed]
29. Mazzoni, P.; Krakauer, J.W. An Implicit Plan Overrides an Explicit Strategy during Visuomotor Adaptation. *J. Neurosci.* **2006**, *26*, 3642–3645. [CrossRef] [PubMed]
30. Weiner, M.J.; Hallett, M.; Funkenstein, H.H. Adaptation to lateral displacement of vision in patients with lesions of the central nervous system. *Neurology* **1983**, *33*, 766–772. [CrossRef] [PubMed]
31. Schlerf, J.E.; Xu, J.; Klemfuss, N.M.; Griffiths, T.L.; Ivry, R.B. Individuals with cerebellar degeneration show similar adaptation deficits with large and small visuomotor errors. *J. Neurophysiol.* **2013**, *109*, 1164–1173. [CrossRef]
32. Taylor, J.A.; Klemfuss, N.M.; Ivry, R.B. An explicit strategy prevails when the cerebellum fails to compute movement errors. *Cerebellum* **2010**, *9*, 580–586. [CrossRef]
33. Bonn-Miller, M.O.; Heinz, A.J.; Smith, E.V.; Bruno, R.; Adamson, S. Preliminary Development of a Brief Cannabis Use Disorder Screening Tool: The Cannabis Use Disorder Identification Test Short-Form. *Cannabis Cannabinoid Res.* **2016**, *1*, 252–261. [CrossRef] [PubMed]
34. Casajuana, C.; Balcells-Olivero, M.M.; López-Pelayo, H.; Miquel, L.; Teixidó, L.; Colom, J.; Nutt, D.J.; Rehm, J.; Gual, A. The Standard Joint Unit. *Drug Alcohol Depend.* **2017**, *1*, 109–116. [CrossRef] [PubMed]
35. Weyer, A.; Abele, M.; Schmitz-Hübsch, T.; Schoch, B.; Frings, M.; Timmann, D.; Klockgether, T. Reliability and validity of the scale for the assessment and rating of ataxia: A study in 64 ataxia patients. *Mov. Disord.* **2007**, *22*, 1633–1637. [CrossRef] [PubMed]

36. Crean, R.D.; Crane, N.A.; Mason, B.J. An evidence based review of acute and long-term effects of cannabis use on executive cognitive functions. *J. Addict. Med.* **2011**, *5*, 1–8. [CrossRef] [PubMed]
37. Taylor, J.A.; Ivry, R.B. Flexible cognitive strategies during motor learning. *PLoS Comput. Biol.* **2011**, *7*, e1001096. [CrossRef] [PubMed]
38. Taylor, J.A.; Krakauer, J.W.; Ivry, R.B. Explicit and implicit contributions to learning in a sensorimotor adaptation task. *J. Neurosci.* **2014**, *34*, 3023–3032. [CrossRef] [PubMed]
39. Beason-Held, L.L.; Goh, J.O.; An, Y.; Kraut, M.A.; O'Brien, R.J.; Ferrucci, L.; Resnick, S.M. Changes in brain function occur years before the onset of cognitive impairment. *J. Neurosci.* **2013**, *33*, 18008–18014. [CrossRef]
40. Nakamura, A.; Cuesta, P.; Kato, T.; Arahata, Y.; Iwata, K.; Yamagishi, M.; Kuratsubo, I.; Kato, K.; Bundo, M.; Diers, K.; et al. Early functional network alterations in asymptomatic elders at risk for Alzheimer's disease. *Sci. Rep.* **2017**, *7*, 6517. [CrossRef]
41. Nestoros, J.N.; Vakonaki, E.; Tzatzarakis, M.N.; Alegakis, A.; Skondras, M.D.; Tsatsakis, A.M. Long lasting effects of chronic heavy cannabis abuse. *Am. J. Addict.* **2017**, *26*, 335–342. [CrossRef]
42. Blithikioti, C.; Miquel, L.; Batalla, A.; Rubio, B.; Maffei, G.; Herreros, I.; Gual, A.; Verschure, P.; Balcells-Oliveró, M. Cerebellar alterations in cannabis users: A systematic review. *Addict. Biol.* **2019**. [CrossRef]
43. Morehead, J.R.; Taylor, J.A.; Parvin, D.E.; Ivry, R.B. Characteristics of Implicit Sensorimotor Adaptation Revealed by Task-irrelevant Clamped Feedback. *J. Cogn. Neurosci.* **2017**, *29*, 1061–1074. [CrossRef] [PubMed]

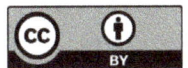 © 2019 by the authors. Licensee MDPI, Basel, Switzerland. This article is an open access article distributed under the terms and conditions of the Creative Commons Attribution (CC BY) license (http://creativecommons.org/licenses/by/4.0/).

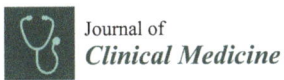

Article

What Do Real Alcohol Outpatients Expect about Alcohol Transdermal Sensors?

Pablo Barrio [1,2,3,*], Lidia Teixidor [1], Magalí Andreu [1] and Antoni Gual [1,2,3]

1. Addictive Behaviors Unit, Clinical Neuroscience Institute, Clinic Hospital, 08036 Barcelona, Spain; lteixidor@clinic.cat (L.T.); magali221292@gmail.com (M.A.); tgual@clinic.cat (A.G.)
2. Department of Psychiatry and Clinical Psychobiology, University of Barcelona, 08036 Barcelona, Spain
3. Grup de Recerca en Addiccions Clínic, Hospital Clínic de Barcelona, IDIBAPS, Universitat de Barcelona, Red de Trastornos adictivos (RETICS), 08036 Barcelona, Spain
* Correspondence: pbarrio@clinic.cat; Tel.: +34-227-5400; Fax: +34-932-275-400

Received: 3 April 2019; Accepted: 3 June 2019; Published: 5 June 2019

Abstract: Objective: Little is known about the potential acceptability of alcohol transdermal sensors among alcohol-dependent outpatients in routine clinical settings. The aim of the present study was to investigate patients' attitudes towards alcohol transdermal sensors, as well as features associated with enhanced acceptability and usability. Methods: A cross-sectional survey among routine alcohol outpatients was conducted. The Drug Attitude Inventory (DAI-10) was adapted to the field of alcohol transdermal sensors for attitudes assessment. Likert-type and multiple-choice questions were used for acceptability and usability evaluation. Results: 68 patients completed the questionnaire, and the DAI-10 mean score was 3 (standard deviation (SD) = 6.5). Internal consistency revealed a Cronbach alpha of 0.613. The score of a single The score of a single Likert-type question about overall perceived value was 7.4 (SD = 2.6). Its correlation with mean DAI-10 scores was $r = 0.633$, with $p < 0.001$. Relapse prevention and a stricter treatment control from therapists were the main reported advantages. Perceived stigma was the main disadvantage. Features increasing device discretion would enhance its acceptability. Conclusions: The data suggest that transdermal sensors could play a role in the clinical treatment of alcohol outpatients and concerns regarding stigma should be taken into account. Future designs should try to minimize size and visibility and stigma concerns should be discussed with patients.

Keywords: alcohol dependence; transdermal sensor; attitudes; stigma

1. Introduction

Alcohol remains a first-order global health problem, with 15 million people affected in the European Union [1]. Recent publications in the United States also warn about an increase in the prevalence of alcohol use disorders during the last decade [2]. The impact it has on both individuals and society is of an enormous dimension, both medically and economically [3,4]. A significant share of these consequences is attributable to the severest form of alcohol use, i.e., alcohol dependence, which is currently considered a chronic disease, with a relapsing–remitting nature. Despite some controversies in the field, abstinence has been the prevailing therapeutic goal in most of the existing settings, being considered the safest and most efficient pathway to early recovery [5,6]. Therefore, for a great majority of professionals dealing with alcohol dependence, monitoring abstinence becomes an indispensable task. Traditional tools for abstinence assessment have consisted of patients' self-reports and alcohol biomarkers. Despite recent improvements, especially in alcohol biomarkers [7,8], there remain some relevant limitations that could be overcome with the use of alcohol transdermal sensors.

Interestingly, in harm reduction or controlled drinking paradigms, alcohol transdermal sensors could also be of special utility, given the importance of quantifying the amount of alcohol ingested when patients chose to reduce their intake instead of abstaining. In quantifying the amount of alcohol consumed, transdermal sensors seem to be the most sensitive tool. In that sense, they could potentially be the ideal partner to the paradigm of heavy use over time [9], where the emphasis is put quantitatively on the amount of ethanol ingested rather than discretely qualifying patients as abstinent or not. This may suggest that transdermal sensors could be seen as a valuable tool to facilitate and improve digital phenotyping in addiction patients [10,11].

Transdermal sensors have been available for some years now. Their main use has been within the justice system [12]. There are also several studies in the literature assessing the devices' validity and functioning, and there have already been randomized trials to evaluate their efficacy and patients' experiences [13–17]. Together, they suggest that transdermal sensors could be effective in helping alcohol patients. They also point out towards good acceptability and feasibility. However, no study has been conducted in real practice, or everyday settings, so little is known about patients' acceptability and attitudes towards such devices in the routine, daily clinical setting of patients undergoing routine treatment with no monetary compensation or legal imperatives. Since they offer an ongoing, 24 h measurement of alcohol through sweat, it could be hypothesized that patients could see them under an autonomy-restricting perspective. However, this has not been evaluated in a formal study. Therefore, it seems important, in order to better understand and anticipate patients' acceptance toward these devices, to assess their attitudes towards alcohol transdermal sensors. Ideally, gathering end-users' perspectives and preferences should facilitate device implementation in routine settings, and therefore enable maximum reach among real patients.

The aim of the present study, conducted among patients who have never used a transdermal device, was therefore two-fold: firstly, to investigate patients' attitudes towards alcohol transdermal sensors, as well as their perceived utility; and secondly, to investigate what features of transdermal sensors would enhance patients' acceptance and usability.

2. Methods

2.1. Study Design and Subjects

We performed a cross-sectional survey among alcohol-dependent patients attending the outpatient service of the Addictive Behaviors Unit of the Clinic Hospital of Barcelona. Subjects were specifically recruited among those attending the routine urine screening program. Ethics consent was granted from the Hospital Clinic Ethics Committee. Informed written consent was obtained from all participants prior to participation in the study.

2.2. Instrument

For this study, a specific questionnaire was designed and all questions were in Spanish. The questionnaire consisted of 3 main parts. The first was aimed at evaluating patients' perceived utility and preferences regarding transdermal sensors. It consisted of 3 multiple choice and 7 Likert-type questions. The second part was designed to obtain patients' beliefs and attitudes towards alcohol transdermal sensors as part of their treatment. Given the lack of similar research for this specific subject, we took advantage of the extensive literature regarding the Drug Attitude Inventory-10 [18], which was initially designed to test attitudes of patients with schizophrenia towards medication in order to correlate it to medication adherence. It consists of ten items; each one is scored with either 1 or −1, depending on whether the response signals a positive attitude towards medication or not. To avoid response bias, half of the items are worded positively, and half negatively. We therefore kept the same wording and the same order of the questions. Its score ranges from −10 to 10. We adapted its ten items to the present study, replacing the concept of medication by that of alcohol transdermal sensors. While such an adaptation of the Drug Attitude Inventory (DAI-10) has not been previously validated in the literature, two previous studies with alcohol patients (one cohort attending Alcoholics Anonymous groups and another cohort obtained from the same outpatient population of this study) performed a similar adaptation of the DAI-10, showing good psychometric properties [19,20]. In addition, we still considered it a good approach to capture patients' attitudes, given the lack of more specific, validated instruments for our study aims. The third was devised to gather basic sociodemographic characteristics. At the beginning of the questionnaire, pictures of the existing transdermal devices were printed (the WristTAS and the SCRAM). Patients received no monetary compensation for participation in the study.

2.3. Procedure

The professional responsible for receiving patients and their urine specimens was an experienced nurse in the addiction field. Within a four-week period at the beginning of 2018, while the nurse received patients, patients were offered the option of participating in the questionnaire. To be included, patients had to be adults diagnosed with an alcohol use disorder and be attending the urine screening program. The main exclusion criteria were the presence of cognitive decline (either based on the nurse's clinical judgment or patient history) and being in a state of intoxication. Patients with any other condition that, in the opinion of the investigators, could have compromised the validity of responses were not offered participation (e.g., an altered psychopathological state). Patients were reassured that all data provided would be kept totally anonymous. Once completed, questionnaires were kept safe until the end of the study, at which point they were analyzed.

2.4. Statistical Analysis

A descriptive analysis of sociodemographic data was conducted. The mean and the standard deviation were used for continuous variables; percentages were used for qualitative variables. Regarding the adapted version of the DAI-10, an internal consistency analysis was carried out with Cronbach's alpha. Concurrent validity was assessed via bivariate correlations between the DAI-10 total score and a 0 to 10 Likert scale measure assessing the potential perceived value of alcohol transdermal sensors as part of patients' treatment. Finally, in order to evaluate if attitudes were influenced by any specific variable, we conducted a lineal regression model with DAI-10 scores as the dependent variable and age, sex, level of instruction, therapeutic objective, and length of urine testing as predictors. Analyses were conducted with SPSS (IBM Corp. Released 2015. IBM SPSS Statistics for Windows, Version 23.0., IBM Corp, Armonk, NY, USA).

3. Results

During the study period, a total of 110 patients attended the urine screening program. Of that, 80 subjects were offered participation in the study (reasons for exclusion: intoxication of 11 patients, cognitive decline of eight patients, other reasons were not specified for 11 patients). A total of eight patients declined participation and four subjects accepted but did not return a questionnaire. That left a total of 68 patients completing the questionnaire. The mean age of the sample was 52.9 years (standard deviation (SD) 12.3). The 66% majority were men, and 39% of the sample were currently employed. Regarding education status, 14% had primary education, 28% had secondary education, 28% had a technical qualification, and 30% had a university qualification. Most of the patients (72%) underwent screening twice a week, 20% once a week, and 8.2% less than once a week. Most of the patients (78%) reported abstinence to be their therapeutic objective. Only a small minority (18%) reported drinking reduction as their aim. Patients had been attending the screening program for an average of 11 months (SD 10.5).

The main advantages and disadvantages attributed to transdermal sensors by patients and their frequencies can be seen in Table 1. Three patients spontaneously reported a decrease in human contact as a potential downside of transdermal sensors. Factors associated with enhanced acceptability and its rating from patients in a scale from 0 to 5 can be seen in Table 2. For both tables, a sex-specific analysis was also conducted. The main difference observed was for stigma, women presenting almost a 2-fold percentage of response compared to men.

Table 1. Advantages and disadvantages attributed to transdermal sensors.

Advantages	Percentage of Responders (Both Sexes)	Male Responders	Female Responders	p-Value (Male vs. female)
To accomplish treatment goals	56%	54.8%	61.9%	0.415
To prevent relapse	41%	31%	57.1%	0.08
To show professionals I do not drink	28.8%	28.6%	28.8%	0.631
To show my family I do not drink	28.8%	23.8%	38.1%	0.700
To have stricter control from my therapists	41%	40.5%	42.9%	0.545
Disadvantages	**Percentage of Responders**			
Stigma associated with device	46%	36.6%	66.7%	0.049
Feeling in control all the time	23%	19.5%	24%	0.368
Physical discomfort	41.5%	39%	42.9%	0.550

Table 2. Features associated with enhanced acceptability (rated from 0 (lowest) to 5 (highest)).

Characteristics	Mean (SD) Both Sexes	Males	Females	p-Value (Male vs. female)
The sensor has a small size	4.2 (1.4)	4.1 (1.5)	4.3 (1.2)	0.627
The sensor is discrete	4.3 (1.4)	4.1 (1.5)	4.4 (1.1)	0.553
Information is never shared without my permission	2.1 (2.1)	1.9 (2.1)	2.5 (2)	0.984
Information is displayed in a web or app where I can always see it	4.1 (1.5)	3.9 (1.7)	4.4 (1.1)	0.920
I can erase the information I want whenever I want	2.0 (3.4)	2.1 (3.8)	1.8 (2.1)	0.725

In a 0 to 10 scale, patients reported a mean score of 6.6 (SD 3.4) regarding the acceptance of a transdermal sensor if their therapist prescribed it. Regarding the adapted DAI-10 questionnaire, the mean score was 3.0 (SD 6.5). Internal consistency, measured with Cronbach's alpha, was 0.613, indicating fair reliability. The question about the overall perceived value of alcohol transdermal sensors showed a mean of 7.4 (SD 2.6). The correlation between this and the DAI-10 score, as a means to investigate concurrent validity, was $r = 0.633$, with $p < 0.001$. The regression model revealed no significant predictor of DAI-10 scores. The differences according to sex regarding the percentage of positive responses to each DAI-10 item can be seen in Figure 1.

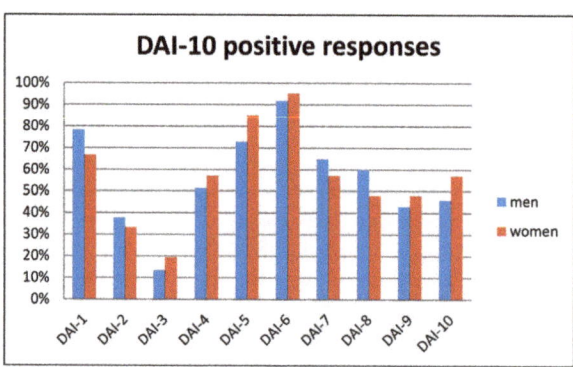

Figure 1. Percentage of positive responses to the Drug Attitude Inventory (DAI-10) questionnaire for each item and according to sex.

Table 3 reports preferences regarding different kinds of devices for transdermal sensors. As can be seen, almost all patients preferred a device similar to a nicotine patch (63%), while the rest of the options were far less frequently preferred.

Table 3. Preferred devices for transdermal sensor implementation.

Device	Percentage of Responders (Both Sexes)	Male Responders	Female Responders
Nicotine patch	63%	63%	62%
Subcutaneous implant	10%	12.5%	4.8%
Wrist-watch or similar device	13%	15%	9.5%
Dental implant	2%	2.5%	0%

4. Discussion

In this study, we aimed to investigate patients' attitudes towards alcohol transdermal sensors. Globally, we believe the results suggest that patients perceive alcohol transdermal sensors as a potentially useful and valuable treatment device.

The adapted version of the DAI-10 scored above average among our sample. Similarly, the overall perceived value as rated in a 0 to 10 scale was high (7.4), and the correlation between both was rather high and clearly significant, suggesting a good concurrent validity. Additionally, the internal consistency of the adapted questionnaire, measured with Cronbach's alpha, was fair. These results suggest the tentative conclusion that the results of the adapted DAI-10 questionnaire could be considered to be reasonably valid.

Looking at patients' responses, the majority stated that preventing relapse and accomplishing their therapeutic goals regarding alcohol were the main functions of transdermal sensors. What is also interesting to note is the significant proportion of respondents that reported "showing professionals or their family that they do not drink" as a main function of transdermal sensors. It suggests that transdermal sensors could play an important role in patients' interaction with both professionals and their social network.

In line with the most frequently reported inconvenience of transdermal sensors (i.e., stigma associated with wearing it), the features that could most enhance the device's acceptability were precisely those that seemed to be designed to reduce the device's visibility (small size and discreteness). Further supporting these findings, the most preferred physical device was a patch similar to the ones used for nicotine replacement therapy. In line with our findings, previous reports about transdermal sensors have also emphasized stigma and embarrassment as major concerns reported by patients [21,22]. What is also worth mentioning is that patients' responses suggest that providing continuous feedback about the information gathered by the device is also essential in order to enhance patients' acceptability and usability.

The results from the previous survey by Alessi and colleagues [17], which was conducted among patients who wore a real sensor, suggest that stigma and embarrassment were not major concerns. This is in sharp contrast to our results. The difference could be explained by the different sample selection and study design procedures, since all patients in the aforementioned survey were gathered from studies conducted with contingency management procedures, and the majority of subjects belonged to non-clinical samples, suggesting a potential selection bias. For example, in one of the studies patients were heavy drinkers not seeking treatment. That means that social desirability and the wish to abstain might have been quite different in both samples. Another potential explanation could be the fact that patients wore the SCRAM as a foot bracelet. This could be considered a discrete device and therefore stigma concerns would have been reduced.

Looking at patients' responses, it seems that physical discomfort is also a main preoccupation among patients. It is probable that similar recommendations to the ones for dealing with stigma and embarrassment could be given. These were reduced size and visibility, which should also increase comfort with the device.

Overall, and in line with the increasing importance that patient-centered care is gaining in medical settings [23], we expect this study to offer relevant insights into patients' perspectives, motives, and attitudes towards alcohol transdermal sensors. We expect knowledge about patients' needs and worries to be increased, so that when, in the near future, they are offered to incorporate transdermal sensors into their treatment program, they can be offered this in a more realistic, friendly, and efficient manner.

Turning to the limitations of the present study, a key issue in interpreting all studies using questionnaires is social desirability [24]. Addiction itself is especially prone to such bias [25,26]. Therefore, although the questionnaires were completely anonymous, the presence of a social desirability bias cannot be totally ruled out.

Other relevant limitations should also be taken into account when interpreting our findings. First, we developed a new questionnaire. Although it was based on an extensively validated one (the DAI-10), it must be acknowledged that our study was not focused on questionnaire validation; therefore, more measurements could have been obtained in order to better validate it. That being said, the internal reliability and the concurrent validity were fair. Another important limitation stems from the fact that all patients belonged to a single outpatient center, a fact that might diminish external validity. Similarly, all patients were recruited from the urine screening program, so the question remains as to whether similar or different results would be observed in other clinical settings. It is also important to mention that the nature of this study was mainly descriptive. However, we tried to find some predictors of patients' attitudes towards transdermal sensors, but found no significant predictors, a fact that could partly be due to insufficient statistical power. Also relevant is the fact that no systematic screening instrument for the detection of cognitive decline or other excluding conditions was used. The clinical nature of the study also precluded an extensive evaluation of patients' clinical characteristics. Finally, four questionnaires were not fully completed and, therefore, we had a minor proportion of missing data, which we excluded from analysis.

5. Conclusions

Though our data suggest that concerns about stigma and embarrassment should be taken into account when planning the implementation of transdermal sensors in routine settings (more notably for female patients), our findings, together with those of previous studies, encourage further efforts to bring transdermal sensors to routine, clinical samples of alcohol-dependent patients.

Future designs of transdermal sensors should aim at reduced size and visibility, thus lowering stigma concerns. Patients should also be allowed full access to the information provided by the sensor.

Author Contributions: Conceptualization, P.B. and A.G.; Data curation, M.A.; Formal analysis, P.B.; Investigation, L.T.; Supervision, A.G.; Writing—review & editing, M.A. and A.G.

Conflicts of Interest: The authors declare no conflict of interest.

References

1. Wittchen, H.U.; Jacobi, F.; Rehm, J.; Gustavsson, A.; Svensson, M.; Jönsson, B.; Olesen, J.; Allgulander, C.; Alonso, J.; Faravelli, C.; et al. The size and burden of mental disorders and other disorders of the brain in Europe 2010. *Eur. Neuropsychopharmacol.* **2011**, *21*, 655–679. [CrossRef] [PubMed]
2. Grant, B.F.; Chou, S.P.; Saha, T.D.; Pickering, R.P.; Kerridge, B.T.; Ruan, W.J.; Huang, B.; Jung, J.; Zhang, H.; Fan, A.; et al. Prevalence of 12-Month Alcohol Use, High-Risk Drinking, and *DSM-IV* Alcohol Use Disorder in the United States, 2001–2002 to 2012–2013. *JAMA Psychiatry* **2017**, *74*, 911. [CrossRef] [PubMed]
3. Barrio, P.; Reynolds, J.; García-Altés, A.; Gual, A.; Anderson, P. Social costs of illegal drugs, alcohol and tobacco in the European Union: A systematic review. *Drug Alcohol Rev.* **2017**, *34*, 135–143. [CrossRef] [PubMed]
4. Miquel, L.; Rehm, J.; Shield, K.D.; Vela, E.; Bustins, M.; Segura, L.; Colom, J.; Anderson, P.; Gual, A. Alcohol, tobacco and health care costs: A population-wide cohort study (n = 606,947 patients) of current drinkers based on medical and administrative health records from Catalonia. *Eur. J. Public Health* **2018**, *28*, 674–680. [CrossRef] [PubMed]
5. Owen, P.; Marlatt, G.A. Should abstinence be the goal for alcohol treatment? Affirmative viewpoint. *Am. J. Addict.* **2001**, *10*, 289–291. [CrossRef]

6. Miquel, L.; Gual, A.; Vela, E.; Lligoña, A.; Bustins, M.; Colom, J.; Rehm, J. Alcohol Consumption and Inpatient Health Service Utilization in a Cohort of Patients With Alcohol Dependence After 20 Years of Follow-up. *Alcohol Alcohol.* **2016**, *9*, 227–233. [CrossRef]
7. Wurst, F.M.; Thon, N.; Yegles, M.; Schrück, A.; Preuss, U.W.; Weinmann, W. Ethanol metabolites: Their role in the assessment of alcohol intake. *Alcohol. Clin. Exp. Res.* **2015**, *39*, 2060–2072. [CrossRef]
8. Barrio, P.; Teixidor, L.; Ortega, L.; Lligoña, A.; Rico, N.; Bedini, J.L.; Vieta, E.; Gual, A. Filling the gap between lab and clinical impact: An open randomized diagnostic trial comparing urinary ethylglucuronide and ethanol in alcohol dependent outpatients. *Drug Alcohol Depend.* **2018**, *183*, 225–230. [CrossRef]
9. Rehm, J.; Marmet, S.; Anderson, P.; Gual, A.; Kraus, L.; Nutt, D.J.; Room, R.; Samokhvalov, A.V.; Scafato, E.; Trapencieris, M.; et al. Defining substance use disorders: Do we really need more than heavy use? *Alcohol Alcohol.* **2013**, *48*, 633–640. [CrossRef]
10. Insel, T.R. Digital Phenotyping. *JAMA* **2017**, *318*, 1215. [CrossRef]
11. Skinner, A.L.; Attwood, A.S.; Baddeley, R.; Evans-Reeves, K.; Bauld, L.; Munafò, M.R. Digital phenotyping and the development and delivery of health guidelines and behaviour change interventions. *Addiction* **2017**, *112*, 1281–1285. [CrossRef] [PubMed]
12. McKnight, A.S.; Fell, J.C.; Auld-Owens, A. *Transdermal Alcohol Monitoring: Case Studies*; The National Academies of Sciences, Engineering, and Medicine: Washington, DC, USA, 2012.
13. Barnett, N.P.; Meade, E.B.; Glynn, T.R. Predictors of detection of alcohol use episodes using a transdermal alcohol sensor. *Exp. Clin. Psychopharmacol.* **2014**, *22*, 86–96. [CrossRef] [PubMed]
14. Mathias, C.W.; Hill-Kapturczak, N.; Karns-Wright, T.E.; Mullen, J.; Roache, J.D.; Fell, J.C.; Dougherty, D.M. Translating transdermal alcohol monitoring procedures for contingency management among adults recently arrested for DWI. *Addict. Behav.* **2018**, *83*, 56–63. [CrossRef] [PubMed]
15. Simons, J.S.; Wills, T.A.; Emery, N.N.; Marks, R.M. Quantifying alcohol consumption: Self-report, transdermal assessment, and prediction of dependence symptoms. *Addict. Behav.* **2015**, *50*, 205–212. [CrossRef] [PubMed]
16. Barnett, N.P.; Celio, M.A.; Tidey, J.W.; Murphy, J.G.; Colby, S.M.; Swift, R.M. A preliminary randomized controlled trial of contingency management for alcohol use reduction using a transdermal alcohol sensor. *Addiction* **2017**, *112*, 1025–1035. [CrossRef]
17. Alessi, S.M.; Barnett, N.P.; Petry, N.M. Experiences with SCRAMx alcohol monitoring technology in 100 alcohol treatment outpatients. *Drug Alcohol Depend.* **2017**, *178*, 417–424. [CrossRef]
18. Hogan, T.P.; Awad, A.G.; Eastwood, R. A self-report scale predictive of drug compliance in schizophrenics: Reliability and discriminative validity. *Psychol. Med.* **1983**, *13*, 177–183. [CrossRef]
19. Barrio, P.; Teixidor, L.; Ortega, L.; Balcells, M.; Vieta, E.; Gual, A. Patients' Knowledge and Attitudes Towards Regular Alcohol Urine Screening. *J. Addict. Med.* **2017**, *11*, 300–307. [CrossRef]
20. Terra, M.B.; Barros, H.M.T.; Stein, A.T.; Figueira, I.; Athayde, L.D.; da Silveira, D.X. Internal consistency and factor structure of the adherence scale for alcoholics anonymous. *Estud. Psicol.* **2011**, *28*, 107–113.
21. Greenfield, T.K.; Bond, J.; Kerr, W.C. Biomonitoring for Improving Alcohol Consumption Surveys: The New Gold Standard? *Alcohol Res.* **2014**, *36*, 39–45.
22. Marques, P.; McKnight, S. *Evaluating Transdermal Alcohol Measuring Devices*; National Highway Traffic Safety Administration: Washington, DC, USA, 2007.
23. Bradley, K.A.; Kivlahan, D.R. Bringing patient-centered care to patients with alcohol use disorders. *JAMA* **2014**, *311*, 1861–1862. [CrossRef] [PubMed]
24. Van De Mortel, T.F.; Van De Mortel Rn, T.F. Faking it: Social desirability response bias in self-report research. *Aust. J. Adv. Nurs. Aust. J. Adv. Nurs. Aust. J. Adv. Nurs.* **2008**, *25*, 40–48.
25. Davis, C.G.; Thake, J.; Vilhena, N. Social desirability biases in self-reported alcohol consumption and harms. *Addict. Behav.* **2010**, *35*, 302–311. [CrossRef] [PubMed]
26. Zemore, S.E. The effect of social desirability on reported motivation, substance use severity, and treatment attendance. *J. Subst. Abuse Treat.* **2012**, *42*, 400–412. [CrossRef] [PubMed]

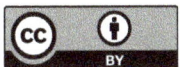 © 2019 by the authors. Licensee MDPI, Basel, Switzerland. This article is an open access article distributed under the terms and conditions of the Creative Commons Attribution (CC BY) license (http://creativecommons.org/licenses/by/4.0/).

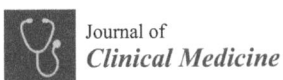

Article

Clinical Improvements in Comorbid Gambling/Cocaine Use Disorder (GD/CUD) Patients Undergoing Repetitive Transcranial Magnetic Stimulation (rTMS)

Stefano Cardullo [1,†], Luis Javier Gomez Perez [1,†], Linda Marconi [1], Alberto Terraneo [1], Luigi Gallimberti [1], Antonello Bonci [1,2,3,4] and Graziella Madeo [1,2,*]

1. Human Science and Brain Research, Novella Fronda Foundation, Piazza Castello, 35141 Padua, Italy; stefano.cardullo@gmail.com (S.C.); luigomper@gmail.com (L.J.G.P.); linda.marconi22@gmail.com (L.M.); alberto.terraneo@gmail.com (A.T.); luigi.gallimberti@studiogallimberti.it (L.G.); antonello.bonci@nih.gov (A.B.)
2. Intramural Research Program, National Institute on Drug Abuse, National Institutes of Health, Baltimore, MD 21224, USA
3. Solomon H. Snyder Department of Neuroscience, Johns Hopkins University School of Medicine, Baltimore, MD 21205, USA
4. Department of Psychiatry and Behavioral Sciences, Johns Hopkins University School of Medicine, Baltimore, MD 21287, USA
* Correspondence: graziemadeo@gmail.com
† Co-first authors.

Received: 24 April 2019; Accepted: 28 May 2019; Published: 30 May 2019

Abstract: (1) Background: Pathological gambling behaviors may coexist with cocaine use disorder (CUD), underlying common pathogenic mechanisms. Repetitive transcranial magnetic stimulation (rTMS) has shown promise as a therapeutic intervention for CUD. In this case series, we evaluated the clinical effects of rTMS protocol stimulating the left dorsolateral prefrontal cortex (DLPFC) on the pattern of gambling and cocaine use. (2) Methods: Gambling severity, craving for cocaine, sleep, and other negative affect symptoms were recorded in seven patients with a diagnosis of gambling disorder (South Oaks Gambling Screen (SOGS) >5), in comorbidity with CUD, using the following scales: Gambling-Symptom Assessment Scale (G-SAS), Cocaine Craving Questionnaire (CCQ), Beck Depression Inventory-II (BDI-II), Self-rating Anxiety Scale (SAS), and Symptoms checklist-90 (SCL-90). The measures were assessed before the rTMS treatment and after 5, 30, and 60 days of treatment. Patterns of gambling and cocaine use were assessed by self-report and regular urine screens. (3) Results: Gambling severity at baseline ranged from mild to severe (mean ± Standard Error of the Mean (SEM), G-SAS score baseline: 24.42 ± 2.79). G-SAS scores significantly improved after treatment (G-SAS score Day 60: 2.66 ± 1.08). Compared to baseline, consistent improvements were significantly seen in craving for cocaine and in negative-affect symptoms. (4) Conclusions: The present findings provide unprecedent insights into the potential role of rTMS as a therapeutic intervention for reducing both gambling and cocaine use in patients with a dual diagnosis.

Keywords: gambling disorder (GD); cocaine use disorder (CUD); craving; repetitive transcranial magnetic stimulation (rTMS); Gambling-Symptoms Assessment Scale (G-SAS); dorsolateral prefrontal cortex (DLPFC)

1. Introduction

Pathological gambling behaviors frequently co-occur with substance use [1]. A prevalence rate of 10.3% has been reported for gambling disorder (GD) diagnosis in substance use disorders

(SUD) patients [2,3], while GD patients have a 57.5% prevalence for substance-related disorder comorbidity [4,5]. Despite the differences observed in cue and stress-related craving, GD shares some of the neurobiological substrates, psychological processes, and behavioral manifestations of SUDs [6–8]. Compelling evidence supports that both GD and SUDs are sustained by impaired neuroplasticity and dysfunctions within reward, stress and cognitive-control systems. These abnormalities underline the core clinical manifestations [9], such as compulsive gambling or compulsive drug consumption, craving, altered reward sensitivity, and impaired self-control and decision-making processes [10]. Moreover, diminished executive functions (e.g., diminished response inhibition, cognitive flexibility) in GD patients compared to healthy controls seem related to differential functioning of the cognitive control circuit involving the dorsolateral prefrontal cortex (DLPFC) and the anterior cingulate cortex (ACC) [11].

Neuromodulation approaches could represent a promising therapeutic intervention for GD [12], able to restore the abnormalities in cognitive motivational-behavioral and executive functions. Non-invasive brain stimulation techniques, like transcranial magnetic stimulation (TMS), may enhance cognitive control through DLPFC stimulation, thus restoring some of the core symptoms of either GD and SUDs [13–16]. Specifically, repetitive TMS (rTMS) stimulating the left DLPFC has been shown to be effective in reducing craving in substance-related disorders [17–20] and to improve cognitive functioning [21]. Currently, a limited number of TMS pilot studies in GD has investigated whether TMS may be a promising treatment for GD, often providing conflicting results. For instance, in a sham-controlled cross-over high-frequency rTMS study targeting the left DLPFC, active rTMS diminished cue-induced craving compared to sham rTMS [22]. Conversely, low-frequency rTMS (1 Hz) over the right DLPFC had similar effects as sham stimulation on craving, even though with a large placebo effect [23]. In another trial involving nine gamblers, a single session of high frequency rTMS reduced desire to gamble, whereas continuous theta burst stimulation (cTBS) reduced blood pressure, with no effects on craving [24]. In this same study no effects on impulsive behavior (delay discounting) and Stroop interference were evident. Yet, the only deep transcranial stimulation pilot study at 1 Hz targeting prefrontal regions had no effects on pathological gambling [25]. This discrepancy might be related to small sample size, variability of study design, stimulation parameters, and protocols [8]. Moreover, most of them investigated the effects of a single TMS session, which is unlikely to influence a complex behavioral pattern, such as gambling. Nevertheless, from these few studies, it appears that TMS has the ability to alter at least some of the working mechanisms underlying pathological gambling. The abundant evidence on neurobiological and behavioral similarities between GD and SUDs [26] and the potential clinical benefit from cumulative rTMS sessions [27] led us to investigate whether gambling symptoms in patients with cocaine use disorder (CUD) may improve following a high frequency rTMS treatment targeting the left DLPFC.

Here, we report a case series of seven treatment-seeking patients with cocaine use disorder (CUD) comorbid with GD who underwent an rTMS treatment stimulating the left DLPFC. We investigated the clinical changes regarding the patterns of cocaine use, gambling, and accompanying withdrawal symptoms during the treatment.

2. Materials and Methods

The study was conducted in accordance with the Declaration of Helsinki and the protocol approved by the Ethics Committee for Psychological Research, University of Padua (Protocol Number: 2551; registration Number: NCT03733821) [28].

2.1. Participants and Treatment

Seven male participants diagnosed as suffering from cocaine use disorder (CUD) were selected based on comorbidity with GD, according to DSM-5 [29], from 87 patients recruited for a retrospective observational study investigating sleep disturbances. All participants, treatment seekers for CUD, provided informed consent and underwent an rTMS protocol at a clinic center for addiction treatment in Padua, Italy. During the screening, patients were assessed for substances of abuse pattern and gambling experiences. Only CUD patients comorbid with GD were selected. GD was determined by a clinical interview with an SUD expert psychiatrist combined with a score equal to or greater than 5 on the South Oaks Gambling Screen (SOGS) [30]. All patients were slot machine players, except one, who mainly played online poker. To exclude contraindications to receive rTMS, a TMS safety screening was administered to all patients in line with international recommendations for TMS safety and ethics [31]. Patients with a lifetime history of other psychiatric diseases, including major depression, schizophrenia, bipolar disorder or other psychoses, current alcohol and other substance use disorders (excluding cocaine, tobacco, and caffeine), personality disorders, and unstable medical illness were also excluded from the initial sample. During treatment, cocaine use was monitored by urine drug tests and relapses were reported. The urine drug testing also screened for morphine, methadone, tetrahydrocannabinol (THC), phencyclidine, amphetamine, and methamphetamine. Pharmacological therapy remained unchanged or was not prescribed during the treatment. rTMS treatment was administered to each patient by a trained clinical physiologist using a medical device (MagPro R30) targeting the left DLPFC. Treatment consisted of twice-daily rTMS sessions for the first five consecutive days of treatment, followed by twice-daily rTMS sessions once a week over eight weeks. Protocol parameters, such as stimulation parameters and motor threshold detection, were defined according to the procedures described by Terraneo et al. [18]. To best identify the DLPFC (Montreal Neurological Institute (MNI) coordinates x: −50, y: 30, z: 36), we used an optical TMS navigator (Localite, St. Augustin, Germany) and a magnetic resonance image (MRI) template. The stimulation parameters were: frequency: 15 Hz; intensity: 100% of the motor threshold; 60 impulses per stimulation train; inter-train interval: 15 s; and 40 total trains for a session duration of 13 min. At each session, adverse events, including seizures, syncopes, neurological complications, or subjective complaints about memory, concentration, pain, headache, vertigo, or fatigue were assessed.

Gambling symptomatology was evaluated by Gambling Symptom Assessment Scale (G-SAS) [32]. The G-SAS is a 12-item self-rated scale designed to assess gambling symptom severity and change during treatment with a score ranging from 0 to 4 [32].

Participants were also assessed for craving, subjective sleep quality, depression, anxiety, and other negative affect symptoms. The Cocaine Craving Questionnaire (CCQ) [33] is a 5-item self-report questionnaire measuring five aspects of craving: current intensity, intensity during the previous 24 h, frequency, responsiveness to drug-related conditioned stimuli, and imagined likelihood of use if in a setting with access to drugs [34]. The 19-item Pittsburgh Sleep Quality Index (PSQI) [35] is the most commonly used retrospective self-report questionnaire measuring the self-perceived quality of sleep [36]. It investigates sleep quality, sleep latency, sleep duration, habitual sleep efficiency, sleep disturbances, use of sleeping medications, and daytime dysfunction [37]. The Beck Depression Inventory-II (BDI-II) [38] is a 21-item self-report questionnaire format with four options under each item, ranging from not present (0) to severe (3), measuring depressive symptoms. The Self-rating Anxiety Scale (SAS) [39], is a 20-item measure developed to assess the frequency of anxiety symptoms based on diagnostic conceptualizations. It consists primarily of somatic symptoms. The Symptoms checklist 90-Revised [40] is a 90-item self-report inventory which assesses psychological distress in terms of nine primary symptom dimensions and three summary scores termed global scores. The Global Severity Index (GSI), the outcome of which we used in this study, is the single best indicator of the current level or depth of an individual's disorder. It combines information concerning the number of symptoms reported with the intensity of perceived distress [41].

The assessments were made at baseline, immediately after completion of the first week of treatment, as well as 30 and 60 days after the beginning of treatment (day 5, day 30, day 60). BDI-II was not included in the assessment on day 5 since it considers changes in the preceding two weeks. Some participants did not complete every scale at every time point, for the main following reasons: clinical response, missing follow-up visit, missing TMS session, and refusal. We included participants who completed outcome measures for at least three time points, including the baseline.

2.2. Statistical Analyses

We used repeated-measures analyses of variance (ANOVA) for testing the effect of treatment over time, followed by the Tukey test for post-hoc comparison analysis between timepoints (day 5, day 30, and day 60). Data were expressed as mean ± SD, unless otherwise specified; α was set at <0.05, two-tailed. All the analyses were performed using RStudio version 1.1.453 [42] with R version 3.5.0 [43] and the package emmeans [44]. G*Power (ver 3.1.9.4) was used to perform a power analysis and estimate the sample size. For the computation of this estimate we considered the effects we observed in a previous pilot study [18]. Considering an Effect size $f(U) = 1.1$, an $\alpha = 0.05$, a power $(1 - \beta) = 0.95$, one group and four measurements, a sample size of seven patients was required.

3. Results

The full demographic and clinical characteristics of the participants are presented in Table 1. The total sample consisted of seven male patients, aged between 30 and 49 (42.14 ± 5.74). Treatment variables are specified in Table 1.

Table 1. Demographic and clinical characteristics of the participants.

Variables	$n = 7$ [1]
Age (years)	42.14 (5.74)
Education (years)	12 (3.19)
Cocaine: Age at first experience (years)	27.71 (9.06)
Cocaine: Age at addiction (years)	37.42 (7.51)
Gambling: Age at first experience (years)	19.14 (5.61)
Gambling: Age at addiction (years)	27 (8.31)
SOGS score	9.14 (1.88)
G-SAS score at baseline	24.42 (6.84)
CCQ score at baseline	24.85 (9.56)
PSQI score at baseline	10 (3.25)
BDI-II score at baseline	22.42 (6.16)
SAS score at baseline	50.71 (4.76)
GSI score at baseline	68.32 (10.2)

[1] Data are presented as mean (standard deviation). SOGS: South Oaks Gambling Screen; G-SAS: Gambling-Symptom Assessment Scale; CCQ: Cocaine Craving Questionnaire; PSQI: Pittsburgh Sleep Quality Index; BDI-II: Beck Depression Inventory-II; SAS: Self-rating Anxiety Scale; GSI: Global Severity Index of the Symptoms checklist 90—Revised.

G-SAS scores significantly improved at each time point after the first week of treatment ($F(3,22) = 16.71$, $p < 0.001$, $R^2 = 0.69$; Figure 1a). Pairwise comparisons showed that G-SAS scores at day 5 were significantly lower than those at baseline ($t(22) = 5.61$, $p < 0.001$). This improvement was maintained at the subsequent timepoints: day 30 ($t(22) = 5.07$, $p < 0.001$) and day 60 ($t(22) = 6.22$, $p < 0.001$). Similarly, craving for cocaine, reflected in CCQ scores, significantly decreased over time ($F(3,24) = 9.52$, $p < 0.001$, $R^2 = 0.54$; Figure 1b). Pairwise comparisons showed a significant improvement from baseline to day 5 ($t(24) = 4.12$, $p < 0.001$) and levels were maintained at day 30 ($t(24) = 4.30$, $p < 0.001$) and at day 60 ($t(24) = 4.60$, $p < 0.001$). No significant differences were found when comparing G-SAS and CCQ scores among day 5, day 30, and day 60. Of seven patients, four did not report any relapse in cocaine and in gambling behaviors during the 60 days of treatment.

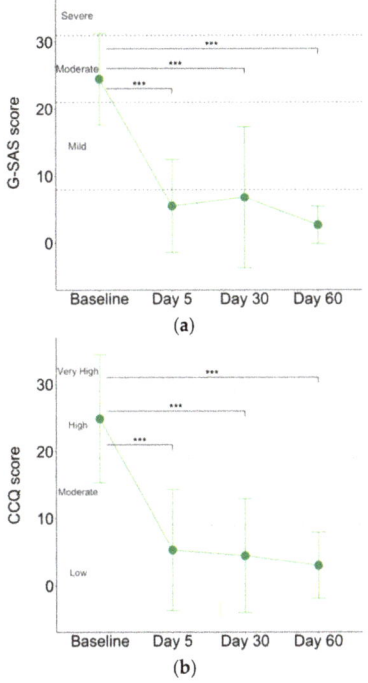

Figure 1. Plot of the means and 95% confidence intervals of (**a**) Gambling-Symptom Assessment Scale (G-SAS) and (**b**) Cocaine Craving Scale (CCQ). *** p value < 0.001.

Similarly, sleep disturbance, depression, anxiety, and the other negative affect symptoms significantly decreased over time as reflected in PSQI ($F(3,24) = 5.40, p < 0.01, R^2 = 0.40$), BDI-II ($F(2,18) = 21.53, p < 0.001, R^2 = 0.70$), SAS ($F(3,23) = 14.19, p < 0.001, R^2 = 0.64$), and GSI ($F(3,24) = 7.04, p < 0.01, R^2 = 0.46$). The secondary outcome improvement was significant at day 5 of the treatment in comparison to the baseline (PSQI: $t(24) = 3.40, p = 0.01$; SAS: $t(25) = 5.68, p < 0.001$; GSI: $t(24) = 3.69, p < 0.01$) and stable overtime: day 30 (PSQI: $t(24) = 3.50, p < 0.01$; BDI-II: $t(18) = 5.40, p < 0.001$; SAS: $t(23) = 4.25, p < 0.01$; GSI: $t(24) = 3.38, p = 0.01$) and day 60 (PSQI: $t(24) = 2.72, p = 0.05$; BDI-II: $t(18) = 5.92, p < 0.001$; SAS: $t(23) = 5.47, p < 0.001$; GSI: $t(24) = 4.05, p < 0.01$).

3.1. Cocaine Use

Five out of seven patients did not use cocaine for the entire duration of the study. One patient used cocaine after the first 15 days of treatment. Another patient used cocaine during the first week and another three times within 60 days of treatment. None of the patients used other drugs included in the urine drug screen.

3.2. Safety

No adverse events were reported.

4. Discussion

To our knowledge, this is the first study reporting clinical improvements in patients with a dual diagnosis of CUD and GD following an rTMS treatment stimulating the left DLPFC.

We evaluated changes in cocaine use and gambling patterns as well as the accompanying symptoms, including sleep disturbances, mood, anxiety, and other negative symptoms [45,46] in seven patients seeking treatment for CUD.

The severity of the gambling symptoms and cocaine craving ranged from moderate to severe at baseline, as assessed by G-SAS and CCQ. G-SAS and CCQ scores dramatically dropped at the end of the first week of treatment and were stable during the following 60 days of treatment. Moreover, four out of seven patients did not show either cocaine use or relapse of gambling behaviors; one patient reported four gambling episodes during the first month of treatment (total 454 €), without any cocaine use; one patient reported a single gambling episode during the first week of treatment (150 €) associated with cocaine use, followed by another three uses within 60 days of treatment; one patient reported several cocaine uses after the first 15 days of treatment but no gambling behavior. The improvement of cocaine-related symptoms is in line with previous findings showing that high-frequency left-DLPFC-rTMS stimulation is effective in diminishing cocaine craving [17,19,47] and intake [18]. Neuroimaging studies have shown common activation abnormalities in regions of the mesolimbic reward system in patients with substance-related disorders and GD [48–52], supporting the concept of a common etiology for both disorders. The repeated exposure to addictive stimuli induces plastic changes within reward pathways leading to the hypersensitivity of the brain reward system to the addictive stimulus itself and addiction-related cues. This process is instrumental for conditioning to occur, since previous neutral stimuli can acquire an incentive salience and promote habit formation with repeated exposure to the cues [53,54]. This shift from goal-directed behavior to more habitual responding specifically involves the dorsal striatum (DS) [54], a region implicated in reward, habit learning, and compulsive behaviors. The shift from prefrontal cortical to striatal control may emphasize maladaptive neuroplasticity changes in both GD and SUDs [8]. Accordingly, we observed clinical improvement of either gambling or cocaine-related symptoms. So far, only a few pilot studies have explored the effects of TMS on gambling urges and behavior [22–24]. One of these studies evaluated the effect of deep TMS over the DLPFC for 15 days reporting an improvement of craving scores as opposed to a retention of gambling behavior in all patients [25]. Conflicting results might reflect differences in stimulation parameters and treatment conditions. Of note, the clinical improvement in our small cohort of patients was maintained for the whole 60 days period of treatment. Moreover, we observed a significant change of accompanying symptoms to addictive behaviors, including sleep disturbances, depression, anxiety, and negative-affect symptoms, as demonstrated by the improvement of PSQI, BDI-II, SAS, and SCL-90-R scores during the treatment period. Several findings already support a beneficial effect of rTMS for primary sleep disorders and for sleep disturbances comorbid with other neuropsychiatric disorders [55–58]. To our knowledge, this is one of the first studies reporting a beneficial effect on accompanying symptoms to addictive behaviors and, thus, the results have to be interpreted cautiously. We can argue that anxiety, depressive, and negative-affect symptoms may indirectly benefit from the improvement of the patterns of use and gambling, including the diminished craving and possibly a better executive function control. In our setting with a small sample size, no control group, or a sham-controlled double blind design, we cannot rule out a possible placebo effect, as previously reported in another study using low frequency rTMS targeting the right DLPFC [23]. However, the longer period of observation and the cumulative rTMS sessions may support a beneficial effect related to the neuromodulatory intervention. Certainly, rigorously conducted clinical trials with sham-controlled double-blind designs are needed to investigate whether TMS protocols have the potential to be effective to treat cognitive dysfunctions, reduce craving, and/or the gambling behavior in patients with GD.

Author Contributions: S.C., L.J.G.P., G.M. conceptualized and designed the study; S.C., L.J.G.P., and L.M. collected the data; S.C. and L.J.G.P. performed data processing and statistical analysis. S.C., L.J.G.P., G.M. wrote the manuscript. G.M., L.G., A.T. supervised the project. G.M., L.G., A.T., A.B. critically revised and edited the manuscript.

Funding: Funding for this study was provided by the Novella Fronda Foundation, Padua, Italy. The Novella Fronda Foundation had no further role in study design; in the collection, analysis, and interpretation of data; in the writing of the report; and in the decision to submit the paper for publication.

Acknowledgments: The authors would like to thank the Zardi-Gori Foundation for the fellowship bursary.

Conflicts of Interest: The authors declare no conflict of interest.

References

1. Petry, N.M.; Stinson, F.S.; Grant, B.F. Comorbidity of DSM-IV Pathological Gambling and Other Psychiatric Disorders. *J. Clin. Psychiatry* **2005**, *66*, 564–574. [CrossRef]
2. Weinstock, J.; Blanco, C.; Petry, N.M. Health correlates of pathological gambling in a methadone maintenance clinic. *Exp. Clin. Psychopharmacol.* **2006**, *14*, 87–93. [CrossRef]
3. Rennert, L.; Denis, C.; Peer, K.; Lynch, K.G.; Gelernter, J.; Kranzler, H.R. DSM-5 gambling disorder: Prevalence and characteristics in a substance use disorder sample. *Exp. Clin. Psychopharmacol.* **2014**, *22*, 50. [CrossRef]
4. Ibáñez, A.; Blanco, C.; Donahue, E.; Lesieur, H.R.; Pérez de Castro, I.; Fernández-Piqueras, J.; Sáiz-Ruiz, J. Psychiatric comorbidity in pathological gamblers seeking treatment. *Am. J. Psychiatry* **2001**, *158*, 1733–1735. [CrossRef]
5. Lorains, F.K.; Cowlishaw, S.; Thomas, S.A. Prevalence of comorbid disorders in problem and pathological gambling: Systematic review and meta-analysis of population surveys. *Addiction* **2011**, *106*, 490–498. [CrossRef]
6. Shaffer, H.J.; LaPlante, D.A.; LaBrie, R.A.; Kidman, R.C.; Donato, A.N.; Stanton, M.V. Toward a Syndrome Model of Addiction: Multiple Expressions, Common Etiology. *Harv. Rev. Psychiatry* **2004**, *12*, 367–374. [CrossRef] [PubMed]
7. Goudriaan, A.E.; Yücel, M.; van Holst, R.J. Getting a grip on problem gambling: What can neuroscience tell us? *Front. Behav. Neurosci.* **2014**, *8*, 141. [CrossRef]
8. Spagnolo, P.A.; Gómez Pérez, L.J.; Terraneo, A.; Gallimberti, L.; Bonci, A. Neural Correlates of Cue-and Stress-induced Craving in Gambling Disorders: Implications for Transcranial Magnetic Stimulation Interventions. *Eur. J. Neurosci.* **2019**, 1–14. [CrossRef] [PubMed]
9. Spagnolo, P.A.; Goldman, D. Neuromodulation interventions for addictive disorders: Challenges, promise, and roadmap for future research. *Brain* **2017**, *140*, 1183–1203. [CrossRef] [PubMed]
10. Koob, G.F.; Volkow, N.D. Neurobiology of addiction: A neurocircuitry analysis. *Lancet Psychiatry* **2016**, *3*, 760–773. [CrossRef]
11. Van Holst, R.J.; van den Brink, W.; Veltman, D.J.; Goudriaan, A.E. Brain imaging studies in pathological gambling. *Curr. Psychiatry Rep.* **2010**, *12*, 418–425. [CrossRef]
12. Volkow, N.D.; Koob, G.F.; McLellan, A.T. Neurobiologic Advances from the Brain Disease Model of Addiction. *N. Engl. J. Med.* **2016**, *374*, 363–371. [CrossRef]
13. Diana, M.; Raij, T.; Melis, M.; Nummenmaa, A.; Leggio, L.; Bonci, A. Rehabilitating the addicted brain with transcranial magnetic stimulation. *Nat. Rev. Neurosci.* **2017**, *18*, 685–693. [CrossRef]
14. Hanlon, C.A.; Canterberry, M.; Taylor, J.J.; DeVries, W.; Li, X.; Brown, T.R.; George, M.S. Probing the Frontostriatal Loops Involved in Executive and Limbic Processing via Interleaved TMS and Functional MRI at Two Prefrontal Locations: A Pilot Study. *PLoS ONE* **2013**, *8*, e67917. [CrossRef]
15. Lantrip, C.; Gunning, F.M.; Flashman, L.; Roth, R.M.; Holtzheimer, P.E. Effects of transcranial magnetic stimulation on the cognitive control of emotion: Potential antidepressant mechanisms. *J. ECT* **2017**, *33*, 73–80. [CrossRef]
16. Möbius, M.; Lacomblé, L.; Meyer, T.; Schutter, D.J.L.G.; Gielkens, T.; Becker, E.S.; Tendolkar, I.; van Eijndhoven, P. Repetitive transcranial magnetic stimulation modulates the impact of a negative mood induction. *Soc. Cognit. Affect. Neurosci.* **2017**, *12*, 526–533. [CrossRef]
17. Politi, E.; Fauci, E.; Santoro, A.; Smeraldi, E. Daily sessions of transcranial magnetic stimulation to the left prefrontal cortex gradually reduce cocaine craving. *Am. J. Addict.* **2008**, *17*, 345–346. [CrossRef] [PubMed]
18. Terraneo, A.; Leggio, L.; Saladini, M.; Ermani, M.; Bonci, A.; Gallimberti, L. Transcranial magnetic stimulation of dorsolateral prefrontal cortex reduces cocaine use: A pilot study. *Eur. Neuropsychopharmacol.* **2016**, *26*, 37–44. [CrossRef]

19. Rapinesi, C.; Del Casale, A.; Di Pietro, S.; Ferri, V.R.; Piacentino, D.; Sani, G.; Raccah, R.N.; Zangen, A.; Ferracuti, S.; Vento, A.E.; et al. Add-on high frequency deep transcranial magnetic stimulation (dTMS) to bilateral prefrontal cortex reduces cocaine craving in patients with cocaine use disorder. *Neurosci. Lett.* **2016**, *629*, 43–47. [CrossRef]
20. Jansen, J.M.; Daams, J.G.; Koeter, M.W.J.; Veltman, D.J.; Van Den Brink, W.; Goudriaan, A.E. Effects of non-invasive neurostimulation on craving: A meta-analysis. *Neurosci. Biobehav. Rev.* **2013**, *37*, 2472–2480. [CrossRef]
21. Schluter, R.; Daams, J.; van Holst, R.J.; Goudriaan, A.E. Effects of Noninvasive Neuromodulation on Executive and Other Cognitive Functions in Addictive Disorders: A Systematic Review. *Front. Neurosci.* **2018**, *12*, 642. [CrossRef] [PubMed]
22. Gay, A.; Boutet, C.; Sigaud, T.; Kamgoue, A.; Sevos, J.; Brunelin, J.; Massoubre, C. A single session of repetitive transcranial magnetic stimulation of the prefrontal cortex reduces cue-induced craving in patients with gambling disorder. *Eur. Psychiatry* **2017**, *41*, 68–74. [CrossRef]
23. Sauvaget, A.; Bulteau, S.; Guilleux, A.; Leboucher, J.; Pichot, A.; Valrivière, P.; Vanelle, J.-M.; Sébille-Rivain, V.; Grall-Bronnec, M. Both active and sham low-frequency rTMS single sessions over the right DLPFC decrease cue-induced cravings among pathological gamblers seeking treatment: A randomized, double-blind, sham-controlled crossover trial. *J. Behav. Addict.* **2018**, *7*, 126–136. [CrossRef]
24. Zack, M.; Cho, S.S.; Parlee, J.; Jacobs, M.; Li, C.; Boileau, I.; Strafella, A. Effects of High Frequency Repeated Transcranial Magnetic Stimulation and Continuous Theta Burst Stimulation on Gambling Reinforcement, Delay Discounting, and Stroop Interference in Men with Pathological Gambling. *Brain Stimul.* **2016**, *9*, 867–875. [CrossRef] [PubMed]
25. Rosenberg, O.; Klein, L.D.; Dannon, P.N. Deep transcranial magnetic stimulation for the treatment of pathological gambling. *Psychiatry Res.* **2013**, *206*, 111–113. [CrossRef]
26. Potenza, M.N.; Steinberg, M.A.; Skudlarski, P.; Fulbright, R.K.; Lacadie, C.M.; Wilber, M.K.; Rounsaville, B.J.; Gore, J.C.; Wexler, B.E. Gambling Urges in Pathological Gambling. *Arch. Gen. Psychiatry* **2003**, *60*, 828–836. [CrossRef]
27. Valero-Cabré, A.; Pascual-Leone, A.; Rushmore, R.J. Cumulative sessions of repetitive transcranial magnetic stimulation (rTMS) build up facilitation to subsequent TMS-mediated behavioural disruptions. *Eur. J. Neurosci.* **2008**, *27*, 765–774. [CrossRef] [PubMed]
28. U.S. National Library of Medicine. ClinicalTrials.gov. Identifier: NCT03733821, Sleep Modifications in Patients with Cocaine Use Disorders Treated with Transcranial Magnetic Stimulation (TMS). Available online: https://clinicaltrials.gov/ct2/show/NCT03733821 (accessed on 29 May 2019).
29. American Psychiatric Association. *Diagnostic and Statistical Manual of Mental Disorders: DSM-5*; American Psychiatric Pub: Washington, DC, USA, 2013; ISBN 9780890425541.
30. Lesieur, H.R.; Blume, S.B. The South Oaks Gambling Screen (SOGS): A new instrument for the identification of Pathological gamblers. *Am. J. Psychiatry* **1987**, *144*, 1184–1188.
31. Rossi, S.; Hallett, M.; Rossini, P.M.; Pascual-Leone, A.; Avanzini, G.; Bestmann, S.; Berardelli, A.; Brewer, C.; Canli, T.; Cantello, R.; et al. Safety, ethical considerations, and application guidelines for the use of transcranial magnetic stimulation in clinical practice and research. *Clin. Neurophysiol.* **2009**, *120*, 2008–2039. [CrossRef]
32. Kim, S.W.; Grant, J.E.; Potenza, M.N.; Blanco, C.; Hollander, E. The Gambling Symptom Assessment Scale (G-SAS): A reliability and validity study. *Psychiatry Res.* **2009**, *166*, 76–84.
33. Weiss, R.D.; Griffin, M.L.; Hufford, C.; Muenz, L.R.; Najavits, L.M.; Jansson, S.B.; Kogan, J.; Thompson, H.J. Early Prediction of Initiation of Abstinence From Cocaine. *Am. J. Addict.* **1997**, *6*, 224–231. [CrossRef]
34. Weiss, R.D.; Griffin, M.L.; Hufford, C. Craving in hospitalized cocaine abusers as a predictor of outcome. *Am. J. Drug Alcohol Abus.* **1995**, *21*, 289–301. [CrossRef]
35. Buysse, D.J.; Reynolds, C.F.; Monk, T.H.; Berman, S.R.; Kupfer, D.J. The Pittsburgh Sleep Quality Index: A new instrument for psychiatric practice and research. *Psychiatry Res.* **1989**, *28*, 193–213. [CrossRef]
36. Mollayeva, T.; Thurairajah, P.; Burton, K.; Mollayeva, S.; Shapiro, C.M.; Colantonio, A. The Pittsburgh sleep quality index as a screening tool for sleep dysfunction in clinical and non-clinical samples: A systematic review and meta-analysis. *Sleep Med. Rev.* **2016**, *25*, 52–73. [CrossRef]
37. Curcio, G.; Tempesta, D.; Scarlata, S.; Marzano, C.; Moroni, F.; Rossini, P.M.; Ferrara, M.; De Gennaro, L. Validity of the Italian version of the Pittsburgh sleep quality index (PSQI). *Neurol. Sci.* **2013**, *34*, 511–519. [CrossRef]

38. Beck, A.T.; Steer, R.A.; Brown, G.K. *Beck Depression Inventory-II*; Psychological Corporation: San Antonio, TX, USA, 1996; ISBN 0158018389.
39. Zung, W.W.K. A Rating Instrument for Anxiety Disorders. *Psychosomatics* **1971**, *12*, 371–379. [CrossRef]
40. Derogatis, L.R. *Symptom Checklist-90-R (SCL-90-R): Administration, Scoring, and Procedures Manual*, 3rd ed.; NCS Pearson: Minneapolis, MN, USA, 1994.
41. Derogatis, L.R.; Rickels, K.; Rock, A.F. The SCL-90 and the MMPI: A step in the validation of a new self-report scale. *Br. J. Psychiatry* **1976**, *128*, 280–289. [CrossRef]
42. RStudio Team. *RStudio: Integrated Development for R*; RStudio, Inc.: Boston, MA, USA, 2016.
43. R Foundation for Statistical Computing Team. *R: A Language and Environment for Statistical Computing*; R Foundation for Statistical Computing: Vienna, Austria, 2018.
44. Lenth, R. Emmeans: Estimated marginal means, aka least-squares means. *R Package Version* **2018**, *1*, 1.
45. Hall, G.W.; Carriero, N.J.; Takushi, R.Y.; Montoya, I.D.; Preston, K.L.; Gorelick, D.A. Pathological gambling among cocaine-dependent outpatients. *Am. J. Psychiatry* **2000**, *157*, 1127–1133. [CrossRef] [PubMed]
46. Wareham, J.D.; Potenza, M.N. Pathological gambling and substance use disorders. *Am. J. Drug Alcohol Abus.* **2010**, *36*, 242–247. [CrossRef]
47. Camprodon, J.A.; Martínez-Raga, J.; Alonso-Alonso, M.; Shih, M.C.; Pascual-Leone, A. One session of high frequency repetitive transcranial magnetic stimulation (rTMS) to the right prefrontal cortex transiently reduces cocaine craving. *Drug Alcohol Depend.* **2007**, *86*, 91–94. [CrossRef] [PubMed]
48. Hudgens-Haney, M.E.; Hamm, J.P.; Goodie, A.S.; Krusemark, E.A.; McDowell, J.E.; Clementz, B.A. Neural correlates of the impact of control on decision making in pathological gambling. *Biol. Psychol.* **2013**, *92*, 365–372. [CrossRef]
49. Limbrick-Oldfield, E.H.; Van Holst, R.J.; Clark, L. Fronto-striatal dysregulation in drug addiction and pathological gambling: Consistent inconsistencies? *NeuroImage Clin.* **2013**, *2*, 385–393. [CrossRef]
50. Miedl, S.F.; Peters, J.; Büchel, C. Altered neural reward representations in pathological gamblers revealed by delay and probability discounting. *Arch. Gen. Psychiatry* **2012**, *69*, 177–186. [CrossRef]
51. Choi, J.S.; Shin, Y.C.; Jung, W.H.; Jang, J.H.; Kang, D.H.; Choi, C.H.; Choi, S.W.; Lee, J.Y.; Hwang, J.Y.; Kwon, J.S. Altered Brain Activity during Reward Anticipation in Pathological Gambling and Obsessive-Compulsive Disorder. *PLoS ONE* **2012**, *7*, e45938. [CrossRef]
52. Tschernegg, M.; Crone, J.S.; Eigenberger, T.; Schwartenbeck, P.; Fauth-Bühler, M.; Lemènager, T.; Mann, K.; Thon, N.; Wurst, F.M.; Kronbichler, M. Abnormalities of functional brain networks in pathological gambling: A graph-theoretical approach. *Front. Hum. Neurosci.* **2013**, *7*, 625. [CrossRef]
53. Everitt, B.J.; Belin, D.; Economidou, D.; Pelloux, Y.; Dalley, J.W.; Robbins, T.W. Review. Neural mechanisms underlying the vulnerability to develop compulsive drug-seeking habits and addiction. *Philos. Trans. R. Soc. Lond. Ser. B Biol. Sci.* **2008**, *363*, 3125–3135. [CrossRef]
54. Everitt, B.J.; Robbins, T.W. Neural systems of reinforcement for drug addiction: From actions to habits to compulsion. *Nat. Neurosci.* **2005**, *8*, 1481. [CrossRef] [PubMed]
55. Jiang, C.G.; Zhang, T.; Yue, F.G.; Yi, M.L.; Gao, D. Efficacy of Repetitive Transcranial Magnetic Stimulation in the Treatment of Patients with Chronic Primary Insomnia. *Cell Biochem. Biophys.* **2013**, *67*, 169–173. [CrossRef]
56. Donse, L.; Sack, A.T.; Fitzgerald, P.B.; Arns, M. Sleep disturbances in obsessive-compulsive disorder: Association with non-response to repetitive transcranial magnetic stimulation (rTMS). *J. Anxiety Disord.* **2017**, *49*, 31–39. [CrossRef]
57. Sánchez-Escandón, O.; Arana-Lechuga, Y.; Terán-Pérez, G.; Ruiz-Chow, A.; González-Robles, R.; Shkurovich-Bialik, P.; Collado-Corona, M.A.A.; Velázquez-Moctezuma, J. Effect of low-frequency repetitive transcranial magnetic stimulation on sleep pattern and quality of life in patients with focal epilepsy. *Sleep Med.* **2016**, *20*, 37–40. [CrossRef] [PubMed]
58. Pellicciari, M.C.; Cordone, S.; Marzano, C.; Bignotti, S.; Gazzoli, A.; Miniussi, C.; De Gennaro, L. Dorsolateral prefrontal transcranial magnetic stimulation in patients with major depression locally affects alpha power of REM sleep. *Front. Hum. Neurosci.* **2013**, *7*, 433. [CrossRef] [PubMed]

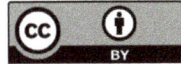

© 2019 by the authors. Licensee MDPI, Basel, Switzerland. This article is an open access article distributed under the terms and conditions of the Creative Commons Attribution (CC BY) license (http://creativecommons.org/licenses/by/4.0/).

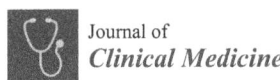

Article

The More You Take It, the Better It Works: Six-Month Results of a Nalmefene Phase-IV Trial

Pablo Barrio [1,*], Carlos Roncero [2], Lluisa Ortega [1], Josep Guardia [3], Lara Yuguero [4] and Antoni Gual [1]

1. Addictive Behaviors Unit, Clinic Hospital, University of Barcelona, Barcelona 08036, Spain; llortega@clinic.cat (L.O.); tgual@clinic.cat (A.G.)
2. Psychiatry Service, University of Salamanca Health Care Complex, Institute of Biomedicine, University of Salamanca, Salamanca 37007, Spain; croncero@saludcastillayleon.es
3. Addictive Behavior Unit, Psychiatry Department, Hospital de la Santa Creu i Sant Pau Barcelona, Barcelona 08041, Spain; jguardia@santpau.cat
4. Addictive Behaviors Unit, Germanes Hospitalàries, Sant Boi, Barcelona 08830, Spain; lyuguero.hbmenni@hospitalarias.es
* Correspondence: pbarrio@clinic.cat; Tel.: +34-932275400

Received: 19 February 2019; Accepted: 3 April 2019; Published: 6 April 2019

Abstract: Background: Alcohol use disorders remain a major health problem. Reduced drinking has been increasingly recognized as a valuable alternative to abstinence. Nalmefene has shown in previous, experimental studies to be a useful tool to aid reduced drinking. However, more data from routine practice settings are needed in order to obtain evidence with high external validity. The aim of this study was to conduct a single-arm phase-IV study with alcohol-dependent outpatients starting with nalmefene for the first time. Here, we present the main effectiveness analysis, scheduled at six months. Methods: This was an observational, multisite, single-arm, phase-IV study conducted among adult alcohol-dependent outpatients who received nalmefene for the first time. The study consisted of four visits: Baseline, 1 month, 6 months, and 12 months. At each visit, drinking variables were obtained from the time-line follow-back regarding the previous month. Satisfaction with medication was also assessed from both patients and professionals with the Medication Satisfaction Questionnaire. A repeated measures mixed model was performed for effective analysis regarding drinking outcomes (reduction in total alcohol consumption and the number of heavy drinking days). Regression analyses were performed in order to find predictors of responses to nalmefene. Results: From a total of 110 patients included, 63 reported data at the six-month visit. On average, patients took nalmefene 69% of days during the month previous to the 6-month assessment. Compared to the one month results, the number of heavy drinking days and total alcohol consumption increased. Still, they were significantly lower than baseline values (outcome evolution over time was from 13.5 to 6.8 to 9.4 days/month, and from 169 to 79 to 116 units/month). A total of 23 patients were considered medication responders. The number of days of taking nalmefene was significantly associated in the regression analysis. Satisfaction was globally high for both professionals and patients and, overall, nalmefene was well-tolerated with no serious adverse events reported. Conclusion: The data provided by this phase-IV study suggest that nalmefene is an effective, well-tolerated treatment for alcohol-dependence in real world, clinical settings.

Keywords: drinking reduction; nalmefene; phase-IV trial; 6 months; observational

1. Introduction

Alcohol remains a first-order global health problem, with 15 million affected people in the EU [1]. Recent publications in the US also warn about an increase in the prevalence of alcohol use disorders during the last decade [2]. The impact it has on both individuals and society is of an enormous dimension, both medically and economically [3,4]. Several strategies have been applied to decrease the burden of the problem, ranging from public health intervention to individualized psychosocial and pharmacological treatment.

In the arena of pharmacological treatments, one of the latest incorporations has been nalmefene. The lack of real-world data, the need to assess adverse events in clinical populations, and the critiques surrounding the drug since its approval led to the need of a phase-IV trial. A single-arm, observational, phase-IV study of nalmefene, including 110 patients, was started in four different sites in Barcelona, Spain, in 2015.

Baseline and one month results [5] suggested nalmefene was effective in reducing alcohol consumption. They also showed that it was well-tolerated with no serious adverse events, and the satisfaction with the drug of both professionals and patients was high.

The study, which was designed to last 12 months, consisted of four assessment points in time (baseline, 1, 6 and 12 months). In this paper we report the results of the main effectiveness analysis which was scheduled at 6 months.

2. Methods

A full description of the methods has been described elsewhere [5]. As a summary, this was an observational, multisite, single-arm, phase-IV study, conducted among adult alcohol-dependent outpatients taking nalmefene for the first time. The study consisted of 4 visits: Baseline, 4 weeks, 6 months, and 12 months.

The main outcome variables of the study were:

(1) Reduction in drinking parameters, measured as a change from baseline in heavy drinking days and total alcohol consumption (units in the previous 28 days). The data were derived from the previous month's timeline follow-back. As the study was conducted in Spain, one drink was considered to contain 10 g of pure ethanol.

(2) Patient and clinician satisfaction, as measured by the Medication Satisfaction Questionnaire (MSQ) [6,7]. Secondary outcomes included changes in drinking risk-level according to the WHO definitions (very high-risk: More than 100 g of alcohol per day in men and more than 60 in women; high-risk: 60–100 g per day in men, 40–60 g per day in women; medium-risk: 40–60 g per day in men, 20–40 g per day in women; low-risk: 1–40 g per day in men, 1–20 g per day in women). Liver enzymes were also analyzed.

Other collected variables at baseline included previous history of drug use, psychiatric history, family history of drug and alcohol use, and concomitant or changes in psychiatric medication during the study period. At the study visit, the number of days that patients took nalmefene was also recorded.

Responders to medication were defined in the same manner as in the 1-month publication (a reduction in daily alcohol consumption of at least 70% or downshift of two categories in the drinking risk-level, according to the World Health Organization (WHO), or a shift to low-risk category)

For effectiveness analysis, the repeated measures linear mixed procedure was used for both heavy-drinking days and total alcohol consumption as main outcomes. Age, sex, and number of days taking nalmefene were entered as fixed effects. We also included the presence of any psychiatric or addictive comorbidity as covariates. For each main outcome, regression coefficients (b), t-values and p-values were calculated. Statistical significance was set at 0.05. Missing data at 6 months for outcome variables was addressed with the conservative approach of baseline observation carried forward (BOCF). Days of medication intake were imputed to 0 for missing values. A descriptive analysis of the Medication Satisfaction Questionnaire (MSQ) was conducted. A satisfaction analysis and a logistic regression analysis for the detection of significant predictors of medication responders were conducted. Included variables were sex, age, number of days taking nalmefene, presence of comorbid drug use, and presence of psychiatric comorbidity. A descriptive analysis of adverse events was also conducted.

The study protocol, final approved informed consent document, and all supporting information were submitted to and approved by the institutional review boards of all participating centers. All participants provided written informed consent before taking part in study procedures. The study was conducted in accordance with the International Conference on Harmonization and Good Clinical Practice and the principles of the Declaration of Helsinki.

3. Results

3.1. Sample

From a total of 110 patients included at baseline, 47 were lost to the follow-up at six months, leaving a total of 63 patients reporting drinking outcomes at six months. Of these, 34 patients were still taking nalmefene. Accordingly, drug interruption was reported by 29 patients (eight due to low efficacy, four due to the achievement of the reduction aim, one due to adverse reactions, two due to the change to an abstinence aim, and 14 due to other reasons). No overdoses were reported. Of the 34 patients still on nalmefene, complete abstinence was reported by six subjects.

In patients still on nalmefene, the mean number of days of patients taking the drug over the previous month was 19.3 (SD = 11.6). More than half of the patients (57%) took it on a daily basis. Basal characteristics of participants can be observed in Table 1.

Table 1. Baseline sociodemographic and clinical characteristics of included patients.

Characteristic [a]	Phase-IV (n = 110)
Age, years	44.4 (9.4)
Sex male	73 (66.4)
Higher education	30 (27,3)
Organic comorbidity [b]	30 (27,3)
Age at the onset of drinking problems	23 (12,4)
Drinking Risk Level	
Low	50 (45.5)
Medium	18 (16.4)
High	24 (21.8)
Very High	18 (16.3)
g-Glutamyltransferase (IU/L)	84 (128.2)
Alanine aminotransferase (IU/L)	29.2 (15.5)
Aspartate aminotransferase (IU/L)	30,8 (17.6)
Previously treated for alcohol-dependence	51 (46.4)
Previous pharmacological treatment	35 (32,2)
Years of alcohol-dependence untreated	17.5 (12,7)
Previously treated for alcohol-withdrawal	33 (30)
Personal history of psychiatric problems	40 (36.4)
Family history of alcohol problems	53 (48.2)
Addictive comorbidities [c] (past or present)	72 (65.5)
Percentage of days taking study medication	70 (64)
Accepts use of alcohol app	52 (47.1)
Monthly heavy drinking days (baseline)	13.5 (11)
Mean alcohol consumption (grams per day; baseline)	60.4 (74,6)

a: Data are expressed as n (%) for categorical variables and mean (SD) for continuous variables; b: defined as the presence of diabetes, hypertension, high blood cholesterol or any other significant medical condition; c: defined as any substance use disorder (except nicotine dependence), past or current, as clinically evaluated in the first visit of the study.

3.2. Efficacy

Both drinking outcomes increased, compared to month 1, but were still significantly reduced when compared to baseline values. The mean number of heavy-drinking days over the last 4 weeks was 9.4 (SD = 10.8) and the total alcohol consumption in units, also over the last 4 weeks, was 116.4 (SD = 171.8). Evolution over time of these parameters can be seen in Figure 1. As a sensitivity analysis, evolution over time, according to per protocol analysis, is provided in Figure 2. Per protocol analysis was conducted using only available data, that is, patients lost to follow-up were not included in this analysis.

The repeated measures linear mixed model revealed a significant effect in both outcomes at time 1 (first month). Given the increase in both outcomes at time 2 (month 6), no further significant changes were observed. The rest of the covariates were not statistically significant.

A total of 23 patients (21%) were considered medication responders. The only significant predictor found was the number of days with medication intake (OR = 1.058, CI 95% 1.001–1.118).

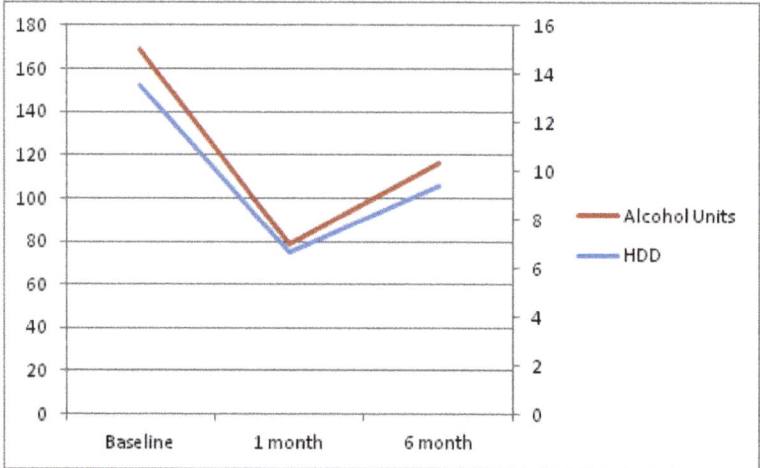

Figure 1. The change over time of study outcomes according to intention-to-treat analysis. The left axis shows alcohol units over the last 4 weeks. The right axis shows heavy-drinking days over the last 4 weeks. HDD: heavy drinking days.

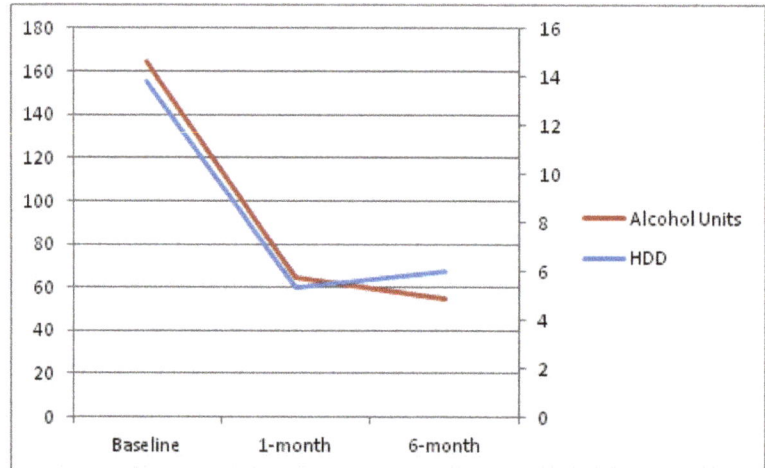

Figure 2. The change over time of study outcomes, according to per protocol analysis. The left axis shows alcohol units over the last 4 weeks. The right axis shows heavy-drinking days over the last 4 weeks. HDD: heavy drinking days.

3.3. Satisfaction

Figure 3 displays the satisfaction of professionals and patients with nalmefene at six months, as recorded by the MSQ. In the logistic regression analysis, the the number of days taking study medication revealed a significant effect upon patient satisfaction (OR = 1.074, CI 95% 1.021–1.130).

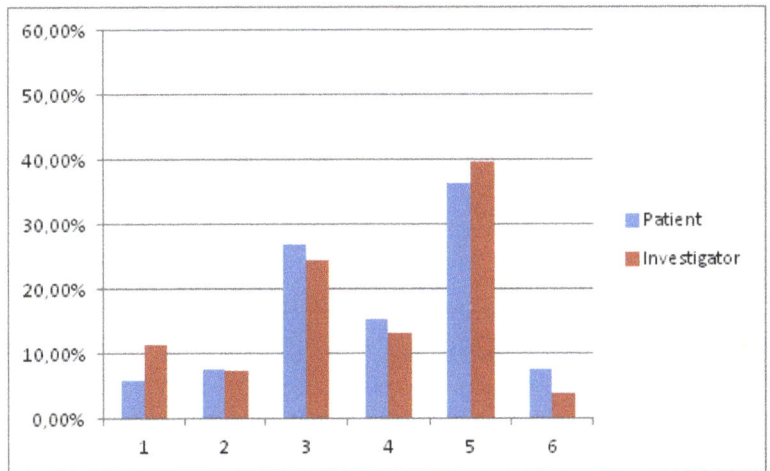

Figure 3. The satisfaction with treatment according to the Medication Satisfaction Questionnaire. 1: Extremely dissatisfied; 2: Very dissatisfied; 3: Somewhat dissatisfied; 4: Neither satisfied nor dissatisfied; 5: Somewhat satisfied; 6: Very satisfied; 7: Extremely satisfied.

3.4. Safety

At six months, no new drug-related adverse events were notified. That left a total of 29 patients with medication-related adverse events during the first month of treatment. Most events were mild, and no serious adverse events were recorded. Additionally, no overdose was observed or notified.

4. Discussion

The main 6 month effectiveness analysis of this phase-IV trial suggests that nalmefene is effective in reducing alcohol-use when used in real-world, clinical settings. Similar to the 1 month results, nalmefene was well-tolerated and no significant, severe, or life-threatening reactions were observed. There are, however, relevant observations to be made in comparison with previous 1 month results.

Both heavy-drinking days and total alcohol consumption increased for the whole sample, suggesting nalmefene loses some efficacy over time. It is important to bear in mind that this is, in fact, a common phenomenon to many addiction treatments, whether pharmacological or psychosocial. On the other hand, we took the conservative approach of baseline observation carried forward (BOCF) to deal with missing data, a fact that could have decreased our statistical power.

It is important to note the relatively small number of patients still taking nalmefene at six months (31% approximately). While low-efficacy and adverse reactions might explain an important share of medication drop-outs, it is also possible that patients who are offered nalmefene are more prone to treatment abandonment, since it has been shown that patients still drinking, and those who aim at reduction objectives, are at greater risk of treatment drop-outs [8–10].

Taken together, we believe these observations should remind professionals that patients who are prescribed nalmefene are especially prone to abandon treatment, and that efforts should also be directed toward increasing treatment retention.

Worth mentioning is a similar, recent study [11] conducted among outpatients in routine settings that showed a significant decrease of drinking outcomes at 24 weeks. Similar to our sample, and other previous experimental studies with nalmefene [12], psychiatric comorbidity was high. Interestingly, and contrary to our findings, improvements were seen over the six-month period. All taken together, recent evidence suggests that nalmefene is indeed effective for alcohol use disorder patients in routine settings, where comorbidity is frequent.

In trying to find differential characteristics between responders and non-responders to treatment, as measured by reductions in alcohol consumption parameters and changes in drinking risk categories, only the number of days taking nalmefene yielded significant effects.

Regarding satisfaction data, a slight decrease in comparison to one month results was observed, probably mimicking the decreased effectiveness at six months. Interestingly, the number of days taking medication was the only covariate associated with increased satisfaction. While it could be interpreted as a consequence, rather than a cause of increased satisfaction, and similar to the regression analysis, which was conducted in order to find predictors of treatment response, we believe this finding suggests that nalmefene might work better over the long-run if taken daily or with a high degree of frequency, rather than sporadically. Another hypothesis worth considering when analyzing this data could be that a higher degree of medication intake is, indeed, a reflection of higher motivation in patients. Therefore, the results obtained in this study are probably not to be entirely attributed to pharmacological effects. It is also fundamental to comment on the fact that we imputed as 0 the days of medication intake in the cases where this variable was missing. While we consider this imputation not unlikely, especially given that nalmefene requires ongoing medical prescription in Spain, it is also true that, in combination with the BOCF imputation for missing drinking outcomes, it could have biased the results obtained, regarding days of medication intake as a significant predictor of both medication response and satisfaction.

Finally, several other limitations apply to this study, such as its observational design and lack of control group, the reduced sample size, and the limited geographical area where the study was conducted.

5. Conclusions

Nalmefene seems to provide further effectiveness at 6 months, in spite of it being reduced, as compared to the first month, after initiating treatment. Our results suggest that a more frequent intake might be related to better outcomes, both in terms of satisfaction and reduced drinking.

Author Contributions: Conceptualization, A.G. and P.B.; methodology, A.G. and P.B.; formal analysis, P.B.; investigation, P.B., C.R., J.G., L.Y. and L.O.; writing—original draft preparation, P.B.; writing—review and editing, P.B.,C.R.,L.O., L.Y. and J.G.; funding acquisition, A.G.

Funding: This study was funded by Lundbeck. The sponsor was involved in the study design, but not in data collection, analysis, manuscript writing, or decision of submitting the article for publication.

Conflicts of Interest: P.B., C.R., J.G., and A.G. have received honoraria from Lundbeck. P.B. has also received honoraria from Pfizer. C.R. has also received honoraria from Janssen-cilag, Otsuka, Server, GSK, Rovi, Astra, MSD and Sanofi. L.Y. L.O. have no conflict of interest to declare.

References

1. Wittchen, H.U.; Jacobi, F.; Rehm, J.; Gustavsson, A.; Svensson, M.; Jönsson, B.; Olesen, J.; Allgulander, C.; Alonso, J.; Faravelli, C.; et al. The size and burden of mental disorders and other disorders of the brain in Europe 2010. *Eur. Neuropsychopharmacol.* **2011**, *21*, 655–679. [CrossRef] [PubMed]
2. Grant, B.F.; Chou, S.P.; Saha, T.D.; Pickering, R.P.; Kerridge, B.T.; Ruan, W.J.; Huang, B.; Jung, J.; Zhang, H.; Fan, A.; et al. Prevalence of 12-Month Alcohol Use, High-Risk Drinking, and *DSM-IV* Alcohol Use Disorder in the United States, 2001–2002 to 2012–2013. *JAMA Psychiatry* **2017**, *74*, 911. [CrossRef] [PubMed]
3. Barrio, P.; Reynolds, J.; García-Altés, A.; Gual, A.; Anderson, P. Social costs of illegal drugs, alcohol and tobacco in the European Union: A systematic review. *Drug. Alcohol Rev.* **2017**. [CrossRef] [PubMed]

4. Miquel, L.; Rehm, J.; Shield, K.D.; Vela, E.; Bustins, M.; Segura, L.; Colom, J.; Anderson, P.; Gual, A. Alcohol, tobacco and health care costs: A population-wide cohort study (n = 606947 patients) of current drinkers based on medical and administrative health records from Catalonia. *Eur. J. Public Health* **2018**. [CrossRef] [PubMed]
5. Barrio, P.; Ortega, L.; Guardia, J.; Roncero, C.; Yuguero, L.; Gual, A. Who Receives Nalmefene and How Does It Work in the Real World? A Single-Arm, Phase IV Study of Nalmefene in Alcohol Dependent Outpatients: Baseline and 1-Month Results. *Clin. Drug. Investig.* **2017**. [CrossRef] [PubMed]
6. Kalali, A. Patient Satisfaction with, and Acceptability of, Atypical Antipsychotics. *Curr. Med. Res. Opin.* **1999**, *15*, 135–137. [CrossRef] [PubMed]
7. Vernon, M.K.; Revicki, D.A.; Awad, A.G.; Dirani, R.; Panish, J.; Canuso, C.M.; Grinspan, A.; Mannix, S.; Kalali, A.H. Psychometric evaluation of the Medication Satisfaction Questionnaire (MSQ) to assess satisfaction with antipsychotic medication among schizophrenia patients. *Schizophr. Res.* **2010**, *118*, 271–278. [CrossRef] [PubMed]
8. Haug, S.; Schaub, M.P. Treatment outcome, treatment retention, and their predictors among clients of five outpatient alcohol treatment centres in Switzerland. *BMC Public Health* **2016**, *16*, 581. [CrossRef] [PubMed]
9. Haug, S.; Eggli, P.; Schaub, M.P. Drinking Goals and Their Association With Treatment Retention and Treatment Outcomes Among Clients in Outpatient Alcohol Treatment. *Subst. Use Misuse* **2016**, 1–9. [CrossRef] [PubMed]
10. Meyer, A.; Wapp, M.; Strik, W.; Moggi, F. Association Between Drinking Goal and Alcohol Use One Year After Residential Treatment: A Multicenter Study. *J. Addict. Dis.* **2014**, *33*, 234–242. [CrossRef] [PubMed]
11. Di Nicola, M.; De Filippis, S.; Martinotti, G.; De Risio, L.; Pettorruso, M.; De Persis, S.; Giovanni, A.; Maremmani, I.; di Giannantonio, M.; Janiri, L. Nalmefene in Alcohol Use Disorder Subjects with Psychiatric Comorbidity: A Naturalistic Study. *Adv. Ther.* **2017**, *34*, 1636–1649. [CrossRef] [PubMed]
12. Van den Brink, W.; Sørensen, P.; Torup, L.; Mann, K.; Gual, A.; SENSE Study Group. Long-term efficacy, tolerability and safety of nalmefene as-needed in patients with alcohol dependence: A 1-year, randomised controlled study. *J. Psychopharmacol.* **2014**, *28*, 733–744. [CrossRef] [PubMed]

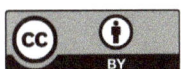 © 2019 by the authors. Licensee MDPI, Basel, Switzerland. This article is an open access article distributed under the terms and conditions of the Creative Commons Attribution (CC BY) license (http://creativecommons.org/licenses/by/4.0/).

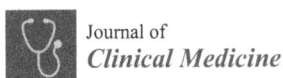

Article

Application of Diagnostic Interview for Internet Addiction (DIA) in Clinical Practice for Korean Adolescents

Hyera Ryu [1], Ji Yoon Lee [1], A Ruem Choi [1], Sun Ju Chung [1], Minkyung Park [1], Soo-Young Bhang [2], Jun-Gun Kwon [3], Yong-Sil Kweon [4,*] and Jung-Seok Choi [1,5,*]

1. Department of Psychiatry, SMG-SNU Boramae Medical Center, Seoul 07061, Korea; hyera.ryu12@gmail.com (H.R.); idiyuni91@gmail.com (J.Y.L.); choiar90@gmail.com (A.R.C.); sunjujung1991@gmail.com (S.J.C.); reneedrv@gmail.com (M.P.)
2. Department of Psychiatry, Eulji General Hospital, Seoul 01830, Korea; dresme@daum.net
3. I Will Center, Seoul Metropolitan Boramae Youth Center, Seoul 07062, Korea; jun@boramyc.or.kr
4. Department of Psychiatry, Uijeongbu St. Mary's Hospital, The Catholic University of Korea College of Medicine, Gyeonggi 11765, Korea
5. Department of Psychiatry and Behavioral Science, Seoul National University College of Medicine, Seoul 03080, Korea
* Correspondence: yskwn@catholic.ac.kr (Y.-S.K.); choijs73@gmail.com (J.-S.C.); Tel.: +82-31-1661-7500 (Y.-S.K.); +82-2-870-2177 (J.-S.C.)

Received: 4 January 2019; Accepted: 2 February 2019; Published: 6 February 2019

Abstract: The increased prevalence of Internet Gaming Disorder (IGD) and the inclusion of IGD in DSM-5 and ICD-11 emphasizes the importance of measuring and describing the IGD symptoms. We examined the psychometric properties of the Diagnostic Interview for Internet Addiction (DIA), a semi-structured diagnostic interview tool for IGD, and verified the application of DIA in clinical practice for Korean adolescents. The DIA is conducted in a manner that interviews both adolescents and their caregivers, and each item has a standardized representative question and various examples. It consists of 10 items based on the DSM-5 IGD diagnostic criteria, which is cognitive salience, withdrawal, tolerance, difficulty in regulating use, loss of interest in other activities, persistent use despite negative results, deception regarding Internet/games/SNS use, use of Internet/games/SNS to avoid negative feelings, interference with role performance, and craving. The study included 103 adolescents divided into three subgroups (mild risk, moderate risk, and addicted group) based on the total score of DIA. Demographic and clinical characteristics were compared among the DIA subgroups using the chi-square test and analysis of variance (ANOVA), and correlation analysis was used to examine the associations of IGD symptoms with clinical variables (e.g., impulsivity, aggression, depression, anxiety, self-esteem). The DIA total score was significantly correlated with Internet and smartphone addiction, depression, state anxiety, self-esteem, impulsivity, aggression, and stress. Furthermore, the moderate risk and addicted group showed significantly higher levels of Internet and smartphone addiction, anxiety, depression, impulsivity, aggression, stress, and lower self-esteem compared with the mild risk group. The Junior Temperament and Character Inventory (JTCI), which measures temperament and character traits, revealed that the mild risk group had higher levels of persistence and self-directedness than did the addicted group. Our findings confirmed the psychometric properties of DIA and the application of the DIA classifications in Korean adolescents.

Keywords: internet gaming disorder; semi-structured diagnostic interview; psychometric properties; adolescents

1. Introduction

The prevalence of Internet addiction has steadily increased, from 10.4% in 2011 to 12.5% in 2014 in Korea [1], and the prevalence of Internet gaming disorder (IGD) is about 6% in Korean adolescents [2]. The American Psychiatric Association (APA) included IGD as a condition worthy of future study in Section III of the 5th edition of the Diagnostic and Statistical Manual of Mental Disorders (DSM-5), and the draft of 11th revision of the International Classification of Diseases (ICD-11), released in 2018, included the definition of gaming disorder (GD) [3,4]. The growing prevalence of IGD and its recognition as a possible behavioral addiction has increased the importance of describing and measuring the symptoms and severity of the condition. In this context, several researchers have noted that unifying the terminology and developing measurement tools based on the DSM-5 IGD diagnostic criteria are necessary to integrate concepts related to IGD [5–8].

As part of this effort, two self-report questionnaires, the Internet Gaming Disorder Test (IGD-20) [9] and the Internet Gaming Disorder Scale-Short Form (IGDS9-SF) [10], were developed based on the DSM-5 IGD diagnostic criteria. Although self-report questionnaires are cost-effective and easy to administer, the tool has some limitations. Jeong et al. (2018) recently found a discrepancy between self-report data and the clinical diagnosis of IGD in adolescents due to underreporting as a result of social desirability effects, which is a limitation of self-report questionnaires [11]. Therefore, semi-structured diagnostic interviews tools are needed to measure IGD symptoms more accurately in adolescents.

Several structured and the semi-structured interviews have been developed to assess IGD symptoms. The checklist for the Assessment of Internet and Computer Game Addiction (AICA-C) is a semi-structured interview that assesses six criteria (craving, tolerance, withdrawal, loss of control, preoccupation, and negative consequences) [12]. The Structured Clinical Interview for Internet Gaming Disorder (SCI-IGD) is a 12-item structured interview based on DSM-5 criteria and IGD-related clinical experience [13]. However, these tools were developed for middle school students and are only interviewed for adolescents without including their caregivers. The Diagnostic Interview for Internet Addiction (DIA) was developed to evaluate internet, games, and SNS addiction according to the DSM-5 diagnostic criteria, both children/adolescents and their caregivers are interviewed. It consists of 10 items, as 'craving' was added to the 9 DSM-5 criteria for IGD (cognitive salience, withdrawal, tolerance, difficulty in regulating use, loss of interest in other activities, persistent use despite negative results, deception regarding Internet/games/social network site (SNS) use, the use of Internet/games/SNS to avoid negative feelings, and interference with role performance). Each item is rated on a 4-point scale (0: No information; 1: No symptoms; 2: Subthreshold; and 3: Threshold level), and the number of items with a score of 3 (threshold) is calculated as the DIA total score. Previous studies have classified the severity of IGD as mild risk, moderate risk, plain addicted, and severe addicted based on the total number of IGD criteria met [14]. Thus, we adopted the previous categories for the DIA subgroups and verified the application of the DIA classifications in clinical practice by comparing IGD-related psychiatric symptoms among the subgroups.

Several studies have shown that IGD is related to internalizing (e.g., depression, anxiety, stress, and self-esteem) and externalizing (e.g., impulsivity and aggression) problems in adolescents [15–17]. Depression is the most common symptom associated with IGD in all age groups, and several studies have found that individuals with IGD experienced more severe depression and anxiety symptoms than did non-addicted individuals [17–21]. A longitudinal study found that depression and anxiety were negative outcomes of Internet gaming [22]. Lam et al. (2009) found that stress-related variables such as family dissatisfaction and recent stressful events were associated with IGD symptoms in adolescents [23]. Moreover, low self-esteem, impulsivity, and aggression are risk factors for IGD in adolescents [22,24,25]. Several studies have found positive correlations between IGD symptoms and personality traits (e.g., sensation seeking, neuroticism, high impulsivity, and high aggressiveness) and negative correlations with extraversion, responsibility, reward dependence, complacency, and self-directedness [25–29]. Thus, we examined the relationship between DIA total scores and internalizing/externalizing problems in adolescents, and compared the various characteristics among the DIA severity subgroups.

We examined the psychometric properties of the DIA in Korean adolescents and verified the application of the DIA classification in clinical practice by comparing the clinical characteristics among subgroups.

2. Materials and Methods

2.1. Participants and Procedure

We screened children and adolescents (aged 7–18 years) who used excessively internet games and/or smartphones in Clinic I-CURE Centers. All participants were screened using questionnaires pertaining to Internet and smartphone addiction (e.g., the Korean Scale for Internet Addiction for adolescents (K-scale); the Korean Smartphone Addiction Scale (S-scale); and the Internet Addiction Proneness Scale for Adolescents (O_A), which is completed by caregivers). Subjects who scored above the cutoff for addiction on at least one screening questionnaire were enrolled in the study. We enrolled 166 participants between August 2015 and December 2017. Of these, 47 children were excluded because the sample size of children was small and there were differences between the questionnaires in children and adolescents (e.g., BDI versus CDI, etc.), and 16 adolescents with intelligence quotient scores <80 or missing data were excluded from the study. The final analysis included 103 subjects between the ages of 13 and 18 years. In this study, the interviewers consisted of a master's-level of clinical psychology and every interviewer was trained by addiction and/or child-adolescents psychiatry specialists. A flow chart of the study is shown in Figure 1.

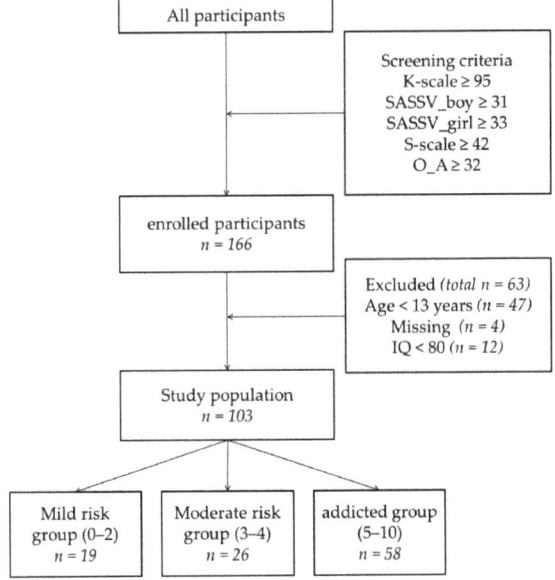

Figure 1. Study flow chart. NOTE: The screening cut-off values shown are those for adolescents; children were excluded from this analysis, and their scores are not reported here. The study participants were divided into subgroups according to their total DIA score. K-scale = Korean Scale for Internet Addiction for adolescents; SAS-SV = Smartphone Addiction Scale-short form version; S-scale = Korean Smartphone Addiction scale; O_A = Internet Addiction Proneness Scale for Adolescents checked by caregivers.

2.2. Measurements

2.2.1. Diagnostic interview for Internet Addiction (DIA)

The DIA is a semi-structured diagnostic interview tool consisting of 10 items based on the DSM-5 Section III IGD diagnostic criteria; it is used to assess Internet, games, and SNS addiction symptoms (i.e., cognitive salience, withdrawal, tolerance, difficulty in regulating use, loss of interest in other activities, persistent use despite negative results, deception regarding Internet/gaming/SNS use, use of Internet/gaming/SNS to avoid negative feelings, interference with role performance, and craving). In this study, the internal consistency coefficient of DIA was 0.72.

DIA interviews take about 10–20 min for each subject and their caregivers. Each item has a standardized representative question and various examples, so clinicians can more easily evaluate the score. For example, to assess 'regulation difficulty in regulating use', there is a representative question: "Do you feel you should reduce the Internet/Games/SNS, but you can't reduce the time you spend doing Internet/Games/SNS?" Detailed examples are provided as follows: "I often do more Internet/Games/SNS than I originally thought", "I often don't do other activities I was planning because of the Internet/Games/SNS", "I try to stop the Internet/games/SNS but it is difficult to break". Table 1 shows the standardized interview script for each item. After interviewing the subjects and caregivers, the clinician calculated the total score to determine whether subjects were addicted to the Internet, games, and/or SNS. Each item was rated on a 4-point scale (0: No information; 1: No symptoms; 2: Subthreshold; 3: Threshold level), and the number of items with a score of 3 was calculated as the total DIA score (range, 0–10).

Table 1. Examples of standardized interview script in Diagnostic Interview for Internet Addiction.

Item	Standardized Representative Questions
1. cognitive salience	"Even if you do not have Internet/Games/SNS, do you spend a lot of time thinking about Internet/Games/SNS or planning what to do next?"
2. withdrawal	"Do you experience restlessness, irritability, depression, anxiety, sadness etc. when you reduce, stop, or not allowed Internet/Games/SNS?"
3. tolerance	"Do you want to spend more Internet/Gaming/SNS time, find more interesting things, or use better equipment such as cell phones, computers to make you feel as fun as before?"
4. difficulty in regulating use	"Do you feel you should reduce the Internet/Games/SNS, but you can't reduce the time you spend doing Internet/Games/SNS?"
5. loss of interest in other activities	"Because of the Internet/Games/SNS, would you be less interested in participating in other leisure activities such as hobbies or meet friends?"
6. persistent use despite negative feelings	"Despite negative consequences, such as lack of sleep time, late school or work, spend too much money, debate with other people, or neglect important things, do you continue the Internet/Games/SNS?"
7. deception regarding Internet/gaming/SNS use	"Do you lie or hide how much time you spend on the Internet/Games/SNS for your family or friends?"
8. use of Internet/gaming/SNS to avoid negative feelings	"Do you use Internet games to avoid/relieve negative feelings?" "Do you use the game to forget unpleasant moods (e.g., helplessness, depression, guilty, anxiety, etc.)?"
9. interference with role performance	"Have you ever been troubled or fallen out by the use of Internet /Games/SNS in your important interpersonal, career, and academic settings?"
10. craving	"Do you have a strong desire to do activities such as internet/ Games/SNS?" "If you want to play internet/Games/SNS, is it hard to tolerate?"

2.2.2. Internet and Smartphone Addiction Scales

The Korean Scale for Internet Addiction for adolescents (K-scale), Smartphone Addiction Scale-short form version (SAS-SV), Smartphone Addiction scale (S-scale), Young's Internet Addiction Test (YIAT), and the Internet Addiction Proneness scale for adolescents (O_A) were used to measure Internet and smartphone addiction symptoms. The K-scale, developed by the National Information Society Agency [30], is a 40-item questionnaire with scores on each item ranging from 1 (not at all) to 4 (always). The SAS-SV is a 10-item scale in which each item is rated on a 6-point Likert scale. Scores above the cutoff values of 31 for males and 33 for females indicate high-risk use [31]. The S-scale is a 15-item questionnaire that measures the level of smartphone addiction on a 4-point Likert scale [32]. The YIAT, developed by Young (1998) [33] and validated in Korean by Kim et al. (2003) [34], consists of 20 items, with higher scores indicating more severe Internet addiction. The O_A consists of 15 items [32]. The internal consistency coefficient of all scales was higher than 0.91 in our study.

2.2.3. Clinical Measurements

We examined internalizing and externalizing problems associated with Internet and smartphone addiction using questionnaires to assess depression, anxiety, self-esteem, impulsivity, aggression, stress, temperament, and personality traits.

The Beck Depression Inventory-II (BDI-II), developed by Beck et al. [35], is a 21-item questionnaire that measures the severity of depression, with higher scores reflecting more severe symptoms. The BDI-II was validated for Korean adolescents by Lee et al. [36], and the Cronbach's alpha was 0.56 in this study. The State–Trait Anxiety Inventory-X1 (STAI-X1) is a 20-item tool that measures state anxiety [37]. The Cronbach's alpha was 0.98 in our study. The Rosenberg Self-Esteem Scale (RSES) [38], which is also translated in Korean, measures perceived self-esteem and self-acceptance, with higher scores reflecting high self-esteem. The Barratt Impulsiveness Scale-II (BIS-II), which consists of 23 items and three subscales (cognitive, motor, and non-planning impulsivity), was developed by Barratt and White [39] and translated into Korean by Lee [40]. The Cronbach's alpha was 0.99. The Korean version of the Aggression Questionnaire (AQ) consists of 27 items, as two of the original 29 items were excluded [41,42]. The AQ measures physical and verbal aggression, anger, and hostility. The Cronbach's alpha was 0.98. The Daily Hassles Questionnaire (DHQ) measures stress related to parents, family environment, friends, school, teachers, and school life. It was developed by Rowlison and Felner [43] and modified and validated in Korean adolescents by Han and Yoo [44]. Finally, we used the Junior Temperament and Character Inventory (JTCI) to assess four temperaments (novelty seeking, harm avoidance, reward dependence, and persistence) and three character traits (self-directedness, cooperativeness, and self-transcendence) in adolescents. The Korean version of the JTCI consists of 82 items, each with 'yes' or 'no' response options.

2.3. Statistical Analysis

The chi-square test and analysis of variance (ANOVA) including post-hoc test (Bonferronni method) were used to compare demographic and clinical characteristics among the DIA subgroups and to assess the application of the DIA subgroup classifications in clinical practice. The psychometric properties of the DIA were examined using internal consistency analysis and Pearson's correlation analysis to assess the association of IGD symptoms (DIA) with Internet and smartphone addiction (K, SAS-SV, S, YIAT, O_A), impulsivity (BIS-11), aggression (AQ), depression (BDI), anxiety (STAI), self-esteem (RSES), stress (DHQ), and temperament/character traits (JTCI). All statistical tests were performed using SPSS software version 21.0 (SPSS, Inc., Chicago, IL, USA).

2.4. Ethical Approval

All subjects and their caregivers gave their informed consent for inclusion before they participated in the study. The study was conducted in accordance with the Declaration of Helsinki, and the protocol was approved by the Institutional Review Board (IRB) for human subjects of Uijeonbu St. Mary's Hospital (UC15ONMI0072), Eulji University Eulji Hospital (EMCS2015-05-020-001) and SMG-SNU Boramae Medical Center (16-2016-4).

3. Results

3.1. Demographic Characteristics

The study included 103 adolescents (mean age, 14.35 ± 1.43 years; 70.9% males) and their caregivers (mean age 46.57 ± 7.69 years; 7.6% males). The Korean Wechsler Intelligence Scale for Children-fourth edition (K-WAIS-IV, 100.03 ± 13.52) was administered to 64 subjects under 16 years of age, and the Korean version of the Wechsler Adult Intelligence Scale, 4th edition (K-WISC-IV, 107.13 ± 12.51) was administered to the remaining subjects. Subjects with DIA total scores of 0–2 were categorized as mild risk, those with scores of 3–4 were moderate risk, and those with scores of 5–10 were classified as addicted. We found no significant differences in sex, age, caregiver's age, or IQ among the three subgroups (mild risk, moderate risk and addicted).

3.2. Psychometric Properties of the Diagnostic Interview for Internet Addiction

The convergent validity of the DIA was assessed by comparing total DIA scores with scores on other scales measuring Internet and smartphone addiction. The correlation coefficients between the DIA and the other scales were as follows: K-scale, 0.426 ($p < 0.01$); SAS-SV, 0.205 ($p < 0.05$); S-scale, 0.234 ($p < 0.05$); Y-IAT, 0.390 ($p < 0.01$); and O_A, 0.343 ($p < 0.01$; Table 2).

Table 2. Correlation analysis between Diagnostic Interview for Internet Addiction and Internet and Smartphone related scale.

	DIA	K	SAS-SV	S	YIAT	O_A
DIA	1					
K	0.426 **	1				
SAS-SV	0.205 *	0.638 **	1			
S	0.234 *	0.733 **	0.885 **	1		
YIAT	0.390 **	0.845 **	0.706 **	0.744 **	1	
O_A	0.343 **	0.084	−0.223 *	−0.146	0.047	1

* $p < 0.05$, ** $p < 0.01$. Note. $n = 103$. DIA = Diagnostic Interview for Internet Addiction; K = Korean Scale for Internet Addiction; SAS-SV = Smartphone Addiction Scale-Short form Version; S = Korean Smartphone Addiction scale; YIAT = Young's Internet Addiction Test; O_A = Internet Addiction Proneness Scale for Adolescents.

Additionally, the correlation analysis performed to examine construct validity revealed significant relationships of the DIA score with the BDI-II ($r = 0.285$, $p < 0.01$), STAI_X1 ($r = 0.294$, $p < 0.01$), RSES ($r = -0.312$, $p < 0.01$), BIS-II ($r = 0.278$, $p < 0.01$), AQ ($r = 0.256$, $p < 0.05$), and DHQ ($r = 0.283$, $p < 0.01$) scores (Table 3). These findings suggest that the presence of several IGD symptoms is associated with higher levels of depression, anxiety, impulsivity, aggression, stress, and low self-esteem.

Table 3. Correlation analysis between the Diagnostic Interview for Internet Addiction and Clinical symptoms.

	DIA	BDI-II	STAI_X1	RSES	BIS-II	AQ	DHQ
DIA	1						
BDI-II	0.285 **	1					
STAI_X1	0.294 **	0.758 **	1				
RSES	−0.312 **	−0.708 **	−0.739 **	1			
BIS-II	0.278 **	0.390 **	0.422 **	−0.540 **	1		
AQ	0.256 *	0.429 **	0.387 **	−0.369 **	0.380 **	1	
DHQ	0.283 **	0.538 **	0.595 **	−0.465 **	0.287 **	0.506 **	1

* $p < 0.05$, ** $p < 0.01$. Note. $n = 103$. DIA = Diagnostic Interview for Internet Addiction; BDI-II = Beck Depression Inventory-II; STAI_X1 = State-Trait Anxiety Inventory X−1; RSES = Rosenberg Self-Esteem Scale; BIS = Barratt Impulsiveness Scale-II; AQ = Aggression Questionnaire; DHQ = Daily Hassles Questionnaire.

3.3. Comparison of Clinical Variables among the Diagnostic Interview for Internet Addiction Subgroups

The participants were divided into three subgroups (mild risk, moderate risk, addicted) according to their DIA total score. Comparisons of the clinical variables (internalizing/externalizing problems and temperament and character traits) among the DIA subgroups are shown in Table 4. We found significant differences in Internet and smartphone addiction, depression, anxiety, self-esteem, impulsivity, aggression, and stress among the subgroups on all of the scales except the SAS-SV. The moderate risk and addicted group had significantly higher levels of Internet and smartphone addiction, anxiety, depression, impulsivity, aggression, and stress and lower self-esteem compared with the mild risk group. Moreover, scores on the JTCI, which measures temperament and character traits, revealed that the mild risk group had significantly higher levels of persistence, self-directedness, and cooperativeness than the addicted group did.

Table 4. Differences in Internet Gaming Disorder symptoms and Clinical variables between Diagnostic Interview for Internet Addiction subgroups.

	Mild Risk M (SD)	Moderate Risk M (SD)	Addicted M (SD)	Total M (SD)	F (Post Hoc)
K	58.15 (13.53)	75.57 (18.73)	78.74 (19.98)	74.14 (20.03)	8.807 ** (1<2,3)
S	28.52 (7.45)	35.11 (7.86)	34.46 (9.50)	33.53 (9.01)	3.848 * (1<2,3)
YIAT	32.76 (10.50)	49.69 (14.13)	50.71 (16.77)	47.14 (16.52)	9.383 ** (1<2,3)
O_A	37.57 (8.00)	40.36 (7.40)	43.22 (6.31)	41.47 (7.20)	5.185 * (1<3)
BDI-II	6.47 (5.79)	15.69 (11.59)	16.18 (12.90)	14.21 (12.04)	5.267 * (1<2,3)
STAI_X1	36.47 (9.60)	44.32 (11.71)	45.83 (12.19)	43.63 (12.05)	4.613 * (1<3)
RSES	30.52 (4.38)	26.88 (4.98)	26.31 (6.33)	27.27 (5.85)	3.937 * (1>3)
BIS	48.31 (6.61)	57.52 (10.32)	56.81 (9.49)	55.34 (9.78)	6.864 * (1<2,3)
AQ	50.36 (12.51)	62.56 (12.62)	62.29 (17.83)	60.05 (16.28)	4.468 * (1<2,3)
DHQ	55.84 (15.55)	70.76 (15.70)	70.77 (17.43)	67.87 (17.52)	6.145 ** (1<2,3)
JTCI_P	54.55 (6.42)	47.68 (7.58)	45.22 (8.71)	47.86 (8.66)	8.743 ** (1>2,3)
JTCI_SD	55.88 (10.80)	48.68 (10.39)	46.15 (10.81)	48.89 (11.21)	5.292 * (1>3)
JTCI_C	56.88 (11.70)	51.20 (8.84)	48.81 (10.10)	51.17 (10.47)	4.065 * (1>3)

* $p < 0.05$, ** $p < 0.01$. Note. No. of mild risk group = 19; No. of moderate risk group = 26; No. of addicted group = 58. Bonferroni post-hoc test results are reported. DIA = Diagnostic Interview for Internet Addiction; K = Korean Scale for Internet Addiction; S = Korean Smartphone Addiction scale; YIAT = Young's Internet Addiction Test; O_A = Internet Addiction Proneness Scale for Adolescents; BDI-II = Beck Depression Inventory-II; STAI_X1 = State-Trait Anxiety Inventory X−1; RSES = Rosenberg Self-Esteem Scale; BIS = Barratt Impulsiveness Scale-II; AQ = Aggression Questionnaire; DHQ = Daily Hassles Questionnaire; JTCI_P = Junior Temperament and Character Inventory_Persistence; SD = Self-Directedness; C = Cooperativeness.

4. Discussion

In this study, we examined the psychometric properties of the DIA and verified the application of the DIA severity classifications in Korean adolescents. The main findings and implications of our study are as follows.

First, in this study, the reliability and validity of DIA were verified. The Cronbach alpha of DIA was 0.72, which means that the DIA meets the internal consistency reliability. Also, we found positive associations between the total DIA scores and scores on other Internet and smartphone addiction scales in Korean adolescents. These findings support the convergent validity of the DIA and are consistent with those of previous studies investigating the relationship between IGD symptoms and Internet/smartphone addiction scales [9,10,45]. In particular, Cho et al. (2014) found that the self-diagnostic Internet addiction scale based on the DSM-5 criteria for IGD was positively correlated with the K-scale, which measures Internet addiction, in Korean middle school students (ages 13 and 14 years) [45]. Kim et al. (2016) reported similar findings in adults [46].

We assessed the construct validity of the DIA by examining the relationship of DIA results with depression, anxiety, stress, impulsivity, aggression, and self-esteem. We found that the subjects who reported more severe IGD symptoms as measured by the DIA had higher levels of depression, anxiety, stress, impulsivity, and aggression. Several studies have shown a relationship between IGD symptoms and psychiatric comorbidity; in particular, one review paper found 92% studies described a significant correlation between IGD symptoms and anxiety and 89% studies with depression [47]. Depression is strongly associated with IGD symptoms, and is the most significant factor associated with the development of online gaming addiction in adolescents [18,48–50]. Gentile et al. (2011) reported that depression and anxiety levels increased in adolescents who became and remained problematic gamers, and Mehroof et al. (2010) found that state anxiety was significantly associated with online gaming addiction [16,22]. Moreover, Internet addiction may contribute to stress. Individuals who experience anxiety and stress have difficulty communicating and interacting with others in healthy and positive ways [51,52]. Furthermore, several studies have shown that impulsivity and aggression are related to Internet addiction in adolescents and increase vulnerability to IGD [22,53–55]. We found a negative correlation between the total DIA score and self-esteem, suggesting that more severe IGD symptoms are associated with lower self-esteem. Similarly, several studies have found a significant relationship between low self-esteem and IGD symptoms such that low self-esteem has been shown to predict the emergence of Internet addiction [25]. Therefore, in this study, the psychometric properties of the DIA were verified by examining the reliability and validity of DIA.

In the context of the application of the DIA classifications in clinical practice for Korean adolescents, we found that subjects in the moderate risk and addicted group had lower self-esteem and significantly higher levels of Internet and smartphone addiction, anxiety, depression, impulsivity, aggression, and stress than did the mild risk group. These findings are similar to those of previous studies mentioned above [16,18,22,47–55], suggesting that early intervention is required when the total DIA score is 3 or above. This is because adolescents who were included in the moderate risk group reported internalizing and externalizing problems similar to the addicted group in DIA.

Previous studies have found associations between Internet addiction and personality traits (e.g., sensation seeking, reward dependence, and self-directedness) [26–28]. Similarly, we found that persistence, self-directedness, and cooperativeness as measured by the JTCI were significantly higher in the mild risk group than in the addicted group. In previous studies of the relationship between personality traits and IGD symptoms, Montag et al. (2011) found that IGD scores were negatively correlated with self-directedness and cooperativeness, and Jimenez-Murcia et al. (2014) found that low self-directedness predicted high IGD scores in video game users [56,57]. These findings indicate that subjects who are in the mild risk group, as classified by the DIA, tend to persist in behavior without sustained reinforcement and are able to control their behavior, unlike those who are in the internet/games/SNS addicted group. Moreover, several studies have shown that previous reports of a relationship between IGD symptoms and novelty seeking, a personality feature linked to impulsivity [58], were inconsistent [16,59,60]. It may be that IGD symptoms are unrelated to novelty seeking, or they may be associated with both high and low novelty seeking, leading to the appearance of no relationship. We found no significant differences in novelty seeking among the DIA subgroups in the present study. These findings suggest that impulsive people may not derive fulfillment or enjoyment from games such as the massively multiplayer online role-playing games (MMORPGs), depending on their psychological profile. Indeed, Billieux et al. (2015) found that the behaviors of online gamers were heterogeneous; individuals with IGD had various psychological profiles, including with regard to novelty seeking, and IGD symptoms differed according to these profiles [61].

Our study has several limitations. First, our subjects were screened using an Internet/smartphone addiction scale. Thus, it may be difficult to generalize our findings to non-clinical populations because our study did not include a control group. In addition, the proportion of the addicted group was about 80% or more, because the internet/games/SNS high-risk users were recruited in this study. Therefore, additional analysis (e.g., factor analysis, ROC curve etc.) should be made to propose a cut-off score of DIA or to make it more useful in a clinical setting. Second, previous studies have shown that the severity of IGD differs among game genres [62,63]. Lope-Fernandez et al. (2014) reported that subjects who played MMORPGs spent more time playing and had significantly higher scores on the

IGD-20 [64]. We did not investigate differences in game genres; further research is needed to examine the DIA subgroups according to the game media type (e.g., internet, games, SNS etc.), various game genres, gaming patterns, and causes of use.

Despite these limitations, we examined the psychometric properties of the DIA, a semi-structured tool, and investigated the relationship between DIA total score and a wide range of clinical characteristics. In addition, although the DSM-5 diagnostic criteria for IGD require the presence of five or more symptoms, our findings suggest that early intervention and continuous observation are advisable for individuals with three or more symptoms according to the DIA.

Author Contributions: Study concept and design: H.R. and J.-S.C.; collection of data: H.R. and J.G.K.; analysis and interpretation of data: H.R., J.Y.L., A.R.C., S.J.C. and M.P.; statistical analysis: H.R.; writing–original draft: H.R., and J.-S.C.; study supervision: J.-S.C., Y.-S.K., and S.Y.B.; access to data: All authors.

Funding: This research was funded by the Korean Mental Health Technology R&D Project, Ministry for Health and Welfare, Republic of Korea (HM14C2603) and the National Research Foundation of Korea (2014M3C7A1062894).

Conflicts of Interest: The authors declare no conflicts of interest.

References

1. Korean National Information Society Agency. *A Survey on Internet Addiction*; Korean National Information Society Agency Report: Seoul, Korea, 2015.
2. Yu, H.; Cho, J. Prevalence of internet gaming disorder among Korean adolescents and associations with non-psychotic psychological symptoms, and physical aggression. *Am. J. Health Behav.* **2016**, *40*, 705–716. [CrossRef] [PubMed]
3. World Health Organization. *The ICD-11 Classification of Mental and Behavioural Disorders: Diagnostic Criteria for Research*; World Health Organization: Geneva, Switzerland, 2018.
4. American Psychiatric Association. *Diagnostic and Statistical Manual of Mental Disorders (DSM-5®)*; American Psychiatric Pub.: Arlington, VA, USA, 2013.
5. Griffiths, M.; King, D.; Demetrovics, Z. DSM-5 internet gaming disorder needs a unified approach to assessment. *Neuropsychiatry* **2014**, *4*, 1–4. [CrossRef]
6. King, D.L.; Haagsma, M.C.; Delfabbro, P.H.; Gradisar, M.; Griffiths, M.D. Toward a consensus definition of pathological video-gaming: A systematic review of psychometric assessment tools. *Clin. Psychol. Rev.* **2013**, *33*, 331–342. [CrossRef] [PubMed]
7. Petry, N.M.; O'brien, C.P. Internet gaming disorder and the DSM-5. *Addict* **2013**, *108*, 1186–1187. [CrossRef] [PubMed]
8. Petry, N.M.; Rehbein, F.; Gentile, D.A.; Lemmens, J.S.; Rumpf, H.J.; Mößle, T.; Bischof, G.; Tao, R.; Fung, D.S.; Borges, G. An international consensus for assessing internet gaming disorder using the new DSM-5 approach. *Addiction* **2014**, *109*, 1399–1406. [CrossRef] [PubMed]
9. Pontes, H.M.; Kiraly, O.; Demetrovics, Z.; Griffiths, M.D. The conceptualisation and measurement of DSM-5 Internet Gaming Disorder: The development of the IGD-20 Test. *PLoS ONE* **2014**, *9*, e110137. [CrossRef] [PubMed]
10. Pontes, H.M.; Griffiths, M.D. Measuring DSM-5 Internet gaming disorder: Development and validation of a short psychometric scale. *Comput. Human Behav.* **2015**, *45*, 137–143. [CrossRef]
11. Jeong, H.; Yim, H.W.; Lee, S.-Y.; Lee, H.K.; Potenza, M.N.; Kwon, J.-H.; Koo, H.J.; Kweon, Y.-S.; Bhang, S.-Y.; Choi, J.-S. Discordance between self-report and clinical diagnosis of Internet gaming disorder in adolescents. *Sci. Rep.* **2018**, *8*, 10084. [CrossRef]
12. Wölfling, K.; Beutel, M.; Müller, K. Construction of a standardized clinical interview to assess internet addiction: First findings regarding the usefulness of AICA-C. *J. Addict. Res. Ther.* **2012**, *6*, 1–7. [CrossRef]
13. Koo, H.J.; Han, D.H.; Park, S.-Y.; Kwon, J.-H. The structured clinical interview for DSM-5 Internet gaming disorder: Development and validation for diagnosing IGD in adolescents. *Psychiatry Investig.* **2017**, *14*, 21–29. [CrossRef]
14. Lee, S.-Y.; Lee, H.K.; Jeong, H.; Yim, H.W.; Bhang, S.-Y.; Jo, S.-J.; Baek, K.-Y.; Kim, E.; Kim, M.S.; Choi, J.-S. The hierarchical implications of Internet gaming disorder criteria: Which indicate more severe pathology? *Psychiatry Investig.* **2017**, *14*, 249–259. [CrossRef] [PubMed]

15. Young, K.S.; Rogers, R.C. The relationship between depression and Internet addiction. *Cyberpsychol. Behav.* **1998**, *1*, 25–28. [CrossRef]
16. Mehroof, M.; Griffiths, M.D. Online gaming addiction: The role of sensation seeking, self-control, neuroticism, aggression, state anxiety, and trait anxiety. *Cyberpsychol. Behav. Soc. Netw.* **2010**, *13*, 313–316. [CrossRef] [PubMed]
17. Müller, K.; Janikian, M.; Dreier, M.; Wölfling, K.; Beutel, M.; Tzavara, C.; Richardson, C.; Tsitsika, A. Regular gaming behavior and internet gaming disorder in European adolescents: Results from a cross-national representative survey of prevalence, predictors, and psychopathological correlates. *Eur. Child Adolesc. Psychiatry* **2015**, *24*, 565–574. [CrossRef] [PubMed]
18. King, D.L.; Delfabbro, P.H. The cognitive psychopathology of internet gaming disorder in adolescence. *J. Abnorm. Child Psychol.* **2016**, *44*, 1635–1645. [CrossRef]
19. Whang, L.S.-M.; Lee, S.; Chang, G. Internet over-users' psychological profiles: A behavior sampling analysis on internet addiction. *Cyberpsychol. Behav.* **2003**, *6*, 143–150. [CrossRef]
20. Strittmatter, E.; Kaess, M.; Parzer, P.; Fischer, G.; Carli, V.; Hoven, C.W.; Wasserman, C.; Sarchiapone, M.; Durkee, T.; Apter, A. Pathological Internet use among adolescents: Comparing gamers and non-gamers. *Psychiatry Res.* **2015**, *228*, 128–135. [CrossRef]
21. Wartberg, L.; Kriston, L.; Kramer, M.; Schwedler, A.; Lincoln, T.; Kammerl, R. Internet gaming disorder in early adolescence: Associations with parental and adolescent mental health. *Eur. Psychiatry* **2017**, *43*, 14–18. [CrossRef]
22. Gentile, D.A.; Choo, H.; Liau, A.; Sim, T.; Li, D.; Fung, D.; Khoo, A. Pathological video game use among youths: A two-year longitudinal study. *Pediatrics* **2011**, *127*. [CrossRef]
23. Lam, L.T.; Peng, Z.-W.; Mai, J.-C.; Jing, J. Factors associated with Internet addiction among adolescents. *Cyberpsychol. Behav.* **2009**, *12*, 551–555. [CrossRef]
24. Du, X.; Qi, X.; Yang, Y.; Du, G.; Gao, P.; Zhang, Y.; Qin, W.; Li, X.; Zhang, Q. Altered structural correlates of impulsivity in adolescents with internet gaming disorder. *Front. Hum. Neurosci.* **2016**, *10*, 4. [CrossRef] [PubMed]
25. Ko, C.-H.; Yen, J.-Y.; Yen, C.-F.; Lin, H.-C.; Yang, M.-J. Factors predictive for incidence and remission of internet addiction in young adolescents: A prospective study. *Cyberpsychol. Behav.* **2007**, *10*, 545–551. [CrossRef] [PubMed]
26. Cao, F.; Su, L. Internet addiction among Chinese adolescents: Prevalence and psychological features. *Child Care Health Dev.* **2007**, *33*, 275–281. [CrossRef] [PubMed]
27. Dalbudak, E.; Evren, C.; Aldemir, S.; Coskun, K.S.; Ugurlu, H.; Yildirim, F.G. Relationship of internet addiction severity with depression, anxiety, and alexithymia, temperament and character in university students. *Cyberpsychol. Behav. Soc. Netw.* **2013**, *16*, 272–278. [CrossRef] [PubMed]
28. Van der Aa, N.; Overbeek, G.; Engels, R.C.; Scholte, R.H.; Meerkerk, G.-J.; Van den Eijnden, R.J. Daily and compulsive internet use and well-being in adolescence: A diathesis-stress model based on big five personality traits. *J. Youth Adolesc.* **2009**, *38*, 765. [CrossRef] [PubMed]
29. Müller, K.W.; Koch, A.; Dickenhorst, U.; Beutel, M.E.; Duven, E.; Wölfling, K. Addressing the question of disorder-specific risk factors of internet addiction: A comparison of personality traits in patients with addictive behaviors and comorbid internet addiction. *BioMed. Res. Int.* **2013**. [CrossRef] [PubMed]
30. Korean National Information Society Agency. *A Validation Study of K-Scale as a Diagnostic Tool*; Korean National Information Society Agency Report: Seoul, Korea, 2013.
31. Kwon, M.; Kim, D.-J.; Cho, H.; Yang, S. The smartphone addiction scale: Development and validation of a short version for adolescents. *PLoS ONE* **2013**, *8*, e83558. [CrossRef] [PubMed]
32. Korean National Information Society Agency. *Third Standardization of Korean Internet Addiction Proneness Scale*; NIA IV-RER-11050; Korean National Information Society Agency Report: Seoul, Korea, 2011.
33. Young, K.S. Internet addiction: The emergence of a new clinical disorder. *Cyberpsychol. Behav.* **1998**, *1*, 237–244. [CrossRef]
34. Kim, E.; Lee, S.; Oh, S. The validation of Korean adolescent internet addiction scale (K-AIAS). *Korean J. Clin. Psychol.* **2003**, *22*, 125–139.
35. Beck, A.T.; Steer, R.A.; Brown, G.K. *Beck Depression Inventory-II (BDI-II)*; Psychological Corporation: San Antonio, TX, USA, 1996.

36. Lee, E.-H.; Lee, S.-J.; Hwang, S.-T.; Hong, S.-H.; Kim, J.-H. Reliability and validity of the Beck Depression Inventory-II among Korean adolescents. *Psychiatry Investig.* **2017**, *14*, 30–36. [CrossRef]
37. Spielberg, C.; Gorsuch, R.; Lushene, R.; Vagg, P.; Jacobs, G. *Manual for the State-Trait Anxiety Inventory*; Consulting Psychologists Press: Palo Alto, CA, USA, 1970.
38. Rosenberg, M. *Conceiving the Self*; Basic Books: New York, NY, USA, 1979.
39. Barratt, E.S.; White, R. Impulsiveness and anxiety related to medical students' performance and attitudes. *J. Med. Educ.* **1969**, *44*, 604–607. [PubMed]
40. Lee, H. *Impulsivity Test Scale*; Guidance Korea: Seoul, Korea, 1992.
41. Seo, S.; Kwon, S. Validation study of the Korean version of the aggression questionnaire. *Korean J. Clin. Psychol.* **2002**, *21*, 487–501.
42. Buss, A.H.; Perry, M. The aggression questionnaire. *J. Pers. Soc. Psychol.* **1992**, *63*, 452. [CrossRef] [PubMed]
43. Rowlison, R.T.; Felner, R.D. Major life events, hassles, and adaptation in adolescence: Confounding in the conceptualization and measurement of life stress and adjustment revisited. *J. Pers. Soc. Psychol.* **1988**, *55*, 432. [CrossRef] [PubMed]
44. Han, M.H.; Yoo, A.J. Development of daily hassles scale for children in Korea. *J. Korean Home Econ. Assoc.* **1995**, *33*, 49–64.
45. Cho, H.; Kwon, M.; Choi, J.-H.; Lee, S.-K.; Choi, J.S.; Choi, S.-W.; Kim, D.-J. Development of the Internet addiction scale based on the Internet Gaming Disorder criteria suggested in DSM-5. *Addict. Behav.* **2014**, *39*, 1361–1366. [CrossRef] [PubMed]
46. Kim, N.R.; Hwang, S.S.-H.; Choi, J.-S.; Kim, D.-J.; Demetrovics, Z.; Király, O.; Nagygyörgy, K.; Griffiths, M.; Hyun, S.Y.; Youn, H.C. Characteristics and psychiatric symptoms of internet gaming disorder among adults using self-reported DSM-5 criteria. *Psychiatry Investig.* **2016**, *13*, 58–66. [CrossRef] [PubMed]
47. González-Bueso, V.; Santamaría, J.; Fernández, D.; Merino, L.; Montero, E.; Ribas, J. Association between internet gaming disorder or pathological video-game use and comorbid psychopathology: A comprehensive review. *Int. J. Environ. Res. Public Health* **2018**, *15*, 668. [CrossRef]
48. Laconi, S.; Pires, S.; Chabrol, H. Internet gaming disorder, motives, game genres and psychopathology. *Comput. Human Behav.* **2017**, *75*, 652–659. [CrossRef]
49. Wang, H.R.; Cho, H.; Kim, D.-J. Prevalence and correlates of comorbid depression in a nonclinical online sample with DSM-5 internet gaming disorder. *J. Affect. Disord.* **2018**, *226*, 1–5. [CrossRef]
50. Hyun, G.J.; Han, D.H.; Lee, Y.S.; Kang, K.D.; Yoo, S.K.; Chung, U.-S.; Renshaw, P.F. Risk factors associated with online game addiction: A hierarchical model. *Comput. Human Behav.* **2015**, *48*, 706–713. [CrossRef]
51. Egger, O.; Rauterberg, M. *Internet Behavior and Addiction*; Swiss Federal Institute of Technology: Zurich, Swizerland, 1996.
52. Akin, A.; Iskender, M. Internet addiction and depression, anxiety and stress. *Int. J. Educ. Sci.* **2011**, *3*, 138–148.
53. Ko, C.-H.; Hsieh, T.-J.; Wang, P.-W.; Lin, W.-C.; Yen, C.-F.; Chen, C.-S.; Yen, J.-Y. Altered gray matter density and disrupted functional connectivity of the amygdala in adults with Internet gaming disorder. *Prog. Neuropsychopharmacol. Biol. Psychiatry* **2015**, *57*, 185–192. [CrossRef] [PubMed]
54. Yen, J.-Y.; Liu, T.-L.; Wang, P.-W.; Chen, C.-S.; Yen, C.-F.; Ko, C.-H. Association between Internet gaming disorder and adult attention deficit and hyperactivity disorder and their correlates: Impulsivity and hostility. *Addict. Behav.* **2017**, *64*, 308–313. [CrossRef] [PubMed]
55. Ryu, H.; Lee, J.-Y.; Choi, A.; Park, S.; Kim, D.-J.; Choi, J.-S. The relationship between impulsivity and internet gaming disorder in young adults: Mediating effects of interpersonal relationships and depression. *Int. J. Environ. Res. Public Health* **2018**, *15*, 458. [CrossRef] [PubMed]
56. Montag, C.; Flierl, M.; Markett, S.; Walter, N.; Jurkiewicz, M.; Reuter, M. Internet addiction and personality in first-person-shooter video gamers. *J. Media Psychol.* **2011**, *23*, 163. [CrossRef]
57. Jiménez-Murcia, S.; Fernández-Aranda, F.; Granero, R.; Chóliz, M.; La Verde, M.; Aguglia, E.; Signorelli, M.S.; Sá, G.M.; Aymamí, N.; Gómez-Peña, M. Video game addiction in gambling disorder: Clinical, psychopathological, and personality correlates. *BioMed. Res. Int.* **2014**. [CrossRef] [PubMed]
58. Whiteside, S.P.; Lynam, D.R. The five factor model and impulsivity: Using a structural model of personality to understand impulsivity. *Pers. Individ. Dif.* **2001**, *30*, 669–689. [CrossRef]
59. Khazaal, Y.; Chatton, A.; Rothen, S.; Achab, S.; Thorens, G.; Zullino, D.; Gmel, G. Psychometric properties of the 7-item game addiction scale among French and German speaking adults. *BMC Psychiatry* **2016**, *16*, 132. [CrossRef]

60. Müller, K.; Dreier, M.; Beutel, M.; Wölfling, K. Is Sensation Seeking a correlate of excessive behaviors and behavioral addictions? A detailed examination of patients with gambling disorder and internet addiction. *Psychiatry Res.* **2016**, *242*, 319–325. [CrossRef]
61. Billieux, J.; Thorens, G.; Khazaal, Y.; Zullino, D.; Achab, S.; Van der Linden, M. Problematic involvement in online games: A cluster analytic approach. *Comput. Human Behav.* **2015**, *43*, 242–250. [CrossRef]
62. Stavropoulos, V.; Kuss, D.J.; Griffiths, M.D.; Wilson, P.; Motti-Stefanidi, F. MMORPG gaming and hostility predict Internet addiction symptoms in adolescents: An empirical multilevel longitudinal study. *Addict. Behav.* **2017**, *64*, 294–300. [CrossRef] [PubMed]
63. Lee, M.-S.; Ko, Y.-H.; Song, H.-S.; Kwon, K.-H.; Lee, H.-S.; Nam, M.; Jung, I.-K. Characteristics of Internet use in relation to game genre in Korean adolescents. *Cyberpsychol. Behav.* **2006**, *10*, 278–285. [CrossRef] [PubMed]
64. Lopez-Fernandez, O.; Honrubia-Serrano, M.L.; Baguley, T.; Griffiths, M.D. Pathological video game playing in Spanish and British adolescents: Towards the exploration of Internet Gaming Disorder symptomatology. *Comput. Human Behav.* **2014**, *41*, 304–312. [CrossRef]

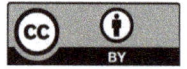

© 2019 by the authors. Licensee MDPI, Basel, Switzerland. This article is an open access article distributed under the terms and conditions of the Creative Commons Attribution (CC BY) license (http://creativecommons.org/licenses/by/4.0/).

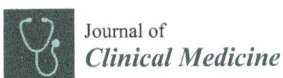

Article

A New Measure for Assessing the Intensity of Addiction Memory in Illicit Drug Users: The Addiction Memory Intensity Scale

Jia-yan Chen [1], Jie-pin Cao [2,3], Yun-cui Wang [1,4], Shuai-qi Li [1,2] and Zeng-zhen Wang [1,2,*]

1. Department of Epidemiology and Biostatistics, School of Public Health, Tongji Medical College, Huazhong University of Science and Technology, Wuhan 430030, China; palachen@hust.edu.cn (J.-y.C.); wangyuncui2017@163.com (Y.-c.W.); omni_slash@163.com (S.-q.L.)
2. Tongji Research Centre of Mental Health, Huazhong University of Science and Technology, Wuhan 430030, China; jiepin.cao@duke.edu
3. School of Nursing, Duke University, Durham, NC 27710, USA
4. School of Nursing, Hubei University of Chinese Medicine, Wuhan 430065, China
* Correspondence: zzhwang@hust.edu.cn; Tel.: +86-27-83657775

Received: 18 October 2018; Accepted: 21 November 2018; Published: 22 November 2018

Abstract: Disrupting the process of memory reconsolidation could be a promising treatment for addiction. However, its application may be constrained by the intensity of addiction memory. This study aimed to develop and initially validate a new measure, the Addiction Memory Intensity Scale (AMIS), for assessing the intensity of addiction memory in illicit drug users. Two studies were conducted in China for item analysis ($n = 345$) and initial validation ($n = 1550$) of the AMIS. The nine-item AMIS was found to have two factors (labelled Visual Clarity and Other Sensory Intensity), which accounted for 64.11% of the total variance. The two-factor structure provided a reasonable fit for sample data and was invariant across groups of different genders and different primary drugs of use. Significant correlations were found between scores on the AMIS and the measures of craving. The AMIS and its factors showed good internal consistency (Cronbach's α: 0.72–0.89) and test-retest reliability (r: 0.72–0.80). These results suggest that the AMIS, which demonstrates an advantage as it is brief and easy to administer, is a reliable and valid tool for measuring the intensity of addiction memory in illicit drug users, and has the potential to be useful in future clinical research.

Keywords: addiction; memory; assessment; substance use disorder

1. Introduction

Addiction memory is conceptualized as a pathological memory related to addictive behaviors [1,2]. Even after long-term abstinence, addiction memory can be reactivated upon re-exposure to substance-related cues and associated with a craving that results in relapse [2,3]. Recently, several studies have found that disrupting the reconsolidation of drug-related memory can reduce craving, attention bias, or drug-using behavior [4–7], indicating that addiction memory can be manipulated during reconsolidation. However, several "boundary conditions" may constrain the application of memory reconsolidation in addiction treatment [8,9]. One of the constraints is the intensity of memory. It has been shown that memories with a higher level of intensity may be more resistant to disruption and require a longer re-exposure (or a shorter time interval between memory acquisition and re-exposure) to induce memory lability [10–12]. Given that, a valid measurement for assessing the intensity of addiction memory is needed before examining the impact of memory intensity on reconsolidation propensity.

Previously, a single-item visual analogue scale (VAS) was used in some studies to assess the vividness of addiction memory [13,14]. Although the VAS has been widely used to evaluate the subjective experience, such as craving [15], this single-item measure may fail to reflect the complex nature of the intensity of addiction memory. Regarding instruments measuring the intensity of addiction memory, we believe that the use of a multi-item scale or questionnaire would be beneficial for research in that it could help to clarify the underlying dimensions [16]. Furthermore, although there have been several scales and questionnaires developed to assess the severity of addiction [17–21], we should note that these instruments were not originally designed to measure the intensity of addiction memory. It is unknown which items or dimensions of the tools may reflect the memory strength, which raises concern about the utility of these indexes in assessing the intensity of addiction memory. Given these concerns, a new measure is needed to evaluate the intensity of addiction memory explicitly.

Studies on the phenomenology of memory, which mainly focus on one's subjective experience retrieved from the memory [22,23], open an opportunity to assess the intensity of addiction memory. Although little is known about the phenomenological characteristics of addiction memory, previous studies have suggested a relationship between addiction memory and autobiographical memory, especially episodic memory [2,3,24]. Similar to the autobiographical memory, addiction memory is related to personal experiences derived from an individual's history of drug use. Thus, research on autobiographical memory can be used as a frame of reference. There have been several studies presenting a diverse variety of phenomenological characteristics of autobiographical memory, such as vividness and sensory details [22,25–30]. Although the classification of phenomenological traits is still under discussion, the characteristics involving the sensory-perceptual information could probably be used as a central measure of memory intensity. The sensory-perceptual details are the primary information retrieved from one's autobiographical (episodic) memories [31]. In the self-memory system, the sensory-perceptual information of autobiographical memory can be directly retrieved when there are event-related cues [31], meaning that the sensory details would be re-experienced when recalling the memory. In that, people may feel a high level of sensory intensity if they retrieve detailed sensory information. Additionally, the visual imagery is presented predominately and correlated with other sensory details (e.g., olfactory, gustatory) in episodic information [32,33]. In sum, a strong memory tends to be visually vivid, full of sensory details. Since the addiction memory is characterized by powerful imprints of the information about psychoactive substances [2,3,24], we infer that the strength of sensory-perceptual information could be used for measuring the intensity of addiction memory.

Although the studies on autobiographical memory provide a research frame for understanding the properties of addiction memory, there is one crucial limitation when applying the measurements of autobiographical memory in assessing the intensity of addiction memory. It should be emphasized that the measures were developed to evaluate the autobiographical memories of individuals about their life events but not specifically their addiction memories. To the best of our knowledge, there is no scale or questionnaire specifically designed for assessing the phenomenological characteristics in the strength of addiction memory. Therefore, our study aimed to fill this gap first through the development and initial validation of a scale specifically for evaluating the intensity of addiction memory in illicit drug users. In our research, a Likert-type scale, which we labelled the Addiction Memory Intensity Scale (AMIS), was initially developed. We conducted two studies: one for item analysis and one for initial validation of the AMIS. We hypothesized that the scale would be a reliable and valid tool for assessing the intensity of addiction memory in illicit drug users.

2. Materials and Methods

2.1. Initial Scale Development

The development of the AMIS began with a review of the literature on the phenomenology of autobiographical memory. Instruments that measured the phenomenological characteristics of autobiographical memory [22,25–30], especially the items involving sensory-perceptual information, were collected as the reference. Regarding the domains of memory intensity, we agree with the previous studies that the strength of sensory-perceptual details can be either considered as one characteristic [27] or classified into visual and non-visual information [22,29]. Therefore, it is prudent to generate different items for visual and non-visual information of addiction memory intensity and to test the factor structure of the AMIS (i.e., whether these two components represent different constructs).

For generating items unique to measuring the intensity of addiction memory, in-depth interviews were conducted with twelve illicit drug users with substance use disorders. The respondents were asked to recall and describe their experiences of using drugs, and then to describe their subjective experience during retrieval of the memories of using drugs. The interview transcripts were reviewed, coded, and classified into the themes of visual and non-visual information via a thematic framework analysis. Forty-four items were then initially generated based on the abovementioned instruments and interviews.

Five psychologists with professional experience in mental health and addiction treatment were invited to a consultation meeting to review the preliminary instrument. Twenty illicit drug users in the drug rehabilitation centers were then interviewed about the understandability and acceptability of the scale and each of the items. Based on the feedback from the psychologists and illicit drug users, items that were ambiguous, repetitive, not understood, or not acceptable were either revised or removed, yielding a 20-item draft of the AMIS. The AMIS draft was piloted in a sample of 345 illicit drug users to evaluate the appropriateness of the items further (see Study-1). The results of Study-1 were used for item selection. After the item selection, a final version of the AMIS was developed, consisting of nine items.

In the present study, the AMIS was specifically developed to measure the intensity of addiction memory in illicit drug users. Given the fact that most of the illicit drug users in China have a low education level, we agree with the previous studies [34–36] that suggest that a fully labelled five-point Likert scale may improve the respondents' ability to discriminate among categories and reduce response bias, without lowering the reliability of the instrument. Therefore, regarding the response options, five-point response categories were labelled (1 = strongly disagree, 2 = disagree, 3 = unsure, 4 = agree, 5 = strongly agree) and used on all the items. The total AMIS score can be obtained by computing the mean of the items; thus, the range of possible scores is from 1 to 5.

2.2. Participants

Two studies were conducted from January 2015 to March 2018 at drug rehabilitation centers in China. Participants were illicit drug users (substance use disorders as diagnosed by the DSM-IV) with the age of at least 18 years old. Illicit drug users who had difficulty in answering the survey as a result of illiteracy, withdrawal symptoms, cognitive disorders, or other psychiatric disorders were excluded from the studies. The study protocols were approved by the Institutional Review Board of the School of Public Health, Tongji Medical College, Huazhong University of Science and Technology (approval file number: [2015]#15). Each participant in the studies provided signed informed consent.

2.2.1. Participants in Study-1

For item analysis, Study-1 was conducted at two drug rehabilitation centers in the city of Wuhan, China. Based on the lists provided by the rehabilitation centers, the illicit drug users were randomly selected by the principal researcher (Z.-Z.W.) using a list of computer-generated random numbers. Ultimately, a total of 345 participants were selected.

2.2.2. Participants in Study-2

For initial validation of the AMIS, Study-2 was conducted at six drug rehabilitation centers in two cities (Wuhan and Zhongshan) in China. To avoid repetition, we excluded the individuals who participated in Study-1. Finally, a total of 1550 participants were recruited at the rehabilitation centers.

2.3. Measurements for Testing Concurrent Validity

In Study-2, the Obsessive Compulsive Drug Use Scale (OCDUS) [37] and a craving visual analogue scale (VAS) were used for concurrent validation since previous studies have indicated that addiction memory is related to craving [38–41]. Given that individuals who experienced a longer term of drug use may undergo more repeated exposures and thus strengthen their intensity of memory [42], the participants' duration of illicit drug use was also used for concurrent validation.

2.3.1. Obsessive Compulsive Drug Use Scale (OCDUS)

The OCDUS was used to measure general craving in the past week. The Chinese version of OCDUS is a 12-item questionnaire and uses a three-factor structure: "interference of drugs," "frequency of craving," and "control of drugs" [37].

2.3.2. Visual Analogue Scale (VAS)

The VAS was used to measure instant craving. The VAS is a 10-cm line with "not at all" on the left and "extremely" on the right. Participants were asked to rate their craving for drugs at present on the VAS.

2.3.3. Duration of Illicit Drug Use

The participants were asked to answer a single question adapted from the Chinese version of Addiction Severity Index-V [17] to report their duration of illicit drug use ("How many years in your life have you regularly used the illicit drugs (e.g., heroin, amphetamines, ketamine, cannabis, cocaine, or more than one substance)?").

2.4. Procedure

The 20-item draft of the AMIS was administered in Study-1. Before answering the scale, participants were instructed to recall memories about their experiences of drug use ("Please recall your experiences of using drugs. Please try your best to recall the experiences in detail, for example, when and where it happened, whom you were with, and what you felt then."). In Study-2, the nine-item AMIS was applied. Participants were given the instruction mentioned above and then completed the scale. Subsequently, they were asked to answer the OCDUS and the VAS. To avoid leaving the participants in a vulnerable state, they were given relaxation techniques after finishing the surveys.

2.5. Data Analysis

The samples available for data analysis numbered 343 in Study-1 and 1420 in Study-2. In Study-1, two participants were unwilling to answer the survey and did not provide any information. Thus, they were excluded from the study. In Study-2, one-hundred-and-thirty questionnaires with missing items were excluded from data analysis. The characteristics of participants who were excluded were not significantly different from those included in the data analysis (Supplementary materials, Table S1). All statistical analyses were performed in SAS 9.4 (SAS Institute Inc., Cary, NC, USA) [43], and the significance level was set at $\alpha = 0.05$ (two-tailed probability).

2.5.1. Study-1: Item Analysis

The critical ratio, item-total correlation, factor loading, and coefficient of stability were calculated for each item. Regarding the coefficient of stability, thirty of the participants were randomly selected using a list of computer-generated random numbers. They were retested two weeks after the first test. The results of the item analysis were used comprehensively for item selection. Items that meet two or more deletion criteria were removed [44]. The deletion criteria were as follows [45]: the critical ratio <3.00, the item-total correlation coefficient <0.40, factor loading <0.45, and coefficient of stability <0.50.

2.5.2. Study-2: Initial Validation of the AMIS

For cross-validation, both exploratory factor analysis (EFA) and confirmatory factor analysis (CFA) were used to validate the factor structure of the AMIS. The sample data were randomly divided into two parts before the factor analyses were conducted. One subset was for EFA ($n = 710$), and the other was for CFA ($n = 710$).

The principal component analysis combined with oblique (direct oblimin) rotation was performed in EFA. The eigenvalue and the scree plot were used to assist in retaining the number of components.

The maximum likelihood estimation was conducted in CFA. The model chi-square statistic, comparative fit index (CFI), standardized root mean square residual (SRMR), root mean square error of approximation (RMSEA), and non-normed fit index (NNFI) were reported. The chi-square statistic was not used as a viable fit index because of its excessive sensitivity to sample size [46,47]. Thereby the acceptable fit-index criteria used in CFA were as follows [46,47]: CFI > 0.90, SRMR < 0.08, RMSEA < 0.10, and NNFI > 0.90. Additionally, the expected cross-validation index (ECVI) was tested to assist model comparison. The model with a lower ECVI value was considered to be better-fitting [46,47].

The impact of gender or primary illicit drug of use on the measurement invariance was tested in a series of multi-group CFAs. The measurement invariance could be justified if [48,49]: the overall fit of the model was acceptable, and the differences in CFI and NNFI between the constrained and unconstrained model were <0.01 and <0.05 respectively. Of the participants recruited, only 1.1% were ketamine users (see Table 1). Due to the insufficient sample size of this subgroup, the ketamine users were excluded from the multi-group CFA models when comparing different primary drugs of use.

Table 1. Characteristics of the participants.

Characteristics	Study-1 ($n = 343$)	Study-2 ($n = 1420$)
Gender (%)		
Male	49.3	50.4
Female	50.7	49.6
Mean age (SD)	35.6 (8.5)	38.4 (9.2)
Education (%)		
Primary school or below	12.5	18.4
Junior high school	55.7	51.1
Senior high school	25.7	24.9
Junior college or above	6.1	5.6
Marital status (%)		
Single	41.1	34.8
Premarital cohabitation	2.3	2.4
Married	38.8	36.0
Divorced or widowed	17.8	26.8
Primary illicit drug of use (%)		
ATS	47.8	43.9
Heroin	26.5	40.1
Ketamine	3.5	1.1
Polydrug use	22.2	14.9
Mean years of illicit drug use (SD)	7.4 (5.9)	10.4 (6.8)

Note: ATS = amphetamine-type stimulants; SD = standard deviation.

The inter-factor correlation and the concurrent validity of the AMIS were estimated using the Pearson correlation coefficient, using a full sample ($n = 1420$). When assessing the correlations between the AMIS and the VAS, the VAS scores were found to follow a non-normal distribution; thus, Spearman correlation coefficients were calculated instead.

To evaluate whether the AMIS could discriminate between the high and moderate-to-low levels of craving, we performed a series of independent-samples t-tests. According to the previous study [50], the participants who scored >5 on the VAS were considered to have a high level of instant desire for drugs. Of the OCDUS, the following cut-off values indicate the high level of related contents: "interference of drugs" >15, "frequency of craving" >15, and "control of drugs" >6 [37].

Cronbach's α coefficient was computed to evaluate the internal consistency of the AMIS in a full sample (n = 1420). Test-retest reliability of the AMIS was obtained from a retest conducted in a subset of sixty participants. The participants were retested two weeks after their first test. The test-retest reliability was assessed using the Pearson correlation coefficient.

3. Results

3.1. Characteristics of the Participants

The characteristics of the participants in our study are shown in Table 1.

3.2. Item Analysis

The results of the item analysis are shown in Table 2. Three items showed an item-total correlation coefficient of <0.40, eleven items showed a factor loading of <0.40, and ten items showed a coefficient of stability of <0.50. Based on the abovementioned criteria for item selection, nine items were ultimately retained in the AMIS.

Table 2. Item analysis of the draft Addiction Memory Intensity Scale (AMIS; n = 343).

Items of the AMIS Draft	Mean (SD)	Critical Ratio	Item-Total Correlation	Factor Loading	Coefficient of Stability	Items Retained
Item-1: recall the images clearly	2.94 (1.19)	6.80	0.46	0.74	0.78	Yes
Item-2: recall the images coherently	2.97 (1.10)	8.84	0.53	0.79	0.71	Yes
Item-3: the sensations and feelings spring to my mind	2.94 (1.17)	6.35	0.45	0.69	0.77	Yes
Item-4: feel what I felt then	2.64 (1.09)	5.82	0.42	0.65	0.72	Yes
Item-5: recall the images as an outsider	3.10 (1.06)	5.52	0.32 *	−0.08 *	−0.06 *	
Item-6: recall the images in detail	3.07 (1.10)	8.94	0.54	0.80	0.81	Yes
Item-7: recall a certain instance at a particular time and place	3.13 (1.11)	6.77	0.45	0.71	0.83	Yes
Item-8: recall the images easily	3.00 (1.12)	9.55	0.57	0.78	0.75	Yes
Item-9: the sensations and feelings are intense	2.31 (1.12)	6.85	0.43	0.51	0.74	Yes
Item-10: the images are far away from me	2.89 (1.09)	4.47	0.34 *	−0.11 *	−0.05 *	
Item-11: the images are dim	2.90 (1.08)	8.41	0.50	0.10 *	0.08 *	
Item-12: recall a merging of many images	3.07 (1.07)	3.56	0.23 *	−0.20 *	0.57	
Item-13: had to search my memory to recall the images	2.99 (1.10)	7.33	0.41	−0.07 *	0.42 *	
Item-14: the evoked physical reactions are weak	2.67 (1.15)	7.77	0.45	−0.02 *	0.19 *	
Item-15: the images are deeply rooted in my mind	2.84 (1.07)	6.03	0.42	0.61	0.65	Yes
Item-16: the images are sketchy	2.94 (1.01)	7.66	0.47	0.03 *	0.31 *	
Item-17: recall the images in pieces	3.05 (1.17)	11.93	0.55	0.08 *	0.41 *	
Item-18: had to search my memory to recall the feelings	3.08 (1.11)	13.61	0.59	0.19 *	0.11 *	
Item-19: relive the experiences without any sensations and feelings	2.76 (1.16)	9.91	0.52	0.08 *	0.38 *	
Item-20: the sensations and feelings are impressive	2.82 (1.17)	14.75	0.65	0.28 *	0.30 *	

Note: * Items that meet the deletion criteria; AMIS = Addiction Memory Intensity Scale; SD = standard deviation.

3.3. Exploratory Factor Analysis (EFA)

Table 3 displays the factor structure of the AMIS. The Kaiser–Meyer–Olkin measure of sampling adequacy (0.90) and Bartlett's test of sphericity (χ^2 = 2910.00, p < 0.001) indicated a suitable correlation matrix for factor analysis. The pattern matrix showed a two-factor structure with each eigenvalue >1 (4.73 and 1.04). The scree plot also suggested this factor solution (Figure 1).

Table 3. Exploratory factor analysis of the Addiction Memory Intensity Scale (AMIS; n = 710) [1].

Items of the AMIS [2]	Factor 1	Factor 2
Factor 1: Visual Clarity (eigenvalue = 4.73, % variance = 52.51)		
Item-7: I can recall a certain instance of using drugs at a particular time and place.	0.85	−0.10
Item-6: I can recall the images of using drugs in detail.	0.82	0.05
Item-1: I can recall the images of using drugs clearly.	0.81	−0.04
Item-2: When I recall the images of using drugs, they emerge coherently.	0.80	0.02
Item-8: I can recall the images of using drugs easily.	0.75	0.06
Item-15: When I recall the images of using drugs, I find that they are deeply rooted in my mind.	0.53	0.31
Factor 2: Other Sensory Intensity (eigenvalue = 1.04, % variance = 11.60)		
Item-9: When I recall my experiences of using drugs, the sensations and feelings are intense.	−0.16	0.91
Item-4: When I recall my experiences of using drugs, I can feel what I felt then.	0.20	0.72
Item-3: When the drugs or drug-related cues are present, the sensations and feelings of using drugs spring to my mind.	0.26	0.59

Note: [1] The pattern matrix was presented; factors were extracted by principal component analysis and were rotated by oblique (direct oblimin) rotation. [2] Numbering reflects the order of items on the original scale. The AMIS was originally developed in Chinese, and the English version presented here was translated only for the publication of our study. AMIS = Addiction Memory Intensity Scale.

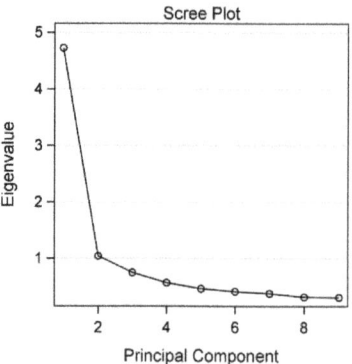

Figure 1. Scree plot based on the principal component analysis (n = 710).

The two-factor solution of the AMIS accounted for 64.11% of the total variance. Factor-1, labelled Visual Clarity, had shown greatest loadings on six items and measured the intensity of one's visual information when retrieving the memories of drug use. Factor-2, labelled Other Sensory Intensity, had shown greatest loadings on three items and evaluated the intensity of one's non-visual sensations and feelings when recalling the experiences of using drugs.

Item-15 was suspected to be a cross-loading item (the difference in factor loading was 0.22, slightly over 0.20). Thus, we tried to delete this item and see how the factor solution and internal consistency were affected. After the factor analysis and sensitivity analysis (Supplementary materials, Table S2), we found that removing this item hardly changed the two-factor structure, but would reduce the internal consistency of the scale. Therefore, item-15 was retained in the AMIS.

3.4. Confirmatory Factor Analysis (CFA)

The two-factor structure of the AMIS from EFA provided an acceptable fit for the other subset of sample data (see Table 4, Model 1). An alternative one-factor model was also constructed to assess the intensity of sensory-perceptual information. All items in this model served as indicators of one single factor. The one-factor model showed an acceptable-to-poor fit to the sample data, with the RMSEA value failed to meet its fit-index criterion (see Table 4, Model 2). Due to the lower ECVI value, the two-factor solution was favored.

Table 4. Confirmatory factor analysis of the Addiction Memory Intensity Scale (AMIS; $n = 710$).

Model	χ^2 (df)	CFI	SRMR	RMSEA	NNFI	ECVI
1. The hypothesized two-factor model	175.88 (25) *	0.95	0.05	0.09	0.93	0.31
2. The alternative one-factor model	218.25 (26) *	0.94	0.05	0.10	0.92	0.36
3. Multi-group model comparing gender	207.28 (50) *	0.95	0.04	0.07	0.93	
4. Multi-group model comparing the primary drug of use	296.46 (95) *	0.94	0.06	0.06	0.93	

Note: * $p < 0.01$; AMIS = Addiction Memory Intensity Scale; CFI = comparative fit index; SRMR = standardized root mean square residual; RMSEA = root mean square error of approximation; NNFI = non-normed fit index; ECVI = expected cross-validation index.

All of the model-fit indexes of the two-factor multi-group models met the acceptance criteria (see Table 4, Model 3 and Model 4). When constraining all parameters to be equal across groups, the differences between the constrained and unconstrained models showed ΔCFIs of <0.01 and ΔNNFIs of <0.05 (across gender: ΔCFI = -0.001, ΔNNFI = 0.007; across primary drug of use: ΔCFI = 0.000, ΔNNFI = 0.006). Also, no significant difference in model fits was observed between the constrained and unconstrained models (across gender: $\Delta\chi^2$ (7) = 10.71, $p = 0.152$; across primary drug of use: $\Delta\chi^2$ (7) = 5.57, $p = 0.591$). These results suggest measurement invariance across the groups.

3.5. Inter-Factor Correlation and Concurrent Validity

There was a moderate, significant correlation between the two factors of the AMIS ($r = 0.65$, $p < 0.001$). The correlations between the AMIS and other measures are shown in Table 5. Significant correlations were found between OCDUS scores, VAS scores, duration of illicit drug use, and AMIS scores.

Table 5. Correlations between the Addiction Memory Intensity Scale and other measures ($n = 1420$).

Measure	Addiction Memory Intensity Scale		
	Total	Visual Clarity	Other Sensory Intensity
OCDUS			
Interference of drugs	0.25 *	0.20 *	0.27 *
Frequency of craving	0.42 *	0.39 *	0.38 *
Control of drugs	0.24 *	0.21 *	0.23 *
VAS	0.20 *	0.14 *	0.25 *
Duration of illicit drug use	0.08 *	0.07 *	0.09 *

Note: * $p < 0.01$. OCDUS = Obsessive Compulsive Drug Use Scale; VAS = Visual Analogue Scale.

3.6. Discriminant Validity

The t-test results showed that, compared to the participants with moderate-to-low levels of craving, those with high levels of craving reported significantly higher scores on the AMIS (Table 6), indicating that the AMIS can discriminate between the high and moderate-to-low levels of craving.

Table 6. Discriminant validity of the Addiction Memory Intensity Scale ($n = 1420$).

Measure	Addiction Memory Intensity Scale (Mean (SD))		
	Total	Visual Clarity	Other Sensory Intensity
OCDUS			
Interference of drugs			
Moderate-to-low	3.3 (0.8)	3.4 (0.9)	3.0 (0.9)
High	4.1 (0.8)	4.2 (0.8)	4.0 (0.9)
	$t = -11.58, p < 0.001$	$t = -10.10, p < 0.001$	$t = -11.38, p < 0.001$
Frequency of craving			
Moderate-to-low	3.3 (0.8)	3.4 (0.9)	3.0 (0.9)
High	4.4 (0.4)	4.5 (0.5)	4.3 (0.6)
	$t = -23.71, p < 0.001$	$t = -20.51, p < 0.001$	$t = -19.87, p < 0.001$
Control of drugs			
Moderate-to-low	3.3 (0.8)	3.4 (0.9)	3.0 (0.9)
High	4.2 (0.7)	4.2 (0.8)	4.0 (0.9)
	$t = -11.66, p < 0.001$	$t = -11.78, p < 0.001$	$t = -10.93, p < 0.001$
VAS			
Moderate-to-low	3.3 (0.9)	3.4 (0.9)	3.0 (1.0)
High	3.6 (0.8)	3.6 (0.8)	3.5 (0.9)
	$t = -5.10, p < 0.001$	$t = -3.80, p < 0.001$	$t = -6.98, p < 0.001$

Note: OCDUS = Obsessive Compulsive Drug Use Scale; VAS = Visual Analogue Scale.

3.7. Reliability

Respectively, Cronbach's α coefficients for the total, Visual Clarity, and Other Sensory Intensity scores on the AMIS were 0.89, 0.88, and 0.72, suggesting a good internal consistency in the scale.

Results from the retest showed that, between the test and the retest, the Pearson correlation coefficients for the AMIS and its two factors were good (Total: 0.80 ($p < 0.01$); Visual Clarity: 0.75 ($p < 0.01$); Other Sensory Intensity: 0.72 ($p < 0.01$)).

4. Discussion

This study develops and initially validates a new measure to assess the intensity of addiction memory in illicit drug users. The final version of the AMIS consists of nine items and shows a robust two-factor structure. Results of the multi-group CFA suggest measurement invariance of the two-factor structure across groups of different genders and different primary drugs of use. The moderate inter-factor correlation further confirms that the internal structure of the AMIS is reasonable. The validity of the AMIS is supported by other findings that there are significant correlations between the AMIS and other measures of craving and that the AMIS can discriminate between different levels of craving. Additionally, the AMIS and its two factors show good internal consistency and test-retest reliability. These results support the AMIS as a valid and reliable tool for measuring the intensity of addiction memory in illicit drug users.

The AMIS was initially developed to assess the intensity of sensory-perceptual information in addiction memory of the illicit drug users. Two phenomenological characteristics (Visual Clarity and Other Sensory Intensity) were identified in EFA. It is notable that the contents of these two factors are consistent with the theoretical dimensions constructed from our assumption. Thus, it is easy to interpret the factors clinically, as follows: Visual Clarity refers to the intensity of illicit drug users' visual information when retrieving the memories of drug use, while Other Sensory Intensity refers to the strength of their non-visual sensations and feelings. Moreover, Visual Clarity explained 52.51% of the total variance, which was higher than Other Sensory Intensity (11.60%). That is, the clarity of visual information accounts for a percentage of variance in the intensity of addiction memory that is greater than other sensory details. Similar to other studies that demonstrate that visual information predominates in the episodic memories [32,33], the results of our study support the significance of visual clarity in the intensity of addiction memory.

Although researchers have differentiated visual clarity from other sensory intensity [22,29], the two components can also be considered as one characteristic which reveals the strength of all sensory-perceptual details [27]. Thus, we compared the two-factor model to an alternative one-factor model. The two-factor solution showed an acceptable fit to the sample data and, due to its lower ECVI value, was considered to fit the data better. Furthermore, it is indicated in the cross-validation that the two-factor structure would be more stable. Therefore, the two-factor solution was preferred. Based on the results of factor analyses and inter-factor correlation analysis, the Visual Clarity and Other Sensory Intensity factors can be considered two related but distinct characteristics of addiction memory intensity.

Regarding the concurrent validity, scores of the AMIS and its factors showed significant correlations with the measures of craving, which is consistent with previous studies, suggesting that addiction memory is related to craving [38–41]. Although the results provide support for the validation of the AMIS, it should also be noted that there were significant but only modest correlations between the AMIS and the measures of craving. This may be due to the fact that addiction memory is long-lasting and resistant to being extinguished, whereas craving is considered to be a transient, fluctuant state that is sensitive to environmental influences [51–53]. In other words, individuals who retrieve vivid details from their memories of using drugs may, if there are other influences, report a low desire for drug use. In our study, the participants did rate extremely low scores on both the measures of craving (Supplementary materials, Table S3), especially the VAS (over one-third of the participants scored 0). Similar situations can be found in other studies. For example, Anton et al. [54] found that the high ratings on craving diminished when the patients were either hospitalized or successfully participated in treatment. Since the participants in our study were undergoing rehabilitation, it might be the engagement in treatment (which may result in a high self-efficacy or mastery of coping skills) that assisted them to prevent the escalation of desire for drug use. That is, it seems the interaction between craving and environmental influences that interfere with the association between the intensity of addiction memory and the level of craving. Significant correlations were also found between the AMIS scores and the duration of illicit drug use. However, the associations were quite modest, which may suggest that the participants' duration of illicit drug use, as measured in our study, is not particularly related to the intensity of addiction memory. It is possible that there may be other factors, such as the strength of the unconditioned stimulus [9], that moderate the associations between the intensity of addiction memory and the duration of illicit drug use. For example, a higher level of frequency or dose of drug use may elicit a stronger memory of addiction, which means the intensity of addiction memory may vary in degrees of frequency or dose of drug use but not merely depend on the duration of drug use. Future studies are needed to collect the participants' full history of drug use and to explore how the drug use history may affect the intensity of addiction memory.

Our study has several limitations that should be considered. First, the participants in our study were hospitalized in the drug rehabilitation centers and could not provide any information on current illicit drug use. Therefore, only craving was measured to evaluate the concurrent validity of AMIS. Second, although we have taken considerable effort to administer the AMIS to a diverse sample, the final version of the scale is a result of the sample used in the current study. Like other scales, the AMIS focused on a specific population (illicit drug users). Given the commonalities across addictions, the items of the AMIS may be adapted for patients with tobacco dependence, alcohol dependence, and so on. However, based on the current study, it is prudent not to draw an over-interpreted conclusion. Whether the AMIS can be decontextualized to produce such a broader application, is unknown. Moreover, although the measurement invariance indicated an absence of difference across primary illicit drug of use, the samples of illicit drug users in this study were primarily using heroin and amphetamine-type stimulants but no other illicit drugs such as cocaine and cannabis; the sample data was not collected from adolescents or non-Chinese speakers either. Thus, it is unknown whether the results of this study can be generalized to other populations of illicit drug users. Finally, although this study initially validates the utility of the AMIS, the scale should further be validated in reconsolidation-based interventions to see whether it can predict responses to the interventions. Also, since the participants were not followed-up, other studies are required to determine the predictive validity of the AMIS.

Regardless of the limitations, this study presents a promising measure to assess the intensity of addiction memory in illicit drug users. The AMIS allows the clinicians and researchers to gather information regarding the strength of addiction memory from a multidimensional perspective. Measurement invariance of the factor structure indicates that the AMIS can be reliably utilized to evaluate the intensity of addiction memory in, at least, heroin and amphetamine-type stimulant users, and thus enable comparison of the memory intensity across illicit drug users. Furthermore, the AMIS may tailor interventions based on responses to the scale, especially the interventions based on memory reconsolidation, although future studies are needed to validate the responsiveness of the AMIS. Finally, the brief nature of the AMIS makes it easy to administer, so that the clinicians and researchers can use the instrument to measure the intensity of addiction memory efficiently.

5. Conclusions

In conclusion, the present study is the first to develop a scale for measuring the intensity of addiction memory in illicit drug users. The current evidence suggests that the AMIS is a reliable and valid tool with the advantages of being brief and easily applied, and has the potential to be useful in future clinical research.

Supplementary Materials: The following are available online at http://www.mdpi.com/2077-0383/7/12/467/s1. Table S1: Comparison of the participants' characteristics in Study-2; Table S2: Factor loading and internal consistency of the Addiction Memory Intensity Scale if item-15 is deleted; Table S3: Descriptive data for measures in Study-2.

Author Contributions: Conceptualization, J.-y.C., J.-p.C., Y.-c.W., S.-q.L., and Z.-z.W.; Data curation, Z.-z.W.; Formal analysis, J.-y.C. and J.-p.C.; Funding acquisition, J.-y.C. and Z.-z.W.; Investigation, J.-y.C., Y.-c.W., and S.-q.L.; Supervision, Z.-z.W.; Writing–original draft, J.-y.C.; Writing–review and editing, J.-y.C., J.-p.C., Y.-c.W., S.-q.L., and Z.-z.W.

Funding: This research was funded by the National Natural Science Foundation of China (grant number 81573236) and the Joint School Research Award Program for Pedagogy, Social Science, and Medical Science (grant number YX2015002). Neither of the funding organizations had a role in the design of the study; in the collection, analyses, or interpretation of data; in the writing of the manuscript; or in the decision to publish the results.

Acknowledgments: Thanks to all staff members participated in our study for their efforts in the data collection.

Conflicts of Interest: The authors declare no conflict of interest.

References

1. Hyman, S.E. Addiction: A disease of learning and memory. *Am. J. Psychiatry* **2005**, *162*, 1414–1422. [CrossRef] [PubMed]
2. Böning, J. Addiction memory as a specific, individually learned memory imprint. *Pharmacopsychiatry* **2009**, *42*, S66–S68. [CrossRef] [PubMed]
3. Boening, J.A.L. Neurobiology of an addiction memory. *J. Neural Transm.* **2001**, *108*, 755–765. [CrossRef] [PubMed]
4. Lee, J.L.; Di Ciano, P.; Thomas, K.L.; Everitt, B.J. Disrupting reconsolidation of drug memories reduces cocaine-seeking behavior. *Neuron* **2005**, *47*, 795–801. [CrossRef] [PubMed]
5. Xue, Y.X.; Luo, Y.X.; Wu, P.; Shi, H.S.; Xue, L.F.; Chen, C.; Zhu, W.L.; Ding, Z.B.; Bao, Y.P.; Shi, J.; et al. A memory retrieval-extinction procedure to prevent drug craving and relapse. *Science* **2012**, *336*, 241–245. [CrossRef] [PubMed]
6. Das, R.K.; Lawn, W.; Kamboj, S.K. Rewriting the valuation and salience of alcohol-related stimuli via memory reconsolidation. *Transl. Psychiatry* **2015**, *5*, e645. [CrossRef] [PubMed]
7. Luo, Y.X.; Xue, Y.X.; Liu, J.F.; Shi, H.S.; Jian, M.; Han, Y.; Zhu, W.L.; Bao, Y.P.; Wu, P.; Ding, Z.B.; et al. A novel UCS memory retrieval-extinction procedure to inhibit relapse to drug seeking. *Nat. Commun.* **2015**, *6*, 7675. [CrossRef] [PubMed]

8. Dennis, T.S.; Perrotti, L.I. Erasing drug memories through the disruption of memory reconsolidation: A review of glutamatergic mechanisms. *J. Appl. Biobehav. Res.* **2015**, *20*, 101–129. [CrossRef]
9. Treanor, M.; Brown, L.A.; Rissman, J.; Craske, M.G. Can memories of traumatic experiences or addiction be erased or modified? A critical review of research on the disruption of memory reconsolidation and its applications. *Perspect. Psychol. Sci.* **2017**, *12*, 290–305. [CrossRef] [PubMed]
10. Suzuki, A.; Josselyn, S.A.; Frankland, P.W.; Masushige, S.; Silva, A.J.; Kida, S. Memory reconsolidation and extinction have distinct temporal and biochemical signatures. *J. Neurosci.* **2004**, *24*, 4787–4795. [CrossRef] [PubMed]
11. Fernandez, R.S.; Bavassi, L.; Forcato, C.; Pedreira, M.E. The dynamic nature of the reconsolidation process and its boundary conditions: Evidence based on human tests. *Neurobiol. Learn. Mem.* **2016**, *130*, 202–212. [CrossRef] [PubMed]
12. Forcato, C.; Fernandez, R.S.; Pedreira, M.E. The role and dynamic of strengthening in the reconsolidation process in a human declarative memory: What decides the fate of recent and older memories? *PLoS ONE* **2013**, *8*, e61688. [CrossRef] [PubMed]
13. Littel, M.; van den Hout, M.A.; Engelhard, I.M. Desensitizing addiction: Using eye movements to reduce the intensity of substance-related mental imagery and craving. *Front. Psychiatry* **2016**, *7*, 14. [CrossRef] [PubMed]
14. Markus, W.; de Weert-van Oene, G.H.; Woud, M.L.; Becker, E.S.; DeJong, C.A. Are addiction-related memories malleable by working memory competition? Transient effects on memory vividness and nicotine craving in a randomized lab experiment. *J. Behav. Ther. Exp. Psychiatry* **2016**, *52*, 83–91. [CrossRef] [PubMed]
15. Rosenberg, H. Clinical and laboratory assessment of the subjective experience of drug craving. *Clin. Psychol. Rev.* **2009**, *29*, 519–534. [CrossRef] [PubMed]
16. Malhotra, N.K.; Mukhopadhyay, S.; Liu, X.; Dash, S. One, few or many? An integrated framework for identifying the items in measurement scales. *Int. J. Market Res.* **2012**, *54*, 835–862. [CrossRef]
17. Luo, W.; Wu, Z.; Wei, X. Reliability and validity of the Chinese version of the addiction severity index. *J. Acquir. Immune Defic. Syndr.* **2010**, *53*, S121–S125. [CrossRef] [PubMed]
18. Butler, S.F.; Budman, S.H.; McGee, M.D.; Davis, M.S.; Cornelli, R.; Morey, L.C. Addiction severity assessment tool: Development of a self-report measure for clients in substance abuse treatment. *Drug Alcohol Depend.* **2005**, *80*, 349–360. [CrossRef] [PubMed]
19. Caretti, V.; Gori, A.; Craparo, G.; Giannini, M.; Iraci-Sareri, G.; Schimmenti, A. A new measure for assessing substance-related and addictive disorders: The addictive behavior questionnaire (ABQ). *J. Clin. Med.* **2018**, *7*, 194. [CrossRef] [PubMed]
20. Gu, J.; Lau, J.T.; Chen, H.; Liu, Z.; Lei, Z.; Li, Z.; Lian, Z.; Wang, R.; Hu, X.; Cai, H.; et al. Validation of the Chinese version of the opiate addiction severity inventory (OASI) and the severity of dependence scale (SDS) in non-institutionalized heroin users in China. *Addict. Behav.* **2008**, *33*, 725–741. [CrossRef] [PubMed]
21. Miele, G.M.; Carpenter, K.M.; Cockerham, M.S.; Trautman, K.D.; Blaine, J.; Hasin, D.S. substance dependence severity scale (SDSS): Reliability and validity of a clinician-administered interview for DSM-IV substance use disorders. *Drug Alcohol Depend.* **2000**, *59*, 63–75. [CrossRef]
22. Sutin, A.R.; Robins, R.W. Phenomenology of autobiographical memories: The memory experiences questionnaire. *Memory* **2007**, *15*, 390–411. [CrossRef] [PubMed]
23. Tulving, E. Episodic memory: From mind to brain. *Annu. Rev. Psychol.* **2002**, *53*, 1–25. [CrossRef] [PubMed]
24. Müller, C.P. Episodic memories and their relevance for psychoactive drug use and addiction. *Front. Behav. Neurosci.* **2013**, *7*, 34. [CrossRef] [PubMed]
25. Johnson, M.K.; Foley, M.A.; Suengas, A.G.; Raye, C.L. Phenomenal characteristics of memories for perceived and imagined autobiographical events. *J. Exp. Psychol. Gen.* **1988**, *117*, 371–376. [CrossRef] [PubMed]
26. Rubin, D.C.; Schrauf, R.W.; Greenberg, D.L. Belief and recollection of autobiographical memories. *Mem. Cognit.* **2003**, *31*, 887–901. [CrossRef] [PubMed]
27. Talarico, J.M.; LaBar, K.S.; Rubin, D.C. Emotional intensity predicts autobiographical memory experience. *Mem. Cognit.* **2004**, *32*, 1118–1132. [CrossRef] [PubMed]
28. Fitzgerald, J.M.; Broadbridge, C.L. Latent constructs of the autobiographical memory questionnaire: A recollection-belief model of autobiographical experience. *Memory* **2013**, *21*, 230–248. [CrossRef] [PubMed]

29. Boyacioglu, I.; Akfirat, S. Development and psychometric properties of a new measure for memory phenomenology: The autobiographical memory characteristics questionnaire. *Memory* **2015**, *23*, 1070–1092. [CrossRef] [PubMed]
30. Luchetti, M.; Sutin, A.R. Measuring the phenomenology of autobiographical memory: A short form of the memory experiences questionnaire. *Memory* **2016**, *24*, 592–602. [CrossRef] [PubMed]
31. Conway, M.A. Sensory-perceptual episodic memory and its context: Autobiographical memory. *Philos. Trans. R. Soc. Lond. B. Biol. Sci.* **2001**, *356*, 1375–1384. [CrossRef] [PubMed]
32. Conway, M.A. Memory and the self. *J. Mem. Lang.* **2005**, *53*, 594–628. [CrossRef]
33. Greenberg, D.L.; Knowlton, B.J. The role of visual imagery in autobiographical memory. *Mem. Cognit.* **2014**, *42*, 922–934. [CrossRef] [PubMed]
34. Preston, C.C.; Colman, A.M. Optimal number of response categories in rating scales: Reliability, validity, discriminating power, and respondent preferences. *Acta Psychol. (Amst.)* **2000**, *104*, 1–15. [CrossRef]
35. Weijters, B.; Cabooter, E.; Schillewaert, N. The effect of rating scale format on response styles: The number of response categories and response category labels. *Int. J. Res. Mark.* **2010**, *27*, 236–247. [CrossRef]
36. Lee, J.; Paek, I. In search of the optimal number of response categories in a rating scale. *J. Psychoeduc. Assess.* **2014**, *32*, 663–673. [CrossRef]
37. Yang, C.; Wei, W.; Vrana, K.E.; Xiao, Y.; Peng, Y.; Chen, D.; Yu, J.; Wang, D.; Ding, F.; Wang, Z. Validation of the obsessive compulsive drug use scale (OCDUS) among male heroin addicts in China. *Int. J. Ment. Health Addic.* **2016**, *14*, 803–819. [CrossRef]
38. Robbins, T.W.; Ersche, K.D.; Everitt, B.J. Drug addiction and the memory systems of the brain. *Ann. N. Y. Acad. Sci.* **2008**, *1141*, 1–21. [CrossRef] [PubMed]
39. Von der Goltz, C.; Kiefer, F. Learning and memory in the aetiopathogenesis of addiction: Future implications for therapy? *Eur. Arch. Psychiatry Clin. Neurosci.* **2009**, *259*, S183–S187. [CrossRef] [PubMed]
40. Torregrossa, M.M.; Corlett, P.R.; Taylor, J.R. Aberrant learning and memory in addiction. *Neurobiol. Learn. Mem.* **2011**, *96*, 609–623. [CrossRef] [PubMed]
41. Contreras, M.; Billeke, P.; Vicencio, S.; Madrid, C.; Perdomo, G.; Gonzalez, M.; Torrealba, F. A role for the insular cortex in long-term memory for context-evoked drug craving in rats. *Neuropsychopharmacology* **2012**, *37*, 2101–2108. [CrossRef] [PubMed]
42. Forcato, C.; Rodriguez, M.L.; Pedreira, M.E. Repeated labilization-reconsolidation processes strengthen declarative memory in humans. *PLoS ONE* **2011**, *6*, e23305. [CrossRef] [PubMed]
43. SAS Institute Inc. *SAS [Computer Program]*; Version 9.4; SAS Institute Inc.: Cary, NC, USA, 2012.
44. Hao, Y.; Sun, X.; Fang, J.; Wu, S.; Zhu, S. The study of statistical methods used for item selection. *Chin. J. Health Stat.* **2004**, *21*, 209–211.
45. Wu, M.L. *Statistical Analysis Practices in Questionnaire Development*; Chongqing University Press: Chongqing, China, 2010; pp. 158–265.
46. Brown, T.A. *Confirmatory Factor Analysis for Applied Research*; The Guilford Press: New York, NY, USA, 2006; pp. 12–211.
47. O'Rourke, N.; Hatcher, L. *A Step-by-Step Approach to Using SAS for Factor Analysis and Structural Equation Modeling*, 2nd ed.; SAS Institute Inc.: Cary, NC, USA, 2013; pp. 182–246.
48. Little, T.D. Mean and covariance structures (MACS) analyses of cross-cultural data: Practical and theoretical issues. *Multivariate Behav. Res.* **1997**, *32*, 53–76. [CrossRef] [PubMed]
49. Cheung, G.W.; Rensvold, R.B. Evaluating goodness-of-fit indexes for testing measurement invariance. *Struct. Equ. Modeling* **2002**, *9*, 233–255. [CrossRef]
50. Yen, C.F.; Lin, H.C.; Wang, P.W.; Ko, C.H.; Lee, K.H.; Hsu, C.Y.; Chung, K.S.; Wu, H.C.; Cheng, C.P. Heroin craving and its correlations with clinical outcome indicators in people with heroin dependence receiving methadone maintenance treatment. *Compr. Psychiatry* **2016**, *65*, 50–56. [CrossRef] [PubMed]
51. Drummond, D.C.; Litten, R.Z.; Lowman, C.; Hunt, W.A. Craving research: Future directions. *Addiction* **2000**, *95*, 247–255. [CrossRef]
52. Sayette, M.A.; Shiffman, S.; Tiffany, S.T.; Niaura, R.S.; Martin, C.S.; Shadel, W.G. The measurement of drug craving. *Addiction* **2000**, *95*, 189–210. [CrossRef] [PubMed]

53. Tiffany, S.T.; Wray, J.M. The clinical significance of drug craving. *Ann. N. Y. Acad. Sci.* **2012**, *1248*, 1–17. [CrossRef] [PubMed]
54. Anton, R.F.; Moak, D.H.; Latham, P. The obsessive compulsive drinking scale: A self-rated instrument for the quantification of thoughts about alcohol and drinking behavior. *Alcohol. Clin. Exp. Res.* **1995**, *19*, 92–99. [CrossRef] [PubMed]

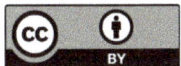

© 2018 by the authors. Licensee MDPI, Basel, Switzerland. This article is an open access article distributed under the terms and conditions of the Creative Commons Attribution (CC BY) license (http://creativecommons.org/licenses/by/4.0/).

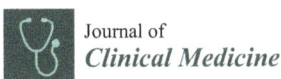

Review

Neurocircuitry of Reward and Addiction: Potential Impact of Dopamine–Glutamate Co-release as Future Target in Substance Use Disorder

Zisis Bimpisidis and Åsa Wallén-Mackenzie *

Department of Organismal Biology, Uppsala University, S-752 36 Uppsala, Sweden
* Correspondence: asa.mackenzie@ebc.uu.se

Received: 9 October 2019; Accepted: 1 November 2019; Published: 6 November 2019

Abstract: Dopamine–glutamate co-release is a unique property of midbrain neurons primarily located in the ventral tegmental area (VTA). Dopamine neurons of the VTA are important for behavioral regulation in response to rewarding substances, including natural rewards and addictive drugs. The impact of glutamate co-release on behaviors regulated by VTA dopamine neurons has been challenging to probe due to lack of selective methodology. However, several studies implementing conditional knockout and optogenetics technologies in transgenic mice have during the past decade pointed towards a role for glutamate co-release in multiple physiological and behavioral processes of importance to substance use and abuse. In this review, we discuss these studies to highlight findings that may be critical when considering mechanisms of importance for prevention and treatment of substance abuse.

Keywords: addiction; reward; transgenic mice; optogenetics; self-administration; cocaine; amphetamine

---

1. Dopamine and Substance Use Disorder

Substance use disorder is a chronic, relapsing neuropsychiatric disease that occurs in a minority of recreational drug users [1]. In vulnerable individuals, the initial elevation of dopamine (DA) upon drug-consumption, which is believed to reflect the reinforcing effects of substances of abuse, will lead to characteristic behavioral patterns related to long-lasting alterations in the glutamatergic system [2–5]. Drug-seeking behavior and objectively reported craving in drug-addicts are both dependent on environmental cues associated with drug intake and can lead to relapse even after many years of abstinence [5,6].

All addictive substances influence the brain DA system which is implicated in reward processing, motivation and behavioral reinforcement [7,8]. The mesolimbic DA system, containing DA neurons located within the ventral tegmental area (VTA) and their projections to the nucleus accumbens (NAc) [9], has been shown to be particularly important for reward processing. DA release in the NAc, in particular in the medial (m) aspect of the shell (Sh) compartment, NAc mSh, has been implicated in the reinforcing properties of both natural and drug rewards [10]. DA modulates the activity of NAc neurons and their response to inputs coming from other limbic areas [1,11,12]. Abusive drugs increase DA levels preferentially in the NAc mSh as compared to the NAc core or the dorsal aspect of the striatum [1,13,14]. While these increases are related to the reinforcing properties of the drugs, the behavioral patterns observed in addicts after chronic drug use are related to more persistent neuroadaptations in the glutamatergic system. It has been shown that the psychostimulant cocaine rapidly induces synaptic plasticity in VTA DA neurons after acute, passive administration [15] and that persistent neuroadaptations can be observed in rats that have self-administered cocaine [16]. Unlike the VTA, synaptic plasticity in medium spiny neurons (MSNs) of the NAc is observed only after long-term cocaine use. Further, any changes in plasticity of the MSNs are contingent to a withdrawal period [17] and occur on MSNs expressing the DA receptor subtype 1 (D1R) [18]. Overall, synaptic changes upon drug administration occur in a time-dependent manner, so that the first changes take place in the VTA, and, after repeated administration, in the NAc, a phenomenon believed to reflect the long-lasting behavioral consequences of chronic drug intake [5]. Comprehensive review articles of putative mechanisms, particular characteristics and regional differences in the context of synaptic plasticity observed in animal models of drug addiction have been published elsewhere and further details are beyond the scope of this review.

2. DA-Glutamate Co-Release in the Mesolimbic System

2.1. DA Neurons in the VTA

Neurons that produce DA and release it into the extracellular space, either in the synapse or along the axon, are commonly referred to as dopaminergic neurons, or simply DA neurons. Molecularly, DA neurons are defined by the presence of the rate-limiting enzyme tyrosine hydroxylase (TH), which enables the production of DA, and the absence of enzymes that convert DA into noradrenalin and adrenalin [19]. Within the ventral midbrain, DA neurons are located in the VTA, substantia nigra *pars compacta* (SNc) and the retrorubral field. The VTA in turn is composed of several subnuclei, at least in rodents: the rostral linear nucleus (RLi), interfascicular nucleus (IF), parabrachial pigmented nucleus (PBP), paranigral nucleus (PN), parainterfascicular nucleus (PIF), and caudal linear nucleus of the raphe (CLi). Also, the rostral-most aspect of the area, which goes under different names, such as VTA rostral and rostro-medial VTA, is most often included when discussing the VTA [9,20–23] (Figure 1).

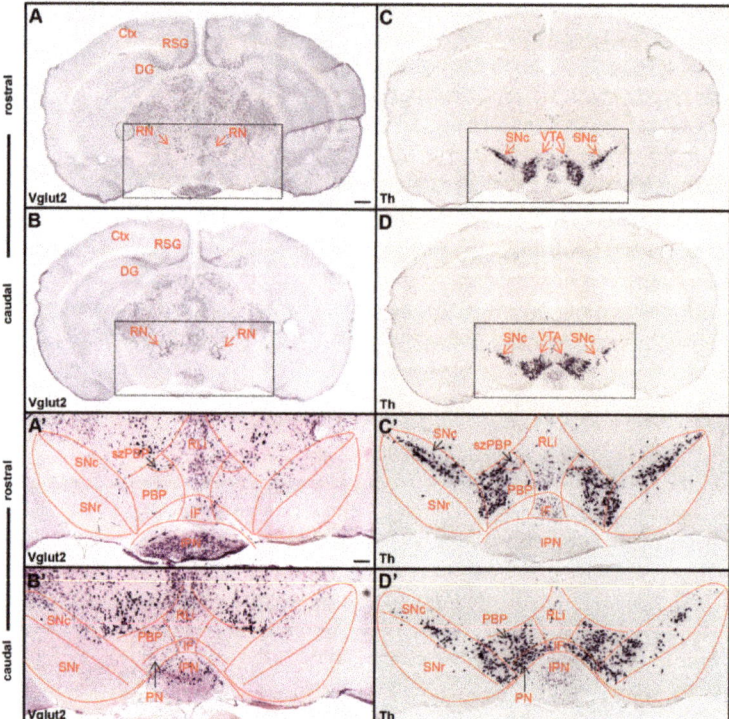

Figure 1. Ample Vglut2 mRNA-positive cells throughout dorsal and ventral midbrain with more sparse expression within the dopaminergic area. Colorimetric in-situ hybridization showing overview

of Vglut2 (**A**,**B**) and Th (**C**,**D**) mRNA in midbrain sections of wildtype adult mouse at two rostro-caudal levels. (**A**,**B**) Vglut2 mRNA is abundant throughout the midbrain with strong signals in e.g., the red nucleus (RN), retrosplenial group of the cortex (RSG) and dentate gyrus (DG), and weaker signals in the ventral tegmental area (VTA) and substantia nigra *pars compacta* (SNc). (**C**,**D**) Th mRNA is selectively localized in dopaminergic neurons of the VTA and SNc; its mRNA signal is implemented to visualize these areas. Dotted square around the VTA and SNc (scale bar 500 mm) presented as closeups in (**A′**–**D′**; scale bar 200 mm). (**C′**,**D′**) SNc, substantia nigra *pars reticulata* (SNr) and subregions of VTA outlined in Th closeups and superimposed on Vglut2 closeups (**A′**,**B′**). (**C′**,**D′**) Th mRNA was strongly localized in the SNc and within the parabrachial pigmented area (PBP) and paranigral nucleus (PN) of the VTA with a weaker signal in the rostral linear nucles (RLi) and caudal aspect of the interfascicular nucleus (IF). (**A′**,**B′**) Within the VTA, Vglut2 mRNA was detected in the PBP, PN, RLi, and IF as well as within the medially-located subzone of the PBP (szPBP) while no Vglut2 mRNA was detected in the GABAergic SNr area. Additional abbreviations: Ctx, Cortex; IPN, interpeducular nucleus. Reprinted from Papathanou et al., 2018 [24].

2.2. Vesicular Glutamate Transporters and the Concept of DA-Glutamate Co-Release

The midbrain DA system was described in the 1960s [25–27] and has been extensively studied since then. In contrast, the glutamatergic system remained more elusive for many years, to a large extent due to the lack of molecular markers that could enable their reliable identification within complex neuronal networks. Around year 2000 came the first reports of identification of the molecules that transport glutamate into presynaptic vesicles, and thereby allow this amino acid to be used as a bona fide neurotransmitter ready to be released into the synapse upon neuronal activation [28–32]. These vesicular glutamate transporters, VGLUTs, which exist in three subtypes (VGLUT1, VGLUT2 and VGLUT3), have been found throughout the brain in various anatomical patterns, and their presence defines a neuron's ability for exocytotic glutamate release upon neuronal depolarization. VGLUTs thereby serve as excellent molecular markers of glutamatergic neurotransmission. Together, VGLUT1 and VGLUT2 cover all classically described glutamatergic neurons. In addition, soon after their discovery, it was found that VGLUTs can be present within neurons assigned to another neurotransmitter phenotype than glutamatergic. For example, VGLUT3 was extensively detected in subtypes of serotonergic and cholinergic neurons, and VGLUT1 in inhibitory neurons (for review, see e.g., [33,34]). The discovery of the VGLUTs thereby opened up for a completely new view of many neuronal systems, as they could be shown to possess the molecular machinery for co-release of glutamate parallel to release of its "first" neurotransmitter, often referred to as the "primary" neurotransmitter. Glutamate co-release is a striking neuronal feature which can help explain some complex physiological features that could not be fully accounted for by the primary neurotransmitter. For example, fast excitatory neurotransmission originating from midbrain DA neurons had been recorded in striatal brain slices and mesencephalic cell cultures using electrophysiological setups, however, it was unknown how DA neurons could give rise to this type of signaling [35–39]. With the finding that some DA neurons contain VGLUT2, originally described in in-vitro cell-based systems [40], and subsequently confirmed in a number of histological studies as described below, a molecular basis for the electrophysiologically measurable fast excitatory post-synaptic currents could be initiated and formed.

Neurons releasing more than one neurotransmitter have been given different names to describe their complexity. Based on the capacity of certain midbrain DA neurons to co-release glutamate, a property in which glutamate is released by a neuron upon depolarization, these neurons have been referred to as co-releasing, but also "bi-lingual", "combinatorial" and "dual-signaling" [19,22,33,34], alluding to their ability to "speak different languages". The ability of neurons to release two or more neurotransmitters has also been referred to as "multiplexed neurochemical signaling", or "multiplexed neurotransmission" [41]. In terms of function, the sorting of vesicular neurotransmitter transporters to subcellular domains will account for the inherent property of co-releasing two or more neurotransmitters which can occur from the same synaptic vesicle, or the same pool of synaptic vesicle within an axon, or from distinct sets of synaptic pools located in different subdomains within axons (reviewed in [33]). The kind of synaptic mechanisms that any given type of co-releasing neuron utilizes needs to be defined experimentally, which can be challenging. While "co-release" generally refers to the release of two or more neurotransmitters from any given neuron, the concept of "co-transmission", which is often used to describe similar phenomena, has been defined more strictly: *"Co-transmission in the strictest sense implies that two neurotransmitters are released at the same time from a common pool of synaptic vesicles within one axon terminal."* [33]. In the context of glutamate co-release from midbrain DA neurons, this type of more narrowly defined "co-transmission" from a common pool of synaptic vesicles within one axon terminal remains to be experimentally identified and defined. Instead, current data rather point towards the co-release of DA and glutamate from different microdomains in axonal terminals. With their discovery that VGLUT2 and VMAT2, the vesicular monoamine transporter, sort to distinct subpopulations of synaptic vesicles within a subset of mesoaccumbens axons in rodents, Zhang and colleagues recently concluded that " ... *our results do not support the hypothesis that axon terminals from these neurons co-release dopamine and glutamate from identical axonal terminals. Rather, our findings indicate that synaptic vesicles that release dopamine or glutamate from mesoaccumbens terminals in both adult rats and adult mice are located in distinct microdomains*" [42]. Based on existing data and current terminology, we have used the term "co-release" throughout this review to broadly describe the concept of DA and glutamate release from the same midbrain neuron without specifying signaling mechanisms.

In summary, while the midbrain DA system has been the focus of attention in the field of reward and addiction for many years, the "subdiscipline" of DA–glutamate co-release is considerably younger. Consequently, the putative role of DA–glutamate co-release in neurocircuitry and behavioral regulation has remained rather unexplored. However, several studies using experimental animals point towards an impact of DA–glutamate co-release in mechanisms of relevance for addiction, suggesting that glutamate co-release is worthwhile to explore for the benefit of new prevention and/or intervention strategies for substance use disorder. Several recent reviews describe DA–glutamate co-release from different research angles, including possible packaging/release mechanisms, putative role of VGLUTs in promoting vesicular packaging of the primary neurotransmitter, post-synaptic effects of the co-released glutamate and more (see e.g., [34,43–45]). In this review, we will focus our attention on behavioral regulation putatively mediated by DA–glutamate co-release as discovered using rodent models. The feature of DA–glutamate co-release may contribute to dopaminergic function in reward mechanisms and may thus be of importance when considering physiological and behavioral consequences of substance use and abuse.

2.3. Expression Patterns of VGLUT2 in the Midbrain DA System and Validation of Glutamate Co-Release

To begin to understand functional implications of DA–glutamate co-release, it is important to know where the neurons that possess this ability are located, as only then can neurocircuitry and behavioral roles be fully delineated. The presence of VGLUT2 within midbrain areas where DA neurons reside have been described in several studies, most in which in-situ hybridization for VGLUT2 mRNA has been combined with the detection of either TH mRNA or TH protein for the visualization of DA neurons. Analyses of mouse and rat midbrains have shown that VGLUT2 mRNA-positive cells are scattered throughout the VTA and the adjacently located SNc with more frequent appearance of VGLUT2/TH co-localizing neurons medially than laterally, primarily in the medial aspect of the VTA [46–48]. VGLUT2-positive neurons in the ventral midbrain have also been described in primates, including humans [49]. In rodents, neurons expressing both the VGLUT2 and TH genes comprise a minority of the total number of cells in the adult VTA expressing either the VGLUT2 or the TH gene [47,50,51]. In two recent studies, we could confirm these previous analyses by showing that the highest density of VGLUT2 neurons in the VTA was found in the RLi, followed by the PBP, PN and IF. In the RLi and within a small spatially-restricted area within the PBP, barely any TH-positive neurons can be found, but here VGLUT2 is high. We have called this VGLUT2-dense area within the PBP "the subzone of the PBP" (szPBP) to distinguish it from the remaining PBP which contains

VGLUT2 at lower density but TH at higher density [23,24] (Figure 1). Thus, the PBP in general has a TH^{high}/VGLUT2^{low} profile, but the szPBP and RLi have the opposite profile, TH^{low}/VGLUT2^{high}.

VGLUT2-TH co-expressing neurons are generally sparse in adulthood, and a temporal regulation between birth and adulthood has been shown [52,53]. When addressing embryogenesis, we could readily identify VGLUT2-TH co-localization already at E12.5 [54] (Figure 2). To address the spatio-temporal profile of VGLUT2 in midbrain DA neurons in more detail, we recently performed a time-study including E14.5, newborn (postnatal day 3, P3) and adult mice (Figure 3) [24]. By co-localizing VGLUT2 mRNA with both TH and dopamine transporter (DAT) mRNAs, we found an interesting temporally dynamic pattern of expression. Almost no co-localization between VGLUT2 with either TH or DAT was detected at E14.5 (Figure 3A–C), while substantial co-localization was observed in the newborn mouse (Figure 3D–F). At P3, VGLUT2 mRNA showed prominent co-localization with both TH and DAT mRNA with higher density of VGLUT2/TH than VGLUT2/DAT double-positive neurons. This is explained by the lower expression of DAT than TH in medial aspects of the VTA, where VGLUT2 is at its highest. In addition, subareas within the VTA showed different amounts of co-localization. Primarily the PBP, but also the PN and IF showed co-localization of VGLUT2 with TH and DAT, respectively. The RLi, which shows the highest levels of VGLUT2 in the VTA, was almost devoid of co-localization of VGLUT2 with either TH or DAT due to the low abundance of these transcripts in this brain nucleus. While readily detected in the newborn mouse, the level of VGLUT2/TH and VGLUT2/DAT double-positive neurons was overall low in all VTA subareas in the adult mouse (Figure 3H,I), confirming previous studies.

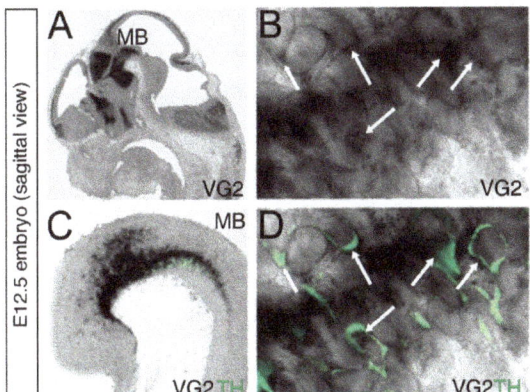

Figure 2. Vglut2 mRNA and Tyrosine hydroxylase (TH) immunoreactivity in midbrain DA neurons. (A–D) In-situ hybridization for Vglut2 (VG2) mRNA (black) combined with fluorescent immunohistochemistry for TH (green) on sagittal sections of an E12.5 embryo. Vglut2 mRNA is detected in multiple regions in the embryo, including the ventral midbrain (MB) where DA neurons develop (A,B). Vglut2 mRNA is co-localized with TH-immunoreactivity in DA neurons within the MB (C,D). Arrows indicate Vglut2-positive cytoplasm (B) and Vglut2/TH double-positive neurons (D) (Magnification: B,D 300x). Reprinted from Birgner et al., 2010 [54].

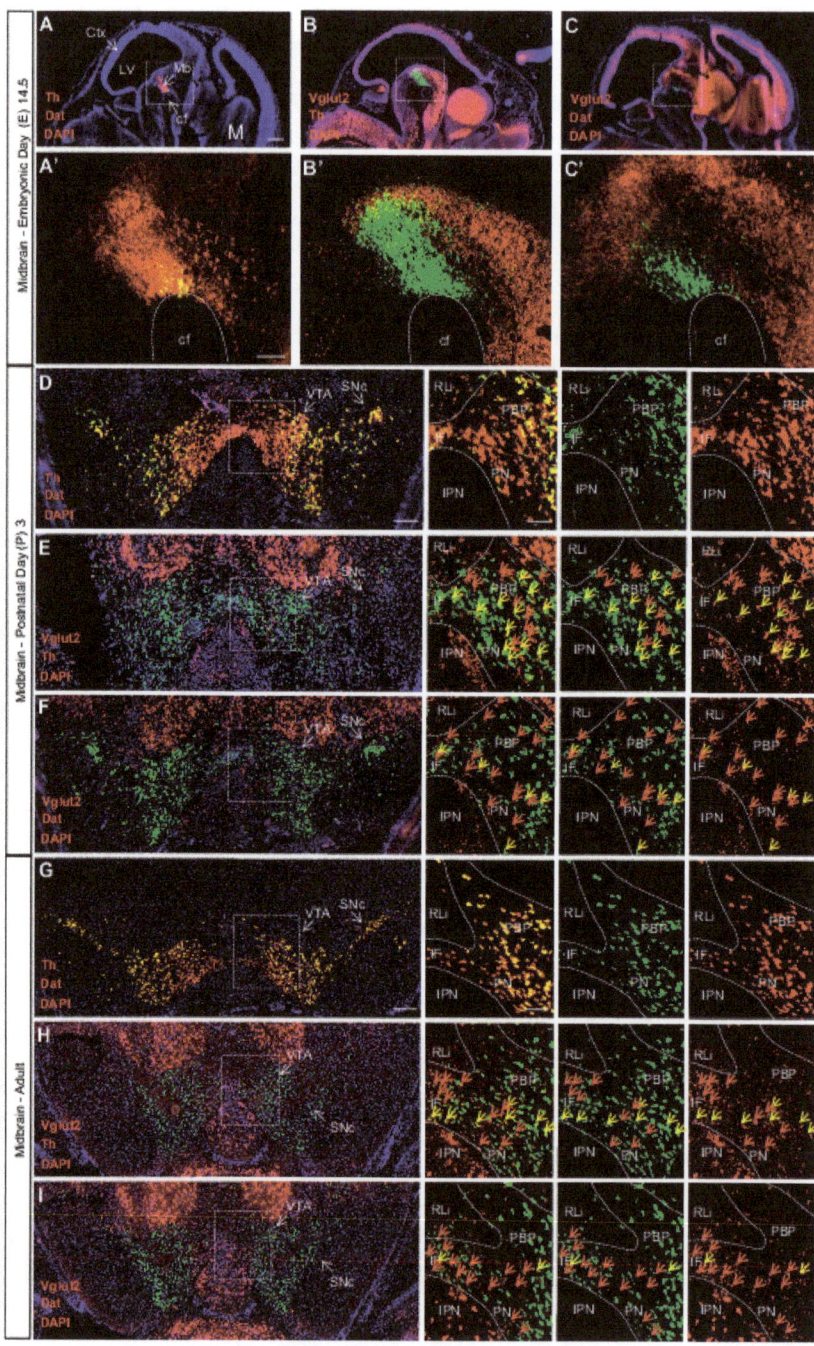

Figure 3. Vglut2, Th and Dat mRNA co-localization within certain VTA dopamine (DA) neurons is sparse at E14.5, peaks around birth and is subsequently down-regulated in adulthood. Double fluorescent in-situ hybridization for Th (red), Dat (green) and Vglut2 (red) mRNA, respectively, on wildtype mouse midbrain sections. (**A–C**) Sagittal sections of E14.5 embryo. Dotted square around the

area of developing midbrain DA neurons (**A–C**) with close-ups in (**A′–C′**). (**A**) Th and Dat mRNA show co-localization (yellow) in the ventral midbrain (scale bar 500 mm). (**A′**) higher magnification of insets (scale bar 100 mm); (**B,B′**) Th and Vglut2 mRNA expression in the midbrain. (**C,C′**) Dat and Vglut2 mRNA show sparse detection in the midbrain. (**D–F**) Coronal sections of ventral midbrain in pups of postnatal day (P) 3. (**D**) Th and Dat show ample co-localization (yellow) in the lateral VTA and SNc (scale bar 250 mm, inset 100 mm). (**E**) Th and Vglut2 mRNA and (**F**) Dat and Vglut2 mRNA prominently co-localize (yellow) at this age in the IF, PBP and PN areas (arrows) but not in the RLi of the VTA. (**G–I**) Coronal sections of the adult midbrain (10 weeks; scale bar 250 mm, inset 100 mm). (**G**) Th and Dat mRNA co-localization (yellow) remains strong; whilst the level of co-localization between (**H**) Th and Vglut2 and (**I**) Dat and Vglut2 mRNAs is lower than at P3 (arrows). Yellow arrows show co-localization green (Dat) and red (Vglut2) channel, red arrows show red (Vglut2) channel (Postnatal Day (P) 3 n = 3; adult n = 3). Abbreviations: cf, cephalic flexture; Ctx, cortex; IF, interfascicular nucleus; IPN, interpeducular nucleus; LV, lateral ventricle; M, medulla; Mb, midbrain; PBP, parabrachial pigmented area; PN, paranigral nuclei; RLi rostral linear nucleus; SNc, Substantia nigra pars compacta; VTA, Ventral tegmental area. Reprinted from Papathanou et al., 2018 [24].

To further the understanding of VGLUT2 expression in developing DA neurons, we have recently addressed VGLUT2 in DA neurons from the time-point around mid-gestation when these neurons are born and can now show that most early differentiating midbrain DA neurons express VGLUT2 at stages E10–11 (Dumas and Wallén-Mackenzie, in press, 2019). Further, we show that this early and abundant VGLUT2-expression is subsequently down-regulated as embryonal development proceeds, providing an explanation for the higher appearance of VGLUT2 in E12.5 than E14.5 described above. By including this novel piece of data into a concept of VGLUT2 expression in midbrain DA neurons, it seems that most, if not all, DA neurons initially express VGLUT2 which is subsequently downregulated during embryonal development to be upregulated in subsets of VTA neurons around birth and again down-regulated in adulthood.

In summary, VGLUT2 co-localizes to a higher extent with TH and DAT in newborn than in adult mice. With the expression of VGLUT2 in DA neurons primarily during early embryogenesis and during a subsequent phase around birth, it is interesting to speculate around putative roles of VGLUT2 in the developing DA neuron. In addition to its temporally regulated expression during the normal life span starting from embryogenesis, it has been shown that VGLUT2 expression levels can be induced in mature organisms upon stress and injury [53,55], suggesting that a glutamate co-releasing phenotype can be acquired, or at least accentuated, at different time-points during life in response to particular experiences. VGLUT2 thus shows an interesting spatio-temporal regulation pattern that may have important implications for behavioral regulation and disorders of the DA system throughout life. Below, we will discuss conditional knockout (cKO) studies in mice that support this observation.

In terms of projections of DA–glutamate co-releasing neurons, DA neurons in the medial aspect of the VTA, where VGLUT2 levels are highest, are known to project to the NAc mSh [10]. Indeed, optogenetics-driven analyses have confirmed previous observations from electrical stimulations in slice and cell culture systems and further shown that that stimulation of DA neurons in the VTA gives rise to excitatory post-synaptic currents in MSNs primarily on the ventral, rather than the dorsal, striatum [56,57]. Perhaps most attention in the DA–glutamate field has been given to MSNs, but also other striatal neurons have been shown to receive input from DA–glutamate co-releasing neurons. Lately, Chuhma and colleagues demonstrated that midbrain DA neurons induce post-synaptic glutamatergic effects in all neuronal types present in the striatum (MSNs, cholinergic interneurons (ChIs also referred as CINs) and fast-spiking interneurons (FSI)), but that the effects are different depending on the anatomical region where the neurons are located, and, specifically for the NAc mSh, most profound on ChIs [58]. While most prominently projecting to the ventral striatum, post-synaptic glutamatergic effects by DA–glutamate co-releasing VTA neurons have also been observed in these same neuronal cell types in the dorsal striatum. Interestingly, ChIs in the dorsomedial parts were shown to be affected differently than those located in the dorsolateral parts [59,60].

Having summarized current knowledge of anatomical positions of DA–glutamate co-releasing neurons in the VTA and their striatal target neurons, the next section will deal with behavioral consequences upon experimentally-achieved disruption of DA–glutamate co-release using transgenics-based approaches in mice.

2.4. Behavioral Consequences upon Disrupted Dopamine–Glutamate Co-Release in Transgenic Mice

The current literature contains several studies in which conditional knockout technology in mice has been used to understand if targeted disruption of VGLUT2 gene expression within DA neurons has any measurable effect on behavioral output. These studies, which are all different implementations of the Cre-LoxP system with the aim to delete glutamate co-release in DA neurons, have in common that they identify significant alterations in responsiveness to natural rewards and/or drugs of abuse (listed in Table 1). Together, these studies strongly implicate the importance of DA–glutamate co-release in mechanisms of relevance to addiction. We will discuss some of these studies in more detail as specific features might be of particular importance when considering DA–glutamate co-release in mechanisms of addiction. We will also go through putative caveats that might be important to bear in mind when interpreting these behavioral data, some of which are based on recent discoveries of so called "off-target" effects in transgenics methodology.

Table 1. List of publications in which dopamine-glutamate co-release has been targeted to probe its putative behavioral roles. Main results summarized. – indicates no change; ↑ increase; ↓ decrease. Abbreviations: RT-PP, real-time place preference; VTA, ventral tegmental area.

Study (Listed in Alphabetical Order)	Strategy to Target DA-Glutamate Co-Release	Test	Effect
Alsiö et al., 2011 [61]	*Vglut2*$^{\it{ff;DAT-Cre}}$	Sucrose preference	lower threshold
		Sucrose self-administration	↑ responding under food restriction
			↑ consumption when fed *ad libitum*
		Cocaine self-administration	↑ for lower doses
			↑ responding for cocaine-associated cues
Birgner et al., 2010 [54]	*Vglut2*$^{\it{ff;DAT-Cre}}$	Rotarod (crude motor coordination)	–
		Beam walking (fine motor coordination)	–
		Elevated plus maze (anxiety)	↑ latency to move
		Multi-variate concentric square field (anxiety and risk analysis)	↑ risk-taking behavior
		Forced swim test (depression)	–
		Radial maze	–
		Acute amphetamine	dose-dependent alterations
Fortin et al., 2012 [62]	*Vglut2*$^{\it{ff;DAT-Cre}}$	Rotarod (crude motor coordination)	↓ motor performance
		Forced swim test (depression)	↓ latency to immobility
		Spontaneous activity in novel environment	↓ horizontal activity
		Acute amphetamine	↓ locomotor responses
		Acute cocaine	↓ locomotor responses

Table 1. Cont.

Study (Listed in Alphabetical Order)	Strategy to Target DA-Glutamate Co-Release	Test	Effect
Hnasko et al., 2010 [63]	$Vglut2^{ff}$;DAT-Cre	Spontaneous locomotion	−
		Rotarod (crude motor coordination)	−
		Acute cocaine	↓ locomotor responses
		Cocaine sensitization	−
		Cocaine conditioned place preference (CPP)	−
Mingote et al., 2017 [64]	$DAT^{IREScre/+}$::GLS1lox/+	Rotarod (crude motor coordination)	−
		Novelty induced locomotion	−
		Elevated plus maze (anxiety)	−
		Fear conditioning	−
		Acute amphetamine	−
		Amphetamine sensitization	↓
		Latent inhibition	↑
Papathanou et al., 2018 [24]	$Vglut2^{ff}$;DAT-CreERT2	Amphetamine and cocaine sensitization	− (baseline AMPA/NMDA ratio altered)
Wang et al., 2017 [65]	$Vglut2^{ff}$;DAT-Cre	RT-PP (optogenetics in VTA)	−
		Self-stimulation (optogenetics in VTA)	no effects on acquisition ↓ responses in higher laser power stimulation

2.5. DAT-Cre-Mediated Gene Targeting of VGLUT2 in Studies Aiming to Unravel the Importance of Glutamate Co-Release in Neurocircuitry of Reward and Addiction

Parallel to findings of VGLUT2 gene expression in midbrain DA neurons, initially detected in the adult rodent VTA [46] and in DA cell cultures [40], our own histological studies identified VGLUT2 in TH-positive neurons of the ventral midbrain of the mouse not only in adulthood but also in the developing embryo already at gestational day 12.5 (E12.5) [54] (Figure 2). Such an early developmental expression suggested to us that VGLUT2 might be important for proper DA cell development, and consequently, for dopaminergic functions at adulthood. At that time, we took two Cre-LoxP approaches to disrupt VGLUT2 in midbrain DA neurons to address if DA–glutamate co-release had any influence on dopaminergic functions. In both approaches, a floxed VGLUT2 mouse line [66,67] was crossed with a Cre-driver transgenic mouse to direct the targeting event to DA neurons: (i) TH-Cre and (ii) DAT-Cre. Both these Cre-drivers are active during embryonal development, from stages around mid-gestation of the mouse embryo. We also tested the "opposite" strategy, to delete the Vesicular monoamine transporter (VMAT2) gene in cells positive for VGLUT2 using a VGLUT2-Cre transgenic mouse line to target a floxed VMAT2 allele. However, this strategy, in which we aimed to delete DA signaling rather than glutamatergic signaling from DA–glutamate co-releasing neurons, resulted in dead pups around birth. We speculated that the neonatal death was due to a breathing phenotype similar to what we observed when deleting VGLUT2 in all cells [66], but caused by monoaminergic rather than glutamatergic loss of function in the breathing circuitry. However, beyond VGLUT2 in midbrain DA neurons, VGLUT2 is expressed in additional monoaminergic neuronal populations in the medulla, including noradrenergic neurons of nuclei A1 and A2 and adrenergic neurons of C1, C2, and C3 nuclei (see e.g., [68,69]), and loss of VMAT2 in these neurons could cause the loss of a series of vital autonomic functions. Further investigations would have been required to fully address the mechanisms for neonatal lethality of targeted deletion of VMAT2 in VGLUT2-neurons, however, we did not perform such studies.

By focusing on gene-targeting of VGLUT2, using the TH-Cre approach to disrupt VGLUT2 expression, we realized early on that TH-Cre will direct targeting to VGLUT2-positive neurons beyond DA neurons, due to an early and non-monoaminergic-selective phase of TH promoter activity [70].

The *Vglut2^{fff;TH-Cre}* cKO mice showed interesting hippocampal phenotypes [70], but were not used in our laboratory for further analysis of DA–glutamate co-releasing neurons. Instead, the approach using DAT-Cre to direct the targeted deletion of VGLUT2 to DA neurons was more promising. *Vglut2^{fff;DAT-Cre}* cKO and control mice were analyzed in several behavioral, electrochemical and biochemical parameters [54]. We found that basal motor and memory functions were normal in these cKO mice, but that their risk-taking behavior was altered. We also found that in both home-cage and novel environments, *Vglut2^{fff;DAT-Cre}* cKO mice showed a greatly blunted overall response to the psychostimulant amphetamine, which exerts strong effects on DA release. Specifically interesting, in a home-cage environment in which all movements were automatically registered, cKO mice showed a strikingly different response than the control with lower total activity at several different doses analyzed (Figure 4). When analyzing horizontal and vertical locomotion parameters separately, it was apparent that the cKO and control mice had strikingly different dose-response curves in terms of behavioral output. At higher doses, locomotion and rearing decreased in the control mice as stereotypic behavior became dominating. Stereotypy was detected as bodily shakings, and in the automated recording of any movement displayed by the mice, these shakings were recorded and contributed to the parameter of total activity. In control mice, the onset of stereotypic behavior thus caused a high level of total activity despite a reduction in locomotion and rearing. In contrast to control mice, cKO mice showed less stereotypy but increased both locomotion and rearing with higher doses. Since both motor function and basal locomotor activity were normal in the cKO mice, these parameters did not contribute to the differential response observed between genotypes. The finding rather suggested that the induction of stereotypic behavior seen at the higher doses in control mice did not at all develop to the same extent in *Vglut2^{fff;DAT-Cre}* cKO mice. The absence of stereotypy likely contributed to the overall lower activity of the cKO mice compared to control mice despite the increase in locomotion and rearing displayed by cKO mice at higher amphetamine doses. In contrast to this remarkable response at higher doses, both locomotion and rearing parameters were lower in cKO than control mice at lower doses, a blunted type of locomotion which might reflect a lower release level of mesostriatal DA in the absence of VGLUT2 in midbrain DA neurons, or which might be directly caused by the reduction of VGLUT2-mediated glutamatergic neurotransmission in the circuitry. In this context, it might be important to bear in mind that VGLUT2 in DA neurons is most abundant during embryonal development (as discussed above), when the DAT-Cre-mediated targeting of VGLUT2 is initiated in the *Vglut2^{fff;DAT-Cre}* cKO mice, suggesting that behavioral manifestations displayed by the cKO mice might be due to neurocircuitry compensations. Developmental adaptations will be further discussed below. In summary, the results of this first study implementing DAT-Cre to disrupt VGLUT2 in DA neurons with the aim to probe the putative importance of DA-glutamate co-release, demonstrated a strikingly altered response curve to amphetamine in the absence of VGLUT2. This finding led us to suggest that VGLUT2 in DAT-Cre neurons is important for the behavioral response to the psychostimulant amphetamine [54]. As described below, this initial finding was substantiated with subsequent studies using additional types of rewards and behavioral paradigms.

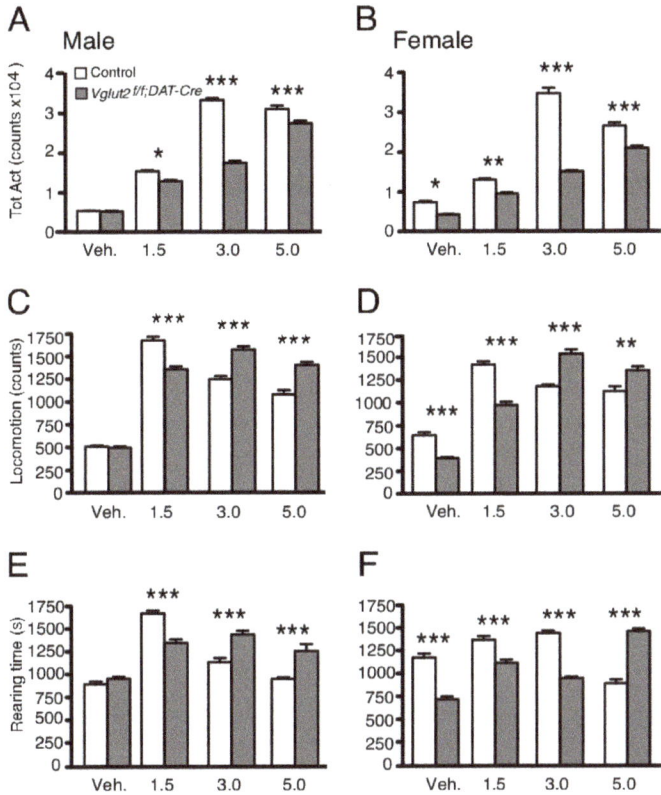

Figure 4. $Vglut2^{ff;DAT-Cre}$ mice show blunted behavioral response to amphetamine, as measured in a home-cage environment. (**A** and **B**) Male and female knockout mice showed a reduced behavioral response to amphetamine as shown by significantly lower total activity at all three doses of amphetamine. (**C** and **D**) Male and female knockout mice display a shift in dose-response to amphetamine-induced locomotion. (**E** and **F**) Male and female knockout mice show a different dose-response profile regarding rearing behavior in response to amphetamine. A right shift in dose-response in locomotion is apparent in the $Vglut2^{ff;DAT-Cre}$ mice. Data were analyzed with one-way ANOVA followed by Tukey's post-hoc test when appropriate. Data are presented as mean ± SEM (n = 9). *, $P < 0.05$; **, $P < 0.01$; ***, $P < 0.001$. Reprinted from Birgner et al., 2010 [54].

Using mouse genetics, several different DAT-Cre transgenic lines and floxed VGLUT2 lines have been produced and combined to create various $Vglut2^{ff;DAT-Cre}$ cKO lines for the study of DA–glutamate co-release. By using different versions of DAT-Cre and floxed VGLUT2 mouse lines, the different $Vglut2^{ff;DAT-Cre}$ cKO lines that exist are not identical but similar, a feature which could be of importance when analyzing the results generated. Also, experimental procedures can vary between laboratories. However, while some discrepancies can been detected when comparing results from different $Vglut2^{ff;DAT-Cre}$ cKO mouse lines and laboratories, overall, the findings point towards the same conclusion which implies DA–glutamate co-release in mechanisms of relevance to addiction. In one important study, Hnasko and colleagues confirmed that midbrain cell cultures from one $Vglut2^{ff;DAT-Cre}$ cKO mouse line lacked VGLUT2 in synaptic boutons of DA neurons and that cKO mice had reduced excitatory post-synaptic potentials (EPSCs) on MSNs of the NAc in response to electrical stimulation of the VTA [63]. Using optogenetic stimulation of DA neurons, Stuber and colleagues subsequently demonstrated that the EPSCs on NAc MSNs were completely abolished in these $Vglut2^{ff;DAT-Cre}$ cKO mice [57]. Behaviorally, *Vglut2^(fff;DAT-Cre)* cKO mice were confirmed to not have deficits in spontaneous locomotion or motor coordination [63], however, one study has reported reductions in spontaneous activity and disturbances in motor coordination in the rotarod motor test in one line of *Vglut2^(fff;DAT-Cre)* cKO mice [62]. Several studies have by now confirmed that *Vglut2^(fff;DAT-Cre)* cKO mice have blunted locomotor activity in response to acutely administered cocaine and amphetamine [54,62,63], but it has also been shown that cKO mice have normal behavioral sensitization after repeated injections of cocaine compared to their control littermates [63]. The cocaine-induced locomotor responses seem to be dissociated from the rewarding effects of cocaine since the cKO mice showed intact conditioned place preference (CPP) to the drug [63].

Following up on these initial studies in which the experimenter delivered drug injections to the rodent, we wished to advance the knowledge further by using operant self-administration methodology to come closer to the situation where the subject itself has the possibility to choose whether or not to administer a rewarding substance. Using the same *Vglut2^(fff;DAT-Cre)* cKO mouse line as in our previous experiments [54], we next analyzed the responses to both natural (sugar) and drug reward in such a self-administration paradigm to investigate how disruption of glutamate co-release from DA neurons is involved in reward processing. In the sugar self-administration test, in which nose-poking in an active nose-poke led to sucrose pellet delivery, *Vglut2^(fff;DAT-Cre)* cKO mice acquired the operant behavior similarly to control mice, but they self-administered significantly more sugar compared to controls. This was particularly evident when the task requirements were higher (FR5: 5 nose-pokes to receive a sucrose pellet) [61]. These responses were selective towards the highly palatable food and resistant to satiety; the cKO mice still consumed more calories from sucrose during the high-requirement task (FR5) compared to littermate controls [61]. When we then tested *Vglut2^(fff;DAT-Cre)* cKO mice in a cocaine self-administration paradigm, the mice displayed increased behavioral responding to receive lower doses of cocaine (Figure 5). Furthermore, during a cue-induced reinstatement phase, where nose-poking would lead only to presentation of cues associated with cocaine intake but not cocaine itself, cKO mice responded significantly more than controls just to receive the cues [61]. Taken together, these results demonstrate that mice lacking the ability to co-release glutamate from DA neurons display distinct patterns of behavior related to reward processing. While *Vglut2^(fff;DAT-Cre)* cKO mice show reduced locomotor activity in response to psychostimulants, specific aspects of the rewarding process associated to these drugs are intact. The animals form normal pavlovian associations in response to cocaine in CPP and they acquire similar rates of cocaine self-administration to control mice. In contrast, *Vglut2^(fff;DAT-Cre)* cKO mice seemed to be more sensitive to sugar and lower doses of cocaine, and strikingly, they were more susceptible to environmental stimuli associated with drug intake as shown by increased response in a cue-induced reinstatement phase during a cocaine self-administration paradigm.

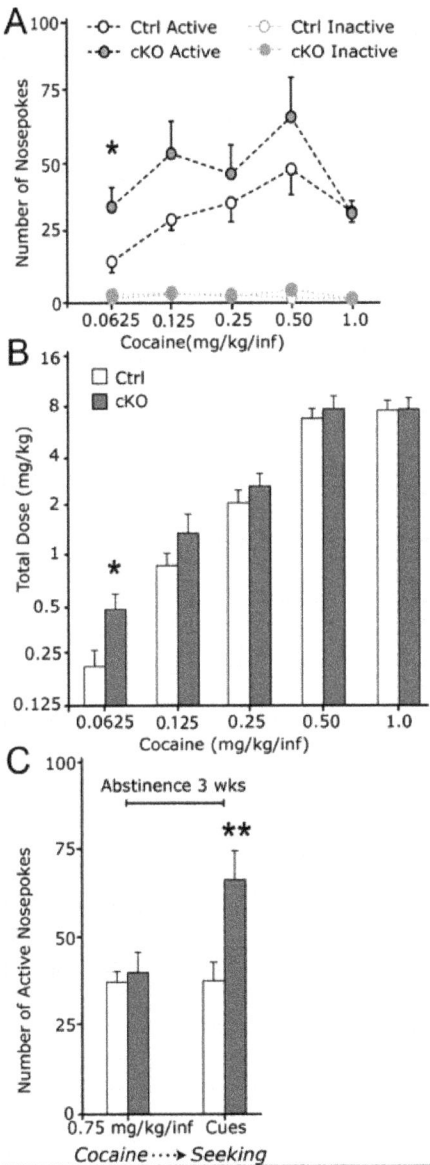

Figure 5. Elevated operant responding for low-dose cocaine and drug-paired cues during extinction in cKO mice. (**A**) Nosepoke response of food-trained mice implanted with indwelling intravenous catheters and allowed to nosepoke for cocaine infusions (controls, $n = 7$; cKO, $n = 7$). (**B**) Total dose self-administered at the different cocaine concentrations in (**A**). (**C**) Cocaine seeking, i.e., responding for light and sound cues previously associated with cocaine in the absence of the drug, of mice from A that had been responding for 0.75 mg/kg per infusion (inf) and subsequently subjected to 21 d of forced cocaine abstinence (controls, $n = 6$; cKO, $n = 5$). Group data represent mean ± SEM. *$p < 0.05$; **$p < 0.01$ versus Ctrl. Reprinted from Alsiö et al., 2011 [61].

To address molecular mechanisms, we next implemented a series of biochemical analyses. We found distinct molecular alterations in certain anatomical areas within the reward system of $Vglut2^{ff;DAT-Cre}$ cKO mice. Interestingly, these alterations could be observed both under baseline conditions and after cocaine administration and might explain the observed behavioral patterns discussed above. $Vglut2^{ff;DAT-Cre}$ cKO mice displayed elevated numbers of D1 receptors (D1R) in dorsal striatal areas and D2 receptors (D2R) in the shell region of the NAc, detected as increased binding of radio-labeled D1R and D2R ligands, respectively [61]. Furthermore, we found that cKO mice showed elevated mRNA levels of the nuclear receptor and immediate early gene Nur77 under baseline conditions in NAc core and dorsal striatal areas. The same elevation was seen in levels of c-Fos mRNA, another immediate early gene commonly used to assess neuronal activation. The elevated levels of Nur77 under baseline conditions in cKO mice were comparable to the ones observed is control mice after cocaine administration (Figure 6) [61]. Nurr77 expression is thought to be tonically inhibited by DA in the striatum and its upregulation to be related with neuroadaptations induced by chronic administration of drugs of abuse [71]. It is possible that the enhanced presence of D2R in the NAc disrupts the DA-mediated tone on Nur77 expression. Noteworthy, the detection of elevated levels of D2R might also reflect an increase in autoreceptors in presynaptic terminals related to decreased DA release. Increased levels of striatal DA receptors and immediate early genes Nur77 and c-Fos might render $Vglut2^{ff;DAT-Cre}$ cKO mice more susceptible to neuroadaptations related to chronic administration of drugs of abuse, or more sensitive to their rewarding properties. This could also be the case for natural rewards. In addition, several studies have identified reduced stimulation-induced DA levels in the striatum of these mice [61–63]. This reduction could be related to disrupted development of the DA system [62] or due to altered intracellular dynamics and reduced synaptic packaging of DA, the "primary" neurotransmitter, due to the absence of VGLUT2 in presynaptic terminals [63,72]. In both scenarios, less DA in the synaptic cleft would result in the cessation of the inhibitory signal to Nur77 expression which in turn may lead to the long-lasting neuroadaptations and behavioral manifestations that have been demonstrated in the studies discussed above. Together, these biochemical analyses demonstrated that gene-targeting of VGLUT2 in DAT-Cre neurons leads to molecular neuroadaptations that are similar to changes observed in control animals only upon systemic administration of addictive drugs (here demonstrated with cocaine). $Vglut2^{ff;DAT-Cre}$ cKO mice showed baseline levels of Nur77 and c-Fos elevated to the extent that cocaine administration did not increase them further, instead, baseline expression was already at the level observed in control mice upon drug administration. Together, the analyses of D1R and D2R availability and levels of immediate early gene expression strongly argue for a potent role of VGLUT2 in maintaining molecular homeostasis: When VGLUT2 is removed in DAT-Cre neurons from embryogenesis, there is a shift in the abundance of a range of molecular players that are important for normal functions of the DA system and this molecular shift is, in turn, likely to contribute to the behavioral manifestations observed in various reward-related experimental paradigms in which the response of the cKO mice differ significantly from that of the control mice.

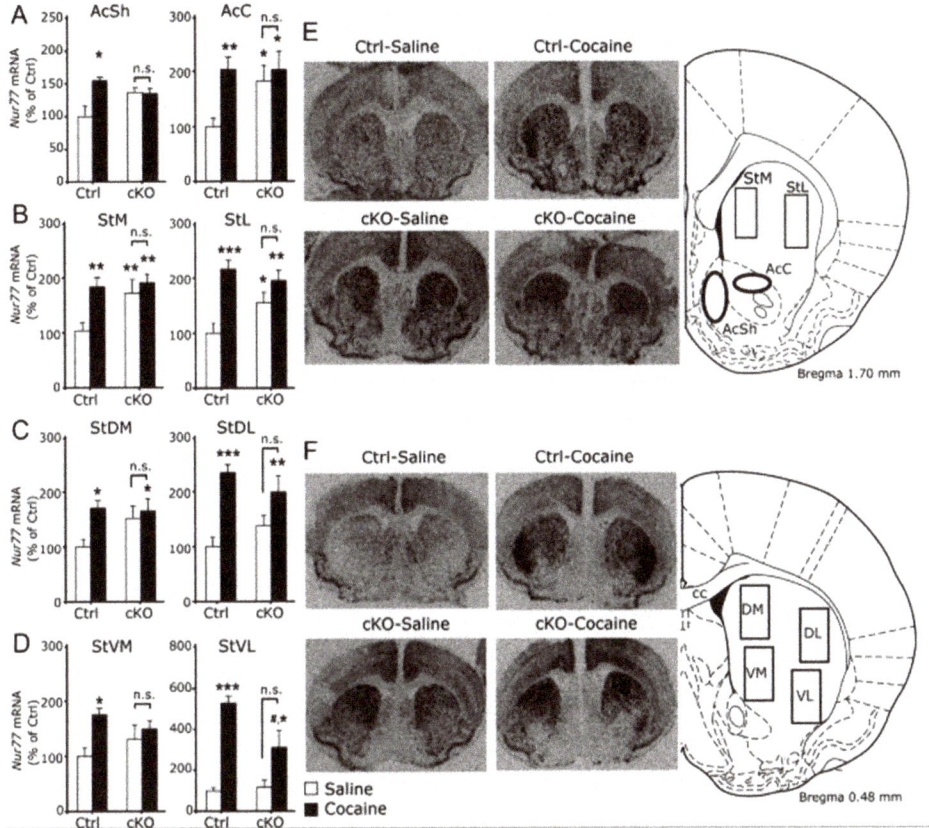

Figure 6. High expression of Nur77 under baseline conditions in cKO mice. (**A–D**) Quantitative in-situ hybridization of Nur77 mRNA levels in Ctrl and cKO mice treated with saline (Ctrl, $n = 6$; cKO, $n = 7$) or cocaine (Ctrl, $n = 5$; cKO, $n = 4$). (**A**) Levels of Nur77mRNAin AcSh and AcC (bregma, 1.70 mm). (**B**) Nur77mRNAlevels in medial (StM) and lateral (StL) rostral striatum (bregma, 1.70 mm). (**C**) Nur77 transcript levels in the caudodorsal striatum (bregma, 0.48 mm). (**D**) Nur77 levels in the caudoventral striatum (bregma, 0.48). (**E,F**) Representative autoradiograms of Nur77 mRNA in-situ hybridization signals in the rostral striatal area (**E**; bregma, 1.70 mm) and in the caudal striatal area (**F**; bregma, 0.48 mm) with schematic illustrations to the right showing the location of the analyzed regions. Group data represent mean ± SEM expressed as percentage of Ctrl (saline). *$p < 0.05$, **$p < 0.01$, and ***$p < 0.001$ versus Ctrl saline group; #$p < 0.05$ versus Ctrl cocaine group. cc, Corpus callosum. Reprinted from Alsiö et al., 2011 [61].

Drug and natural rewards can have several sites of action and influence systems that are not directly related to DA. Experimentally, optogenetic stimulation of the DA system has been used to isolate and dissect out the role of DA neurons in reward responses [73–75]. Previous studies have demonstrated that optogenetic stimulation of VTA DA neurons in mice has potent reinforcing effects on behavior and can induce molecular and behavioral adaptations similar to those observed after cocaine self-administration [76]. In a recent study, $Vglut2^{ff;DAT\text{-}Cre}$ cKO mice were addressed in a collaborative effort to further the understanding of DA-glutamate co-release by using optogenetic approaches to avoid non-selective effects of drug or natural rewards. In this study by Wang et al., we could confirm the reduction of glutamatergic neurotransmission in $Vglut2^{ff;DAT\text{-}Cre}$ cKO mice using both patch-clamp electrophysiology in slice preparations and in-vivo amperometry in the living mouse [65] (see Viereckel et al., [77], for protocol for optogenetics-coupled glutamate electrochemistry in-vivo). By implementing an optogenetics-based intracranial self-stimulation behavioral paradigm, it was found that the acquisition of operant behavior to optogenetically self-stimulate DA neurons in the VTA remained intact in $Vglut2^{\textit{fff;DAT-Cre}}$ cKO mice. However, the rate of responding when parameters of stimulation changed (intensity of stimulation from 8 mW to 32 mW) was lower in $Vglut2^{\textit{fff;DAT-Cre}}$ cKO mice compared to littermate controls [65]. Further, cKO and control mice showed the same level of real-time place preference (RT-PP) for a compartment paired to optogenetic stimulation [65].

To further explore how gene-targeting of VGLUT2 in DAT-Cre neurons might influence dopaminergic function, we recently performed a small pilot study in which $Vglut2^{\textit{fff;DAT-Cre}}$ cKO and control mice were compared in an extended version of the optogenetic self-stimulation paradigm described by Wang et al. [65]. We increased the testing time compared to the previous study [65] and also added several new phases to the program in an attempt to model different aspects of food or drug self-administration: Both fixed and progressive ratios were analyzed, followed through with sessions of forced abstinence, reinstatement, extinction and cue-induced reinstatement, respectively (Figure 7A). Upon stereotaxic surgery to deliver optogenetic DNA constructs to the VTA, mice were first validated in the optogenetic RT-PP paradigm which confirmed the strong RT-PP displayed by both $Vglut2^{\textit{fff;DAT-Cre}}$ cKO and control mice, in accordance with the previous study [65]. Next, the mice were tested in the extended optogenetic self-stimulation program and we could again confirm that cKO and control mice showed the same acquisition rate of the self-stimulation behavior [65]. Further, our extended program found no differences between cKO and control mice upon testing in a single progressive ratio session, in a reinstatement session after a period of forced abstinence or in a 5-day extinction phase where lever-pressing no longer resulted in optogenetic stimulation or cue presentation. However, when the mice were analyzed in a cue-induced reinstatement session, where lever-pressing resulted in cue-light presentation but not laser-stimulation (Figure 7B), cKO mice responded by lever-pressing significantly more vigorously than their littermate controls (Figure 7C & D). While this extended version of the optogenetic self-stimulation program has only been addressed in a modest number of animals, the striking difference observed between cKO and control mice in their behavioral response to cue-presentation should be of interest to address further to fully validate the findings and find out any underlying mechanims.

In summary, taken together with the previous study [65], the presented results here show that the actual acquisition of operant responding in the optogenetics-based self-stimulation paradigm is not different in $Vglut2^{\textit{fff;DAT-Cre}}$ cKO mice compared to control mice. Beyond this observation, by covering several additional behavioral parameters, our pilot study demonstrated that targeted removal of VGLUT2 in DAT-Cre neurons is sufficient to induce profound changes in the animal's response to cues associated with reward delivery. When considering this new result in the context of our previous data pin-pointing that the same transgenic line of $Vglut2^{\textit{fff;DAT-Cre}}$ cKO mice displayed increased behavioral response to cues associated with cocaine, an interesting picture appears: Mice lacking the ability for DA–glutamate co-release demonstrate distinct behavioral disturbances related to increased sensitivity to reward-associated cues. This finding strongly implies a role for DA–glutamate co-release in cue-induced reinstatement which, given its importance for relapse in human addicts, should be of particular interest to explore further in the context of interventive strategies.

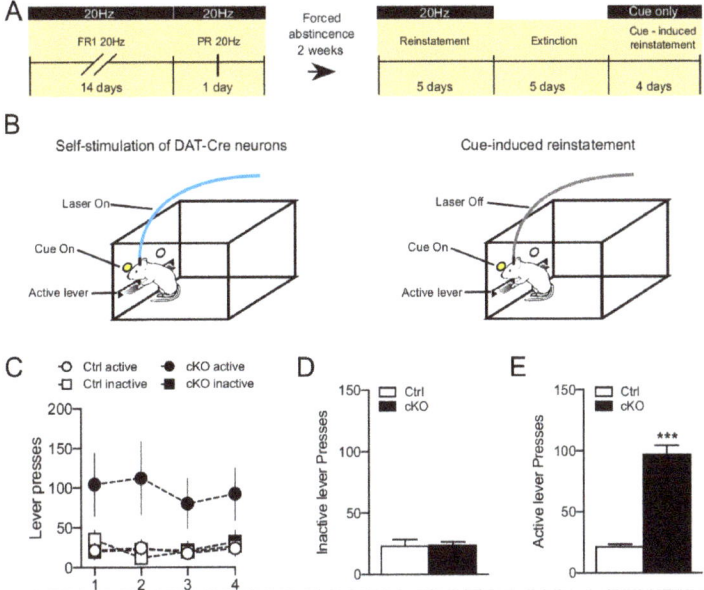

Figure 7. (**A**). Timeline of the intracranial optogenetic self-stimulation (ICSS) experiments. (**B**). Schematic representation of the ICSS procedure and the cue-induced reinstatement phase. (**C**). Active and inactive lever presses during the cue-induced reinstatement period for cKO and control mice. (**D,E**). Average of inactive (**D**) and active (**E**) during the cue-induced reinstatement phase cKO and Ctrl mice. Data are presented as mean ± SEM. *** $p < 0.001$ vs. ctrl. Ctrl $n = 3$, cKO $n = 3$. Original data, Bimpisidis and Wallén-Mackenzie, pilot study, 2019.

2.6. DAT-Cre-Mediated Gene Targeting of Phosphate-Activated Glutaminase (GLS1)

As mentioned above, knocking out VGLUT2 in DA neurons during embryonic development caused reduced release of DA in striatal areas in adulthood [61–63]. This finding might be either the result of disturbances in the development of the DA system when VGLUT2 is no longer present in these neurons [62], due to changes in the presynaptic milieu as a result of VGLUT2 absence [63,72], or both. Mingote and colleagues [64] applied a genetic approach to reduce glutamate release from DA neurons independently of VGLUT2 with the idea to circumvent the effects on DA availability upon VGLUT2 targeting. By using a $DAT^{IREScre/+}$::$GLS1lox/+$ mouse line in which the expression of phosphate-activated glutaminase (GLS1) was disrupted on the heterozygotic level in DAT-Cre neurons, a conditional reduction of glutamate synthesis in DA neurons was achieved. Using this approach, glutamate release from DA neurons was targeted in a frequency-dependent manner; the maintenance of glutamate release was disturbed mainly during high frequencies, normally associated with reward processing. Behaviorally, mice with reduced glutamate synthesis in DA neurons exhibit attenuated amphetamine sensitization and potentiated latent inhibition [64]. Latent inhibition refers to the phenomenon during which animals display attenuated conditioning when they are repeatedly pre-exposed to the conditioned stimulus in neutral settings, a condition thought to model the inability of patients with schizophrenia to show selective attention and to ignore irrelevant stimuli [78]. Attenuated behavioral sensitization and potentiated latent inhibition were previously associated to a mouse line with reduction of glutamate synthesis throughout the brain [78], but Mingote and colleagues narrowed down their observations to prove that the effects are mediated by reduction of glutamate synthesis selectively from DAT-Cre neurons. Indeed, a mouse line with reductions of glutamate synthesis in forebrain areas did not demonstrate the same behavioral manifestations [64]. The role of DA–glutamate co-release in latent inhibition should be of interest to further research in the context of substance use/abuse.

2.7. Some Caveats in the Implementation of Transgenics to Address Neuronal Function

All studies discussed above implemented transgenic approaches that target glutamate co-release from early developmental stages with the common feature of DAT-Cre transgenic mouse lines to drive the recombination of floxed alleles. Since the activity of the endogenous promoters for VGLUT2 [54,70] and DAT [79] both have embryonal onset, it is possible that the observed phenotypes are the result of developmental adaptations resulting from the gene-targeting event of VGLUT2. This possibility has been discussed in the literature cited above, and indeed, it has also been experimentally shown in one $Vglut2^{ff;DAT-Cre}$ mouse line that cKO mice have impaired DA neuron development; the number of midbrain DA neurons and their projections to striatal areas are significantly reduced when VGLUT2 is not present in DAT-Cre neurons [62]. Also, as discussed above, major molecular neuroadaptations occur as a consequence of VGLUT2 gene-targeting with the elevation of D1R and D2R availability and enhanced c-Fos and Nur77 expression levels at baseline conditions. Based on all of these observations, it is highly conceivable that VGLUT2 plays a developmental role in the establishment of the nervous system, a role that stretches beyond its role as pre-synaptic transporter of glutamate into synaptic vesicles. While it has been challenging to dissociate putative developmental adaptations following gene-targeting of VGLUT2 in DA neurons from effects that are solely dependent of loss of vesicular glutamate packaging, issues related to VGLUT2 were avoided using the GLS1-approach presented by Mingote and colleagues [64]. However, not only regulation of VGLUT2 but also the spatio-temporal regulation of the DAT promoter, the sequence of which is used to drive the expression of Cre recombinase in DAT-Cre mice, may also present challenges. Implementation of developmentally regulated promotors always carries the risk of neuroadaptations that might be responsible for behavioral phenotypes, thus leading to misleading conclusions. Furthermore, ectopic expression of Cre recombinase can lead to unwanted targeting [80–82]. In the context of DAT-Cre, we could recently show that several DAT-Cre mouse lines show ectopic expression of Cre recombinase in multiple brain areas that are not associated with monoaminergic neurotransmission. For example, certain amygdaloid subnuclei, septal nuclei and neurons in the lateral habenula, all of which contain VGLUT2 but not DAT, were strongly positive for the DAT-Cre transgenes [82]. Bearing this important observation in mind, it is possible that any results obtained using a DAT-Cre transgene to achieve gene-targeting of a floxed VGLUT2 or GLS1 allele, or any other floxed allele, might be dependent on recombination of the floxed gene in these non-monoaminergic areas. Possible "off-target" effects mediated by DAT-Cre are crucial to consider as they could have consequences on physiological and behavioral output, and hence on conclusions drawn from such experiments. Finding more selective tools to address DA–glutamate co-release in reward and addiction is highly relevant, not least in light of this new revelation.

2.8. DA–Glutamate Co-Release in Neuronal Plasticity within the Ventral Striatum

To address DA–glutamate co-release specifically in the adult mouse and to avoid any developmental effects upon VGLUT2-gene-targeting, we recently applied an inducible knockout approach [24]. In this study, we took advantage of a tamoxifen-inducible DAT-CreERT2 mouse line [83] in which DAT-Cre-expressing neurons will translocate Cre recombinase into the nucleus only upon tamoxifen administration. We could show that the spatial expression pattern of Cre recombinase in the inducible DAT-CreERT2 line is similar to the conventional DAT-Cre line implemented in our previous studies, while the temporal expression is regulated by the time at which the tamoxifen is provided. The new $Vglut2^{ff;DAT-CreERT2}$ cKO mouse line was compared with our previously published $Vglut2^{ff;DAT-Cre}$ cKO mouse line (described above) in a range of experiments in order to have the same VGLUT2 floxed allele targeted by the two different DAT-Cre-drivers. By comparative analysis of $Vglut2^{ff;DAT-CreERT2}$ and $Vglut2^{ff;DAT-Cre}$ cKO mice, we observed that when glutamate co-release was disrupted in adulthood, the mice displayed strikingly different behaviors in response to amphetamine and cocaine compared to mice with a developmentally-induced VGLUT2 targeting event. Unlike the drug-induced locomotor response observed in the $Vglut2^{fff;DAT-Cre}$ cKO mice, which was lower than that shown by control mice, the inducible $Vglut2^{fff;DAT-CreERT2}$ cKO mice displayed a similar level of drug-induced locomotor activity as controls [24]. Additionally, when electrophysiological experiments were performed to investigate how reduced levels of glutamate release from DA neurons might affect the plasticity observed after chronic drug administration, we found that inducible $Vglut2^{fff;DAT-CreERT2}$ mice displayed characteristic increases in markers of synaptic plasticity already under baseline conditions. $Vglut2^{fff;DAT-CreERT2}$ mice showed an increased AMPA/NMDA ratio on D1R-expressing MSNs compared to controls, and these changes were sufficient to occlude further increases normally seen following chronic cocaine administration [24] (Figure 8A). Increased AMPA/NMDA ratio is indicative of the presence of GluR2-lacking subunits of the AMPA receptor that have higher peak conductance and Ca^{2+} permeability and thus higher inward-rectifying properties (expressed as higher rectification index) [1]. While the inducible $Vglut2^{fff;DAT-CreERT2}$ cKO mice showed an increased AMPA/NMDA ratio in baseline conditions, the rectification index of MSNs was unaltered (Figure 8B), reflecting mechanisms others than the replacement of GluR2 in AMPARs [24]. These mechanisms may include net increases in AMPA receptors, decreases in NMDA receptors, or both. Clearly, the mechanisms underlying the observed increases in baseline AMPA/NMDA ratios require further investigation to fully understand this type of regulation. However, already now, these data suggest that deletion of VGLUT2 in mature neurons induced changes in neuronal plasticity already under baseline conditions and that inducible $Vglut2^{fff;DAT-CreERT2}$ cKO mice might have abnormal drug- or other stimuli-induced plasticity. More studies will be needed to find out how these observed changes might be of importance to addiction.

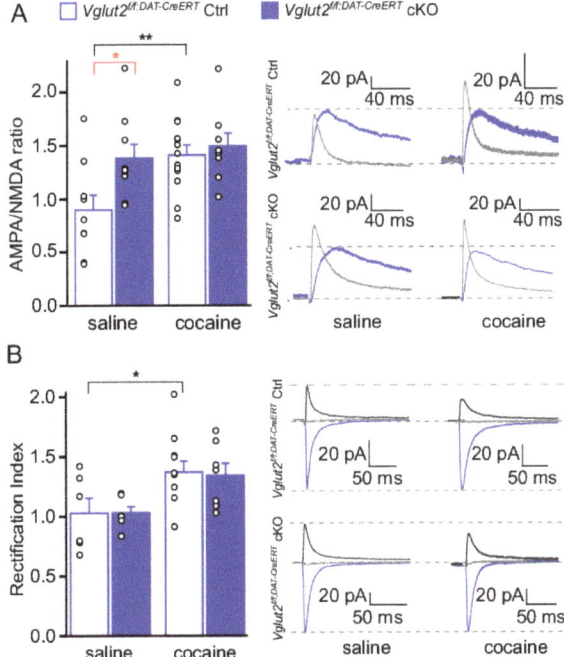

Figure 8. VGLUT2 targeting in mature DA neurons results in an elevated baseline AMPA/NMDA ratio. (**A**) AMPA/NMDA ratio and raw traces of cells from $Vglut2^{fff;DAT-CreERT}$ cKO and ctrl mice treated with saline or cocaine for NMDA current (blue); AMPA current (light gray). (**B**) Rectification index (RI) and

raw traces recorded cells from $Vglut2^{ffDAT-CreERT}$ cKO and ctrl mice treated with saline or cocaine. eKO-DRD1 and eCtrl-DRD1 mice treated with saline or cocaine at −70 mV (blue), 0 mV (light gray) and +40 mV (dark gray). Two-way ANOVA Sidak post hoc (ANOVA ###$p < 0.001$; post hoc between genotype *$p < 0.05$ and post hoc between treatment of same genotype: *$p < 0.05$, **$p < 0.01$, ***$p < 0.001$; RI saline: saline $Vglut2^{ffDAT-CreERT}$ Ctrl, $n = 6$, $Vglut2^{ffDAT-CreERT}$ cKO, $n = 6$; cocaine: $Vglut2^{ffDAT-CreERT}$ Ctrl, $n = 12$; $Vglut2^{ffDAT-CreERT}$ cKO, $n = 7$; AMPA/NMDA ratio saline:: $Vglut2^{ffDAT-CreERT}$ Ctrl, $n = 9$, $Vglut2^{ffDAT-CreERT}$ cKO, $n = 9$; cocaine: $Vglut2^{ffDAT-CreERT}$ Ctrl, $n = 13$, $Vglut2^{ffDAT-CreERT}$ cKO, $n = 7$). Whole-cell patch clamp experiments performed on slices 10 days after last saline or cocaine injection. Reprinted from Papathanou et al., 2018 [24].

In summary, the main take-home message appearing from the various studies knocking out VGLUT2 in DAT-Cre neurons is that detectable neurocircuitry and behavioral changes do indeed occur upon targeted disruption of VGLUT2. No matter which combination of DAT-Cre transgene and floxed VGLUT2 allele that have been combined to probe DA–glutamate co-release, behavioral manifestations all point towards functional aspects of particular interest to reward and substance use/abuse. The availability of VGLUT2 in DA neurons of human individuals [49] might thereby be an important aspect to address in terms of vulnerability and pre-disposition to addiction, as briefly discussed further below.

2.9. Dopamine–Glutamate Co-Release: Implications for Reward Processing

How can all these observations from experimental animals be brought together into a comprehensive model to understand the potential role of DA–glutamate co-release in addiction? Despite the fact that additional studies are necessary in order to fully understand the role of co-release in behavioral regulation even under normal conditions, let alone under conditions of substance abuse, the findings reported in the research field so far can be summarized to form hypotheses related to the observed manifestations.

Drugs that are abused by human individuals can change brain physiology in many ways and eventually lead to characteristic and chronic behavioral patterns clinically known as substance use disorder. An abundance of studies has implicated several major neurotransmitter systems, including the DA and glutamate systems, in these phenomena while the role of combined DA and glutamate effects derived from the same neuron, i.e., DA–glutamate co-release, has only recently begun to be explored. Most studies in the addiction field have focused on the MSNs, as these neurons constitute the majority of neurons in the striatum. Similarly, initial studies of post-synaptic effects of DA–glutamate co-release have mainly been focused on recordings of MSN activity [24,56,57,63]. In the context of MSNs, Adrover and colleagues concluded that acute cocaine administration attenuates the DA neuron-induced EPSCs on MSNs through D2R activation based on the observation that the D2R antagonist sulpiride could reverse these effects [84]. Further, repeated cocaine administrations altered glutamatergic synapses between VTA terminals and NAc shell neurons in a withdrawal-dependent manner. After one day of withdrawal, there were no significant effects on the synapses, but when the VTA-NAc shell synapses were investigated three weeks after the last cocaine injection, a small but significant reduction in probability of neurotransmitter release was observed. This finding might suggest altered plasticity on the presynaptic level on DA–glutamate co-releasing populations, however, through the approach utilized, it cannot be excluded that the observed synapses were solely glutamatergic [85].

As described above, synaptic glutamate release in the striatum exerts different actions in a region- and neuron-type-dependent manner. DA–glutamate co-release has been demonstrated to not show the same distribution pattern throughout the striatum [57,86] and glutamate co-released into the NAc mSh affects ChIs more than MSNs or fast-spiking interneurons [58]. ChIs only constitute about 1–2% of striatal neurons in rodents, but they exert diffuse and profound effects on the physiology of the area [87,88]. ChIs display distinct burst-pause firing patterns and through ACh release, they can modulate presynaptic neurons by acting both at nicotinic and muscarinic ACh receptors [87,89]. Burst-pause firing rates in ChIs coincide with changes in the firing rate of DA neurons in response to reward-related, salient events but they convey different information compared to DA neuron firing [90];

pauses in their synchronous activity is thought to provide an optimal window where DA release due to increases in action potential frequency will have highest efficiency to promote the conveyed messages [11]. The psychostimulant amphetamine which increases DA release in terminal regions, has different effects depending on the region of the striatum and the neuronal type investigated. Thus, it attenuates the "burst-pause" neuronal activity observed on ChIs in the mSh in a dose-dependent manner, as shown by Chuhma et al. [58]. Only high doses affect post-synaptic activity on ChIs in the dorsal striatum while they have little effects on NAc core and on the EPSCs of MSNs in NAc mSh [58]. While the effects of chronic administration of drugs were not investigated in the study by Chuhma and colleagues, these observations indicate that psychostimulants can induce plasticity in different ways depending on anatomical region that in some instances can lead to behavioral abnormalities associated with chronic drug intake.

While it is known that SNc DA neurons project to the dorsal striatum, it has also been well established that VTA DA projections to striatal areas follow a medio-lateral topographical organization in the sense that DA neurons of the medial aspect of the VTA project to the NAc mSh and DA neurons located in the lateral aspect of the VTA project to NAc core [91]. DA neurons in the medial aspect of the VTA, which project mainly to the NAc mSh, are the ones that show the highest VGLUT2 expression levels, as described above. These histological findings have recently been confirmed using novel approaches implementing dual intersectional systems combining promoter activity of both TH and VGLUT2 to achieve selectivity for DA–glutamate co-releasing neurons [44,92]. Using these new approaches, previous results could be confirmed, firmly demonstrating that TH+/VGLUT2+ double-positive cell bodies are located primarily in the medial VTA. Further, identification of NAc mSh projections showed that this region receives the highest percentage of DA–glutamate co-release compared to other parts of the striatum [44,92]. As discussed above, the NAc mSh is a region highly implicated in reward-related behavior and drug addiction.

Based on novel findings that glutamate released by DA neurons mostly affect ChIs in this area, physiological and behavioral effects of DA-glutamate co-release will be discussed in this context. As outlined in a recent comprehensive review by Mingote and colleagues [44], glutamate released from DA neurons modulates the activity of ChIs, initially by increasing their firing rate [58]. This increase is correlated to the release of ACh which acts through nicotinic pre-synaptic receptors to affect DA terminals and further increases DA levels [87,89]. Mingote and colleagues suggest that these subsequent DA increases are necessary to induce behavioral switching, meaning that the organism will be able to engage in alternative behavioral patterns not associated to reward occurrence [44] (Figure 9). This hypothesis is supported by experimental studies on extinction and behavioral observations on $DAT^{IREScre/+}$::$GLS1lox$/+ mice. As discussed above, behavioral studies of these mice showed that they exhibit potentiated latent inhibition compared to control mice [64]. Under normal conditions, control mice would switch their behavior when exposed to conflicting contingencies, but reduced glutamate from DA neurons in the NAc mSh in $DAT^{IREScre/+}$::$GLS1lox$/+ mice induced a potentiation of the preserved response resulting in enhanced latent inhibition [44,64]. Data from our $Vglut2^{f/f;DAT-Cre}$ cKO mice also support this model: $Vglut2^{f/f;DAT-Cre}$ cKO mice will continue operant responding in response to cocaine [61] or optogenetic stimulation cues (Figure 7) during extinction. It is possible that reduction of glutamate release from DA–glutamate co-releasing neurons projecting to NAc mSh prevents disinhibition of downstream circuits which under normal conditions would promote alternative strategies and eventually lead to more efficient reward obtaining behaviors. This is demonstrated through persevered behaviors that can be related to cue-induced relapse in human addicts. For example, pre-clinical studies have demonstrated higher levels of VGLUT2 in terminals of alcohol-preferring rats after alcohol deprivation [93], and severe alcohol use disorder has been associated with polymorphisms in VGLUT2 [94]. While not making a distinction between VGLUT2 in glutamatergic neurons versus DA–glutamate co-releasing neurons in these studies, it is interesting and provoking to consider that alterations in VGLUT2 levels can affect both types of glutamatergic transmission in NAc mSh. Finally, it is possible that disturbed DA–glutamate co-release is responsible for drug-related behavioral manifestations due to overall altered DA tone and consequently to disturbances in behavioral switching.

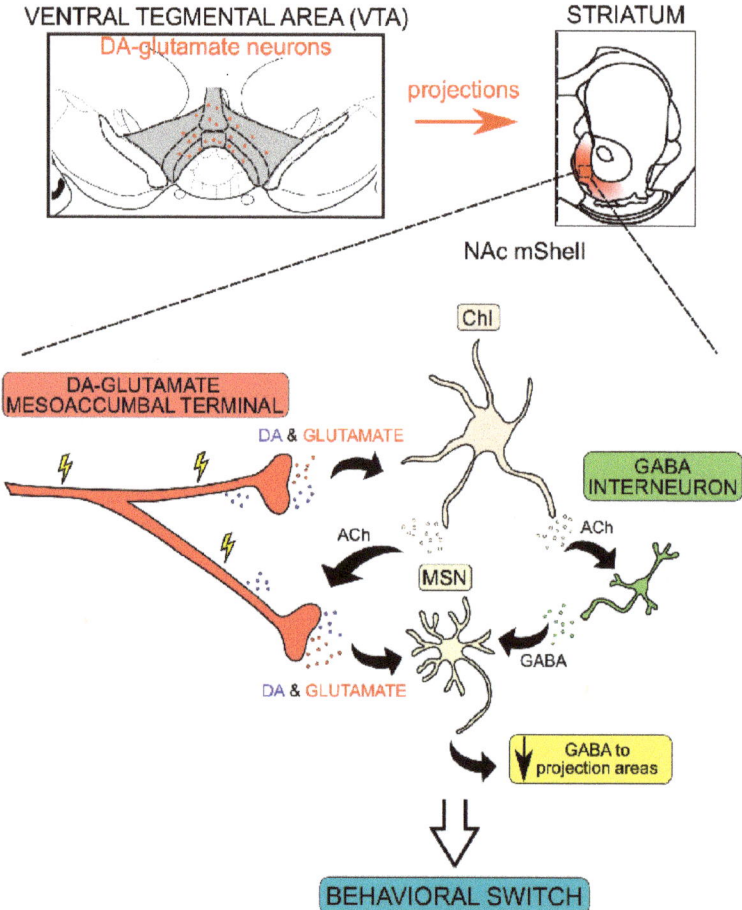

Figure 9. Simplified schematic model of down-stream neurocircuitry effects upon dopamine (DA)–glutamate co-release in the ventral striatal area leading to behavioral output. DA–glutamate co-releasing neurons (red) are located primarily in the medial part of the ventral tegmental area (VTA; gray) from where they project to the nucleus accumbens medial shell (NAc mShell). Burst-firing of these neurons leads to a release of DA and glutamate from mesoaccumbal nerve terminals which subsequently act on DA and glutamate receptors located on cholinergic interneurons (ChIs) and medium spiny neurons (MSNs) in the NAc mShell. DA and glutamate neurotransmission via receptors located on ChIs leads to synchronized activity and acetylcholine (ACh) release. ACh subsequently acts on ACh receptors located in VTA presynaptic terminals to further increase neurotransmitter release. DA and glutamate release, together with increased release of GABA from GABAergic interneurons, also leads to inhibition of the GABAergic MSNs, which in turn leads to disinhibiton of target areas and allows for the occurence of behaviors associated with alternative strategies to obtain reward, a "behavioral switch". Drawing based on original illustration by Mingote et al., 2019 [44].

2.10. Whole-Brain Analysis and Improved Selectivity in Animal Models Should Enhance Current Knowledge of DA-Glutamate Co-Releasing Neurons

While most of the published studies regarding DA–glutamate co-release have focused on the projections from the VTA to the NAc, it has also been reported that co-releasing neurons of the VTA project to a broader set of limbic regions in the rodent brain. The medial prefrontal cortex (mPFC), amygdala and hippocampus have all been shown to receive DA–glutamate co-releasing fibers from the VTA with different synaptic strengths [39,47,86,95–97]. As these brain areas have been strongly implicated in reward processing and drug-induced behavioral adaptations, future studies could aim to investigate the role of DA–glutamate co-release in each of these areas both under normal conditions and in models of disorders, such as addiction and schizophrenia. Furthermore, and consistent with the regional heterogeneity observed within the striatum, neurons of dual DA–glutamate profiles might have different effects on neurocircuitry depending on the target area. For instance, DA neurons projecting to the mPFC have been shown to code for aversive events [98,99] while DA release in the mPFC has the potential to alter dopaminergic and behavioral responses of subcortical areas to both natural stimuli [100] and addictive drugs [101]. For example, one question remaining to be addressed is how mesocortical DA–glutamate co-releasing neurons might influence subcortical responses to salient stimuli. In summary, by opening up for studies covering a brain perspective beyond the striatum, it seems likely that the knowledge of how DA–glutamate co-release affects physiology and behavior of relevance to both health and disease could be increased further.

Another point worth considering to forward current knowledge is the availability of animal models. It has been discussed in the literature how the lack of appropriate animal models has made it challenging to fully address behavioral roles of DA–glutamate co-release [19,22]. While this is indeed true, as outlined above, by implementing Cre-Lox-transgenics in rodents, the results of several different studies converge towards a strong implication for a role of DA–glutamate co-release in reward processing of relevance to addiction [54,61–64]. To now reach further, a higher level of selectivity is on the wish-list. For example, the recently described intersectional approaches ([44,92] and described above) should prove useful for further investigation of DA–glutamate co-release. To advance selectivity when creating new animal models, a first step forward might be to increase the level of anatomical and molecular knowledge of neurons that possess the ability for co-release.

By enhancing current knowledge of molecularly defined subpopulations in the VTA, it may be possible to increase the level of resolution in the anatomical-functional mapping of DA-glutamate co-releasing neurons. In this context, we have recently demonstrated that some, but not all, DA–glutamate co-releasing neurons in the VTA express the NeuroD6 gene, a finding which opens up for subtyping DA–glutamate co-releasing neurons based on molecular profiles beyond TH, DAT and VGLUT2 [102]. Since our identification of VGLUT2 expression in subsets of DA neurons from early embryonal development ([54] and discussed above), we have viewed the VGLUT2-positive DA neuronal population as a distinct subpopulation within the VTA, in accordance with current literature. Based on our initial study [54], we reasoned that the VTA might contain additional subpopulations that, if they could be identified by a molecular profile, could be used to dissect out the causality between distinct neuronal activity in the VTA and behavioral regulation of importance to reward and addiction. To search for additional gene expression patterns that, beyond VGLUT2, might distinguish DA neurons from each other, we performed a microarray analysis followed through with systematic histological validation. Through several steps of analyses, we could identify a number of gene expression patterns that were selective for neuronal groups within the VTA, suggesting that they might represent molecularly definable VTA subpopulations [23]. Similar types of studies have been performed in the pre-clinical DA field focused on Parkinson's disease, which have substantially enriched molecular knowledge of both the VTA and the adjacently located SNc [103,104]. Recently, the advancement of transcriptomics analyses has enabled further gene expression analysis of the VTA and SNc [105,106]. All studies mapping out gene expression patterns in a particular brain location are of particular interest as they provide molecular tools that enable the anatomical-functional dissection of "subpopulations" (or "subgroups" or "subtypes") of neurons.

In our microarray screen comparing gene expression in the VTA and the SNc, we identified the gene encoding the neurogenic basic helix-loop-helix transcription factor NeuroD6 as enriched in the VTA [23]. NeuroD6, which has also been reported by others [105,107,108], was found primarily in DA neurons located in the medial aspect of the VTA, suggesting that NeuroD6 expression represents a distinct subpopulation within the group of medially positioned VTA DA neurons that primarily project to the NAc Sh [23]. We also found that some, but not all, NeuroD6 VTA DA neurons were positive for VGLUT2 (Figure 10). This finding leads us to propose that the DA–glutamate co-releasing phenotype can be dissociated further based on molecular identity. While anatomically interesting, the most important aspect of molecular profiling is when it can be coupled to functional output. To directly test if we could identify a distinct role in behavioral regulation mediated by the newly discovered NeuroD6 VTA subpopulation, we implemented optogenetics using transgenic NeuroD6-Cre mice (also known as NEX-Cre) to direct optogenetic activation selectively to this NeuroD6-positive subpopulation. NeuroD6-Cre mice were compared with DAT-Cre and VGLUT2-Cre mice in a range of optogenetics-based analyses [102]. The experiments provided evidence for both glutamate and DA release in the NAcSh upon optogenetic stimulation in the VTA and could also demonstrate that selective stimulation of NeuroD6 VTA neurons led to significant place preference in a similar, but not identical, manner as when the entire VTA DA neuronal population was activated [102] (Figure 11). Activation of the NeuroD6 VTA subpopulation, with its mixed DA–glutamate co-releasing and non-co-releasing properties, is thereby sufficient to induce a distinct behavioral response [102]. This new finding should be well-worth exploring further in the context of substance use/abuse. This study is an example of how molecular knowledge of distinct VTA neurons can be used to implement available animal models in a new way or to even create new animal models with spatial and temporal selectivity for distinct neuronal subgroups at a level required to advance current knowledge of co-releasing neurons. By establishing direct causality between distinct subgroups of DA–glutamate co-releasing neurons and behavioral regulation of importance to reward and addiction, future studies can use this kind of knowledge to understand how regulation of co-release could be implemented clinically for the benefit of future interventive strategies in substance use disorders.

2.11. Concluding Remarks

This review has summarized the main findings derived from behavioral analyses in genetically modified mice produced with the aim of pin-pointing the putative relevance of DA–glutamate co-release in behavioral regulation. While different kinds of transgenic mouse lines have been generated and analyzed in various methodological paradigms spanning from baseline locomotion to self-administration of abusive substances, all studies share the common conclusion that behaviors of particular interest for addiction are altered when glutamate co-release is disrupted (results summarized in Table 1 and illustrated in Figure 12). Many questions remain to be answered, but so far, the experimental findings point towards glutamate co-release as a putative target in the treatment of substance use disorder, including prevention of relapse. The study of DA–glutamate co-release for clinical purposes would benefit from a higher degree of selectivity in experimental approaches which could aid in determining how this type of signaling could be used as a tool in prevention and treatment of addiction.

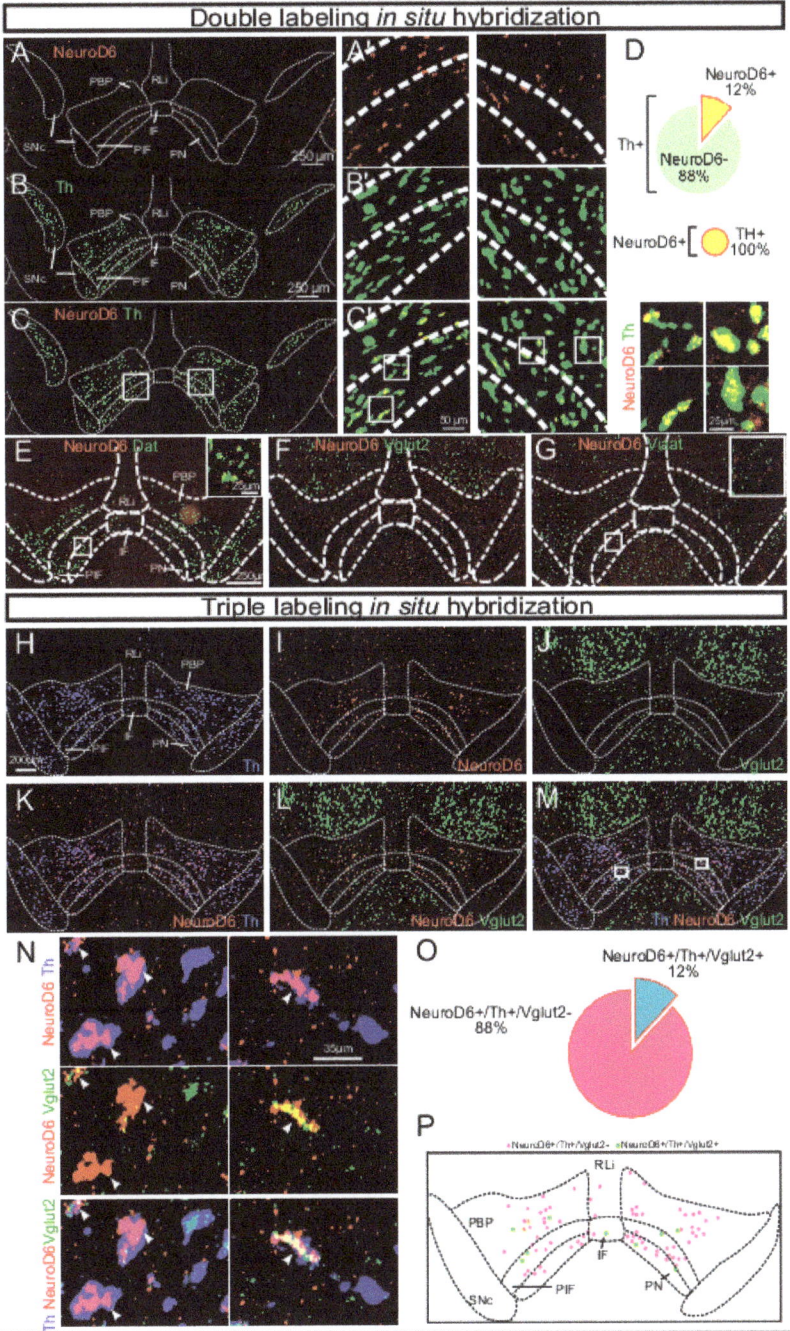

Figure 10. NeuroD6 mRNA is found in a modest population of the VTA and co-localizes with dopaminergic markers and partially with a glutamatergic marker. (**A–G**) Double FISH in the ventral midbrain of adult wild-type mice detecting the following mRNAs. **A**, **A′**, NeuroD6 (red). (**B,B′**) Th (green). (**C,C′**) NeuroD6 (red) and Th (green). Th/NeuroD6 mRNA that overlap are shown in yellow.

Low magnification to the left; close-ups to the right. Schematic outline shows borders for SNc and subregions of VTA: PN, PIF, PBP, IF, RLi. (**D**) Quantification of percentage of NeuroD6-positive cells among all Th VTA cells; all NeuroD6 cells are positive for Th mRNA. (**E**) NeuroD6 (red) and Dat (green), inset with high magnification of Dat/NeuroD6 mRNA overlap (yellow). (**F**) NeuroD6 (red) and Vglut2 (green). (**G**) NeuroD6 (red) and Viaat (green), inset with high magnification of Viaat-negative/NeuroD6-positive (red). (**H–P**) Triple-labeling FISH in the ventral midbrain of adult wild-type mice detecting: (**H**) Th (blue); (**I**) NeuroD6 (red); (**J**) Vglut2 (green) mRNAs and their co-localization: (**K**) NeuroD6/Th; (**L**) NeuroD6/Vglut2; (**M**) Th/NeuroD6/Vglut2. Cellular closeups: (**N**) NeuroD6/Th (top), NeuroD6/Vglut2 (middle), and Th/NeuroD6/Vglut2 (bottom). Arrows point to NeuroD6 mRNA-positive cells. (**O**) Quantification of percentage of NeuroD6+/Th+/Vglut2+ and NeuroD6+/Th+/Vglut2- neurons of the VTA. (**P**) Schematic illustration of distribution pattern of NeuroD6+/Th+/Vglut2+ and NeuroD6+/Th+/Vglut2- neurons within the VTA (same as shown with experimental data in **M**). NeuroD6+/Th+/Vglut2- cells in magenta; NeuroD6+/Th+/Vglut2+ cells in cyan. VTA, ventral tegmental area; SNc, substantia nigra pars compacta; PBP, parabrachial pigmented nucleus; PN, paranigral nucleus; PIF, parainterfascicular nucleus; RLi, rostral linear nucleus; IF, interfascicular nucleus. FISH, fluorescent in situ; Dat, Dopamine transporter; Th, Tyrosine hydroxylase; Vglut2, Vesicular glutamate transporter 2; Viaat, Vesicular inhibitory amino acid transporter. Reprinted from Bimpisidis et al., 2019 [102].

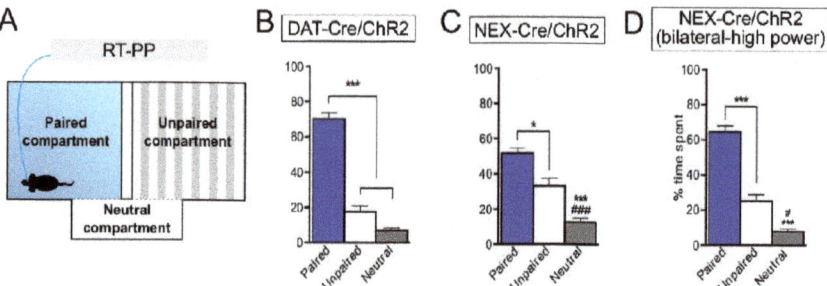

Figure 11. Optogenetic activation of NeuroD6 VTA neurons induces place preference. (**A**) Schematic drawing of the real-time place preference (RT-PP) experimental setup. (**B–D**) average percentage of time spent in each compartment during 4 days of RT-PP ± SEM (bar graphs; right; *$p < 0.05$, ***$p < 0.001$ vs. light-paired compartment; #$p < 0.05$, ##$p < 0.01$, ###$p < 0.001$ vs. unpaired compartment). DAT-Cre, $n = 10$; NEX-Cre, $n = 5$, high-power stimulation of bilaterally-injected NEX-Cre mice, $n = 4$. Reprinted from Bimpisidis et al., 2019 [102].

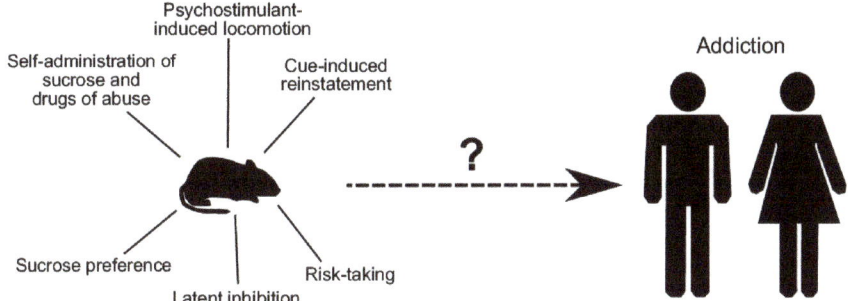

Figure 12. Schematic illustration of behaviors relevant to addiction confirmed in experimental mice to be altered upon disruption of dopamine–glutamate co-release (see text and Table 1). Further studies will be needed to outline how these behaviors relate to typical behaviors of addiction displayed by humans and how dopamine–glutamate co-release can be used as a future target for prevention and treatment.

Author Contributions: Conceptualization and funding acquisition, Å.W.-M.; Writing—original draft, review and editing, Z.B. and Å.W.-M.

Funding: This work was funded by Uppsala University and by grants to ÅWM from the Swedish Research Council (Vetenskapsrådet), Parkinsonfonden, Hjärnfonden and the Research Foundations of Bertil Hållsten, Åhlén and Zoologisk Forskning.

Acknowledgments: Present and previous colleagues in the Mackenzie lab as well as collaborators and colleagues over the world are thanked for contributions to the studies discussed in the text. While we have tried to include all relevant references, we apologize if any citation is wrong or missing. Figures from our own previous work have been reprinted with permission from the publishers.

Conflicts of Interest: The authors declare no conflict of interest.

References

1. Lüscher, C. The Emergence of a Circuit Model for Addiction. *Annu. Rev. Neurosci.* **2016**, *39*, 257–276. [CrossRef]
2. Volkow, N.D.; Morales, M. The Brain on Drugs: From Reward to Addiction. *Cell* **2015**, *162*, 712–725. [CrossRef]
3. Kalivas, P.W. The glutamate homeostasis hypothesis of addiction. *Nat. Rev. Neurosci.* **2009**, *10*, 561–572. [CrossRef]
4. Kourrich, S.; Calu, D.J.; Bonci, A. Intrinsic plasticity: An emerging player in addiction. *Nat. Rev. Neurosci.* **2015**, *16*, 173–184. [CrossRef] [PubMed]
5. Van Huijstee, A.N.; Mansvelder, H.D. Glutamatergic synaptic plasticity in the mesocorticolimbic system in addiction. *Front. Cell. Neurosci.* **2015**, *8*, 1–13. [CrossRef] [PubMed]
6. Volkow, N.D.; Wang, G.J.; Telang, F.; Fowler, J.S.; Logan, J.; Childress, A.R.; Jayne, M.; Ma, Y.; Wong, C. Cocaine cues and dopamine in dorsal striatum: Mechanism of craving in cocaine addiction. *J. Neurosci.* **2006**, *26*, 6583–6588. [CrossRef] [PubMed]
7. Bromberg-Martin, E.S.; Matsumoto, M.; Hikosaka, O. Dopamine in Motivational Control: Rewarding, Aversive, and Alerting. *Neuron* **2010**, *68*, 815–834. [CrossRef] [PubMed]
8. Berridge, K.C.; Robinson, T.E. What is the role of dopamine in reward: Hedonic impact, reward learning, or incentive salience? *Brain Res. Rev.* **1998**, *28*, 309–369. [CrossRef]
9. Björklund, A.; Dunnett, S.B. Dopamine neuron systems in the brain: An update. *Trends Neurosci.* **2007**, *30*, 194–202. [CrossRef]
10. Ikemoto, S. Dopamine reward circuitry: Two projection systems from the ventral midbrain to the nucleus accumbens-olfactory tubercle complex. *Brain Res. Rev.* **2007**, *56*, 27–78. [CrossRef]
11. Threlfell, S.; Cragg, S.J. Dopamine signaling in dorsal versus ventral striatum: The dynamic role of cholinergic interneurons. *Front. Syst. Neurosci.* **2011**, *5*, 1–10. [CrossRef] [PubMed]

12. Volkow, N.D.; Fowler, J.S.; Wang, G. The Addicted Human Brain: Insights from Imaging Studies Find the Latest Version: The Addicted Human Brain: Insights from Imaging Studies. *J. Clin. Investig.* **2003**, *111*, 1444–1451. [CrossRef] [PubMed]
13. Di Chiara, G.; Imperato, A. Drugs abused by humans preferentially increase synaptic dopamine concentrations in the mesolimbic system of freely moving rats. *Proc. Natl. Acad. Sci. USA* **1988**, *85*, 5274–5278. [CrossRef] [PubMed]
14. Pontieri, F.E.; Tanda, G.; Di Chiara, G. Intravenous cocaine, morphine, and amphetamine preferentially increase extracellular dopamine in the "shell" as compared with the "core" of the rat nucleus accumbens. *Proc. Natl. Acad. Sci. USA* **1995**, *92*, 12304–12308. [CrossRef]
15. Ungless, M.A.; Whistler, J.L.; Malenka, R.C.; Bonci, A. Single cocaine exposure in vivo induces long-term potentiation in dopamine neurons. *Nature* **2001**, *411*, 583–587. [CrossRef]
16. Chen, B.T.; Bowers, M.S.; Martin, M.; Hopf, F.W.; Guillory, A.M.; Carelli, R.M.; Chou, J.K.; Bonci, A. Cocaine but Not Natural Reward Self-Administration nor Passive Cocaine Infusion Produces Persistent LTP in the VTA. *Neuron* **2008**, *59*, 288–297. [CrossRef]
17. Kourrich, S.; Rothwell, P.E.; Klug, J.R.; Thomas, M.J. Cocaine experience controls bidirectional synaptic plasticity in the nucleus accumbens. *J. Neurosci.* **2007**, *27*, 7921–7928. [CrossRef]
18. Pascoli, V.; Turiault, M.; Lüscher, C. Reversal of cocaine-evoked synaptic potentiation resets drug-induced adaptive behaviour. *Nature* **2012**, *481*, 71–76. [CrossRef]
19. Morales, M.; Margolis, E.B. Ventral tegmental area: Cellular heterogeneity, connectivity and behaviour. mboxemphNat. Rev. Neurosci. **2017**, *18*, 73–85. [CrossRef]
20. Swanson, L.W. The projections of the ventral tegmental area and adjacent regions: A combined fluorescent retrograde tracer and immunofluorescence study in the rat. *Brain Res. Bull.* **1982**, *9*, 321–353. [CrossRef]
21. Fu, Y.H.; Yuan, Y.; Halliday, G.; Rusznák, Z.; Watson, C.; Paxinos, G. A cytoarchitectonic and chemoarchitectonic analysis of the dopamine cell groups in the substantia nigra, ventral tegmental area, and retrorubral field in the mouse. *Brain Struct. Funct.* **2012**, *217*, 591–612. [CrossRef] [PubMed]
22. Pupe, S.; Wallén-Mackenzie, Å. Cre-driven optogenetics in the heterogeneous genetic panorama of the VTA. *Trends Neurosci.* **2015**, *38*, 375–386. [CrossRef] [PubMed]
23. Viereckel, T.; Dumas, S.; Smith-Anttila, C.J.A.; Vlcek, B.; Bimpisidis, Z.; Lagerström, M.C.; Konradsson-Geuken, Å.; Wallén-Mackenzie, Å. Midbrain Gene Screening Identifies a New Mesoaccumbal Glutamatergic Pathway and a Marker for Dopamine Cells Neuroprotected in Parkinson's Disease. *Sci. Rep.* **2016**, *6*, 1–16. [CrossRef] [PubMed]
24. Papathanou, M.; Creed, M.; Dorst, M.C.; Bimpisidis, Z.; Dumas, S.; Pettersson, H.; Bellone, C.; Silberberg, G.; Lüscher, C.; Wallén-Mackenzie, Å. Targeting VGLUT2 in Mature Dopamine Neurons Decreases Mesoaccumbal Glutamatergic Transmission and Identifies a Role for Glutamate Co-release in Synaptic Plasticity by Increasing Baseline AMPA/NMDA Ratio. *Front. Neural Circuits* **2018**, *12*, 1–20. [CrossRef]
25. Falck, B.; Hillarp, N.-Å.; Thieme, G.; Torp, A. Fluorescence of catechol amines and related compounds condensed with formaldehyde. *J. Histochem. Cytochem.* **1962**, *10*, 348–354. [CrossRef]
26. Dahlström, A.; Fuxe, K. Evidence for the existence of monoamine-containing neurons in the central nervous system. I.Demonstration of monoamines in the cell bodies of brain stem neurons. *Acta Physiol. Scand. Suppl.* **1964**, 1–55.
27. Carlsson, A.; Falck, B.; Hillarp, N.A. Cellular localization of brain monoamines. *Acta Physiol. Scand. Suppl.* **1962**, *56*, 1–28.
28. Bai, L.; Xu, H.; Collins, J.F.; Ghishan, F.K. Molecular and Functional Analysis of a Novel Neuronal Vesicular Glutamate Transporter. *J. Biol. Chem.* **2001**, *276*, 36764–36769. [CrossRef]
29. Bellocchio, E.E.; Reimer, R.J.; Fremeau, J.; Edwards, R.H. Uptake of glutamate into synaptic vesicles by an inorganic phosphate transporter. *Science* **2000**, *289*, 957–960. [CrossRef]
30. Herzog, E.; Bellenchi, G.C.; Gras, C.; Bernard, V.; Ravassard, P.; Bedet, C.; Gasnier, B.; Giros, B.; El Mestikawy, S. The existence of a second vesicular glutamate transporter specifies subpopulations of glutamatergic neurons. *J. Neurosci.* **2001**, *21*, 2–7. [CrossRef]
31. Takamori, S.; Rhee, J.S.; Rosenmund, C.; Jahn, R. Identification of differentiation-associated brain-specific phosphate transporter as a second vesicular glutamate transporter (VGLUT2). *J. Neurosci.* **2001**, *21*, 1–6. [CrossRef]

32. Varoqui, H.; Schäfer, M.K.H.; Zhu, H.; Weihe, E.; Erickson, J.D. Identification of the differentiation-associated Na+/PI transporter as a novel vesicular glutamate transporter expressed in a distinct set of glutamatergic synapses. *J. Neurosci.* **2002**, *22*, 142–155. [CrossRef] [PubMed]
33. El Mestikawy, S.; Wallén-Mackenzie, Å.; Fortin, G.M.; Descarries, L.; Trudeau, L.E. From glutamate co-release to vesicular synergy: Vesicular glutamate transporters. *Nat. Rev. Neurosci.* **2011**, *12*, 204–216. [CrossRef] [PubMed]
34. Trudeau, L.E.; Hnasko, T.S.; Wallén-Mackenzie, Å.; Morales, M.; Rayport, S.; Sulzer, D. The multilingual nature of dopamine neurons. *Prog. Brain Res.* **2014**, *211*, 141–164.
35. Sulzer, D.; Joyce, M.P.; Lin, L.; Geldwert, D.; Haber, S.N.; Hattori, T.; Rayport, S. Dopamine neurons make glutamatergic synapses in vitro. *J. Neurosci.* **1998**, *18*, 4588–4602. [CrossRef]
36. Bourque, M.J.; Trudeau, L.E. GDNF enhances the synaptic efficacy of dopaminergic neurons in culture. *Eur. J. Neurosci.* **2000**, *12*, 3172–3180. [CrossRef]
37. Joyce, M.P.; Rayport, S. Mesoaccumbens dopamine neuron synapses reconstructed in vitro are glutamatergic. *Neuroscience* **2000**, *99*, 445–456. [CrossRef]
38. Chuhma, N.; Zhang, H.; Masson, J.; Zhuang, X.; Sulzer, D.; Hen, R.; Rayport, S. Dopamine Neurons Mediate a Fast Excitatory Signal via Their Glutamatergic Synapses. *J. Neurosci.* **2004**, *24*, 972–981. [CrossRef]
39. Lavin, A.; Nogueira, L.; Lapish, C.C.; Wightman, R.M.; Phillips, P.E.M.; Seamans, J.K. Mesocortical dopamine neurons operate in distinct temporal domains using multimodal signaling. *J. Neurosci.* **2005**, *25*, 5013–5023. [CrossRef]
40. Dal Bo, G.; St.-Gelais, F.; Danik, M.; Williams, S.; Cotton, M.; Trudeau, L.E. Dopamine neurons in culture express VGLUT2 explaining their capacity to release glutamate at synapses in addition to dopamine. *J. Neurochem.* **2004**, *88*, 1398–1405. [CrossRef]
41. Barker, D.J.; Root, D.H.; Zhang, S.; Morales, M. Multiplexed neurochemical signaling by neurons of the ventral tegmental area. *J. Chem. Neuroanat.* **2016**, *73*, 33–42. [CrossRef] [PubMed]
42. Zhang, S.; Qi, J.; Li, X.; Wang, H.L.; Britt, J.P.; Hoffman, A.F.; Bonci, A.; Lupica, C.R.; Morales, M. Dopaminergic and glutamatergic microdomains in a subset of rodent mesoaccumbens axons. *Nat. Neurosci.* **2015**, *18*, 386–396. [CrossRef] [PubMed]
43. Trudeau, L.-E.; El Mestikawy, S. Glutamate Cotransmission in Cholinergic, GABAergic and Monoamine Systems: Contrasts and Commonalities. *Front. Neural Circuits* **2018**, *12*, 113. [CrossRef] [PubMed]
44. Mingote, S.; Amsellem, A.; Kempf, A.; Rayport, S.; Chuhma, N. Dopamine-Glutamate neuron projections to the nucleus accumbens medial shell and behavioral switching. *Neurochem. Int.* **2019**, *129*, 104482. [CrossRef] [PubMed]
45. Hnasko, T.S.; Edwards, R.H. Neurotransmitter Corelease: Mechanism and Physiological Role. *Annu. Rev. Physiol.* **2012**, *74*, 225–243. [CrossRef] [PubMed]
46. Kawano, M.; Kawasaki, A.; Sakata-Haga, H.; Fukui, Y.; Kawano, H.; Nogami, H.; Hisano, S. Particular subpopulations of midbrain and hypothalamic dopamine neurons express vesicular glutamate transporter 2 in the rat brain. *J. Comp. Neurol.* **2006**, *498*, 581–592. [CrossRef]
47. Yamaguchi, T.; Wang, H.-L.; Li, X.; Ng, T.H.; Morales, M. Mesocorticolimbic Glutamatergic Pathway. *J. Neurosci.* **2011**, *31*, 8476–8490. [CrossRef]
48. Yamaguchi, T.; Qi, J.; Wang, H.L.; Zhang, S.; Morales, M. Glutamatergic and dopaminergic neurons in the mouse ventral tegmental area. *Eur. J. Neurosci.* **2015**, *41*, 760–772. [CrossRef]
49. Root, D.H.; Wang, H.L.; Liu, B.; Barker, D.J.; Mód, L.; Szocsics, P.; Silva, A.C.; Maglóczky, Z.; Morales, M. Glutamate neurons are intermixed with midbrain dopamine neurons in nonhuman primates and humans. *Sci. Rep.* **2016**, *6*, 30615. [CrossRef]
50. Yamaguchi, T.; Wang, H.L.; Morales, M. Glutamate neurons in the substantia nigra compacta and retrorubral field. *Eur. J. Neurosci.* **2013**, *38*, 3602–3610. [CrossRef]
51. Morales, M.; Root, D.H. Glutamate neurons within the midbrain dopamine regions. *Neuroscience* **2014**, *282*, 60–68. [CrossRef] [PubMed]
52. Yamaguchi, T.; Sheen, W.; Morales, M. Glutamatergic neurons are present in the rat ventral tegmental area. *Eur. J. Neurosci.* **2007**, *25*, 106–118. [CrossRef] [PubMed]
53. Mendez, J.A.; Bourque, M.J.; Dal Bo, G.; Bourdeau, M.L.; Danik, M.; Williams, S.; Lacaille, J.C.; Trudeau, L.E. Developmental and target-dependent regulation of vesicular glutamate transporter expression by dopamine neurons. *J. Neurosci.* **2008**, *28*, 6309–6318. [CrossRef] [PubMed]

54. Birgner, C.; Nordenankar, K.; Lundblad, M.; Mendez, J.A.; Smith, C.; le Greves, M.; Galter, D.; Olson, L.; Fredriksson, A.; Trudeau, L.-E.; et al. VGLUT2 in dopamine neurons is required for psychostimulant-induced behavioral activation. *Proc. Natl. Acad. Sci. USA* **2010**, *107*, 389–394. [CrossRef]
55. Steinkellner, T.; Zell, V.; Farino, Z.J.; Sonders, M.S.; Villeneuve, M.; Freyberg, R.J.; Przedborski, S.; Lu, W.; Freyberg, Z.; Hnasko, T.S. Role for VGLUT2 in selective vulnerability of midbrain dopamine neurons. *J. Clin. Investig.* **2018**, *128*, 774–788. [CrossRef]
56. Tecuapetla, F.; Patel, J.C.; Xenias, H.; English, D.; Tadros, I.; Shah, F.; Berlin, J.; Deisseroth, K.; Rice, M.E.; Tepper, J.M.; et al. Glutamatergic signaling by mesolimbic dopamine neurons in the nucleus accumbens. *J. Neurosci.* **2010**, *30*, 7105–7110. [CrossRef]
57. Stuber, G.D.; Hnasko, T.S.; Britt, J.P.; Edwards, R.H.; Bonci, A. Dopaminergic Terminals in the Nucleus Accumbens But Not the Dorsal Striatum Corelease Glutamate. *J. Neurosci.* **2010**, *30*, 8229–8233. [CrossRef]
58. Chuhma, N.; Mingote, S.; Moore, H.; Rayport, S. Dopamine neurons control striatal cholinergic neurons via regionally heterogeneous dopamine and glutamate signaling. *Neuron* **2014**, *81*, 901–912. [CrossRef]
59. Chuhma, N.; Mingote, S.; Yetnikoff, L.; Kalmbach, A.; Ma, T.; Ztaou, S.; Sienna, A.C.; Tepler, S.; Poulin, J.F.; Ansorge, M.; et al. Dopamine neuron glutamate cotransmission evokes a delayed excitation in lateral dorsal striatal cholinergic interneurons. *eLife* **2018**, *7*, 1–29. [CrossRef]
60. Cai, Y.; Ford, C.P. Dopamine Cells Differentially Regulate Striatal Cholinergic Transmission across Regions through Corelease of Dopamine and Glutamate. *Cell Rep.* **2018**, *25*, 3148.e3–3157.e3. [CrossRef]
61. Alsiö, J.; Nordenankar, K.; Arvidsson, E.; Birgner, C.; Mahmoudi, S.; Halbout, B.; Smith, C.; Fortin, G.M.; Olson, L.; Descarries, L.; et al. Enhanced Sucrose and Cocaine Self-Administration and Cue-Induced Drug Seeking after Loss of VGLUT2 in Midbrain Dopamine Neurons in Mice. *J. Neurosci.* **2011**, *31*, 12593–12603. [CrossRef] [PubMed]
62. Fortin, G.M.; Bourque, M.-J.; Mendez, J.A.; Leo, D.; Nordenankar, K.; Birgner, C.; Arvidsson, E.; Rymar, V.V.; Berube-Carriere, N.; Claveau, A.-M.; et al. Glutamate Corelease Promotes Growth and Survival of Midbrain Dopamine Neurons. *J. Neurosci.* **2012**, *32*, 17477–17491. [CrossRef] [PubMed]
63. Hnasko, T.S.; Chuhma, N.; Zhang, H.; Goh, G.Y.; Sulzer, D.; Palmiter, R.D.; Rayport, S.; Edwards, R.H. Vesicular glutamate transport promotes dopamine storage and glutamate corelease in vivo. *Neuron* **2010**, *65*, 643–656. [CrossRef] [PubMed]
64. Mingote, S.; Chuhma, N.; Kalmbach, A.; Thomsen, G.M.; Wang, Y.; Mihali, A.; Sferrazza, C.; Zucker-Scharff, I.; Siena, A.C.; Welch, M.G.; et al. Dopamine neuron dependent behaviours mediated by glutamate cotransmission. *eLife* **2017**, *6*, 1–29. [CrossRef] [PubMed]
65. Wang, D.V.; Viereckel, T.; Zell, V.; Konradsson-Geuken, Å.; Broker, C.J.; Talishinsky, A.; Yoo, J.H.; Galinato, M.H.; Arvidsson, E.; Kesner, A.J.; et al. Disrupting Glutamate Co-transmission Does Not Affect Acquisition of Conditioned Behavior Reinforced by Dopamine Neuron Activation. *Cell Rep.* **2017**, *18*, 2584–2591. [CrossRef] [PubMed]
66. Wallén-Mackenzie, Å.; Gezelius, H.; Thoby-Brisson, M.; Nygard, A.; Enjin, A.; Fujiyama, F.; Fortin, G.; Kullander, K. Vesicular Glutamate Transporter 2 Is Required for Central Respiratory Rhythm Generation But Not for Locomotor Central Pattern Generation. *J. Neurosci.* **2006**, *26*, 12294–12307. [CrossRef]
67. Wallén-Mackenzie, Å.; Nordenankar, K.; Fejgin, K.; Lagerström, M.C.; Emilsson, L.; Fredriksson, R.; Wass, C.; Andersson, D.; Egecioglu, E.; Andersson, M.; et al. Restricted cortical and amygdaloid removal of vesicular glutamate transporter 2 in preadolescent mice impacts dopaminergic activity and neuronal circuitry of higher brain function. *J. Neurosci.* **2009**, *29*, 2238–2251. [CrossRef]
68. Stornetta, R.L.; Sevigny, C.P.; Schreihofer, A.M.; Rosin, D.L.; Guyenet, P.G. Vesicular glutamate transporter DNPI/VGLUT2 is expressed by both C1 adrenergic and nonaminergic presympathetic vasomotor neurons of the rat medulla. *J. Comp. Neurol.* **2002**, *444*, 207–220. [CrossRef]
69. Stornetta, R.L.; Sevigny, C.P.; Guyenet, P.G. Vesicular glutamate transporter DNPI/VGLUT2 mRNA is present in C1 and several other groups of brainstem catecholaminergic neurons. *J. Comp. Neurol.* **2002**, *444*, 191–206. [CrossRef]
70. Nordenankar, K.; Smith-Anttila, C.J.A.; Schweizer, N.; Viereckel, T.; Birgner, C.; Mejia-Toiber, J.; Morales, M.; Leao, R.N.; Wallén-Mackenzie, Å. Increased hippocampal excitability and impaired spatial memory function in mice lacking VGLUT2 selectively in neurons defined by tyrosine hydroxylase promoter activity. *Brain Struct. Funct.* **2015**, *220*, 2171–2190. [CrossRef]

71. Campos-Melo, D.; Galleguillos, D.; Sánchez, N.; Gysling, K.; Andrés, M.E. Nur transcription factors in stress and addiction. *Front. Mol. Neurosci.* **2013**, *6*, 1–13. [CrossRef] [PubMed]
72. Aguilar, J.I.; Dunn, M.; Mingote, S.; Karam, C.S.; Farino, Z.J.; Sonders, M.S.; Choi, S.J.; Grygoruk, A.; Zhang, Y.; Cela, C.; et al. Neuronal Depolarization Drives Increased Dopamine Synaptic Vesicle Loading via VGLUT. *Neuron* **2017**, *95*, 1074.e7–1088.e7. [CrossRef] [PubMed]
73. Tsai, H.-C.; Zhang, F.; Adamantidis, A.R.; Stuber, G.D.; Bonci, A.; de Lecea, L.; Deisseroth, K. Phasic firing in dopaminergic neurons is sufficient for behavioral conditioning. *Science* **2009**, *324*, 1080–1084. [CrossRef] [PubMed]
74. Ilango, A.; Kesner, A.J.; Broker, C.J.; Wang, D.V.; Ikemoto, S. Phasic excitation of ventral tegmental dopamine neurons potentiates the initiation of conditioned approach behavior: Parametric and reinforcement-schedule analyses. *Front. Behav. Neurosci.* **2014**, *8*, 155. [CrossRef] [PubMed]
75. Kim, K.M.; Baratta, M.V.; Yang, A.; Lee, D.; Boyden, E.S.; Fiorillo, C.D. Optogenetic mimicry of the transient activation of dopamine neurons by natural reward is sufficient for operant reinforcement. *PLoS ONE* **2012**, *7*, 1–8. [CrossRef]
76. Pascoli, V.; Terrier, J.; Hiver, A.; Lüscher, C. Sufficiency of Mesolimbic Dopamine Neuron Stimulation for the Progression to Addiction. *Neuron* **2015**, *88*, 1054–1066. [CrossRef]
77. Viereckel, T.; Konradsson-Geuken, Å.; Wallén-Mackenzie, Å. Validated multi-step approach for in vivo recording and analysis of optogenetically evoked glutamate in the mouse globus pallidus. *J. Neurochem.* **2018**, *145*, 125–138. [CrossRef]
78. Gaisler-Salomon, I.; Miller, G.M.; Chuhma, N.; Lee, S.; Zhang, H.; Ghoddoussi, F.; Lewandowski, N.; Fairhurst, S.; Wang, Y.; Conjard-Duplany, A.; et al. Glutaminase-deficient mice display hippocampal hypoactivity, insensitivity to pro-psychotic drugs and potentiated latent inhibition: Relevance to schizophrenia. *Neuropsychopharmacology* **2009**, *34*, 2305–2322. [CrossRef]
79. Ang, S.L. Transcriptional control of midbrain dopaminergic neuron development. *Development* **2006**, *133*, 3499–3506. [CrossRef]
80. Lammel, S.; Steinberg, E.E.; Földy, C.; Wall, N.R.; Beier, K.; Luo, L.; Malenka, R.C. Diversity of transgenic mouse models for selective targeting of midbrain dopamine neurons. *Neuron* **2015**, *85*, 429–438. [CrossRef]
81. Stuber, G.D.; Stamatakis, A.M.; Kantak, P.A. Considerations when using cre-driver rodent lines for studying ventral tegmental area circuitry. *Neuron* **2015**, *85*, 439–445. [CrossRef]
82. Papathanou, M.; Dumas, S.; Pettersson, H.; Olson, L.; Wallén-Mackenzie, Å. Off-target effects in transgenic mice: Characterization of Dopamine transporter (DAT)-Cre transgenic mouse lines exposes multiple non-dopaminergic neuronal clusters available for selective targeting within limbic neurocircuitry. *Eneuro* **2019**. [CrossRef]
83. Engblom, D.; Bilbao, A.; Sanchis-Segura, C.; Dahan, L.; Perreau-Lenz, S.; Balland, B.; Parkitna, J.R.; Luján, R.; Halbout, B.; Mameli, M.; et al. Glutamate Receptors on Dopamine Neurons Control the Persistence of Cocaine Seeking. *Neuron* **2008**, *59*, 497–508. [CrossRef] [PubMed]
84. Adrover, M.F.; Shin, J.H.; Alvarez, V.A. Glutamate and dopamine transmission from midbrain dopamine neurons share similar release properties but are differentially affected by cocaine. *J. Neurosci.* **2014**, *34*, 3183–3192. [CrossRef]
85. Ishikawa, M.; Otaka, M.; Neumann, P.A.; Wang, Z.; Cook, J.M.; Schlüter, O.M.; Dong, Y.; Huang, Y.H. Exposure to cocaine regulates inhibitory synaptic transmission from the ventral tegmental area to the nucleus accumbens. *J. Physiol.* **2013**, *591*, 4827–4841. [CrossRef] [PubMed]
86. Mingote, S.; Chuhma, N.; Kusnoor, S.V.; Field, B.; Deutch, A.Y.; Rayport, S. Functional Connectome Analysis of Dopamine Neuron Glutamatergic Connections in Forebrain Regions. *J. Neurosci.* **2015**, *35*, 16259–16271. [CrossRef]
87. Cachope, R.; Mateo, Y.; Mathur, B.N.; Irving, J.; Wang, H.L.; Morales, M.; Lovinger, D.M.; Cheer, J.F. Selective activation of cholinergic interneurons enhances accumbal phasic dopamine release: Setting the tone for reward processing. *Cell Rep.* **2012**, *2*, 33–41. [CrossRef]
88. Descarries, L.; Gisiger, V.; Steriade, M. Diffuse transmission by acetylcholine in the CNS. *Prog. Neurobiol.* **1997**, *53*, 603–625. [CrossRef]

89. Threlfell, S.; Lalic, T.; Platt, N.J.; Jennings, K.A.; Deisseroth, K.; Cragg, S.J. Striatal dopamine release is triggered by synchronized activity in cholinergic interneurons. *Neuron* **2012**, *75*, 58–64. [CrossRef] [PubMed]
90. Morris, G.; Arkadir, D.; Nevet, A.; Vaadia, E.; Bergman, H. Coincident but distinct messages of midbrain dopamine and striatal tonically active neurons. *Neuron* **2004**, *43*, 133–143. [CrossRef]
91. Ikemoto, S.; Bonci, A. Neurocircuitry of drug reward. *Neuropharmacology* **2014**, *76*, 329–341. [CrossRef] [PubMed]
92. Poulin, J.-F.; Caronia, G.; Hofer, C.; Cui, Q.; Helm, B.; Ramakrishnan, C.; Chan, C.S.; Dombeck, D.A.; Deisseroth, K.; Awatramani, R. Mapping projections of molecularly defined dopamine neuron subtypes using intersectional genetic approaches. *Nat. Neurosci.* **2018**, *21*, 1260–1271. [CrossRef] [PubMed]
93. Zhou, F.C.; Sahr, R.N.; Sari, Y.; Behbahani, K. Glutamate and dopamine synaptic terminals in extended amygdala after 14-week chronic alcohol drinking in inbred alcohol-preferring rats. *Alcohol* **2006**, *39*, 39–49. [CrossRef] [PubMed]
94. Comasco, E.; Hallman, J.; Wallén-Mackenzie, Å. Haplotype-tag single nucleotide polymorphism analysis of the Vesicular Glutamate Transporter (VGLUT) genes in severely alcoholic women. *Psychiatry Res.* **2014**, *219*, 403–405. [CrossRef] [PubMed]
95. Hnasko, T.S.; Hjelmstad, G.O.; Fields, H.L.; Edwards, R.H. Ventral Tegmental Area Glutamate Neurons: Electrophysiological Properties and Projections. *J. Neurosci.* **2012**, *32*, 15076–15085. [CrossRef]
96. Gorelova, N.; Mulholland, P.J.; Chandler, L.J.; Seamans, J.K. The glutamatergic component of the mesocortical pathway emanating from different subregions of the ventral midbrain. *Cereb. Cortex* **2012**, *22*, 327–336. [CrossRef]
97. Pérez-López, J.L.; Contreras-López, R.; Ramírez-Jarquín, J.O.; Tecuapetla, F. Direct Glutamatergic Signaling From Midbrain Dopaminergic Neurons Onto Pyramidal Prefrontal Cortex Neurons. *Front. Neural Circuits* **2018**, *12*, 1–10. [CrossRef]
98. Lammel, S.; Ion, D.I.; Roeper, J.; Malenka, R.C. Projection-Specific Modulation of Dopamine Neuron Synapses by Aversive and Rewarding Stimuli. *Neuron* **2011**, *70*, 855–862. [CrossRef]
99. Vander Weele, C.M.; Siciliano, C.A.; Matthews, G.A.; Namburi, P.; Izadmehr, E.M.; Espinel, I.C.; Nieh, E.H.; Schut, E.H.S.; Padilla-Coreano, N.; Burgos-Robles, A.; et al. Dopamine enhances signal-to-noise ratio in cortical-brainstem encoding of aversive stimuli. *Nature* **2018**, *563*, 397–401. [CrossRef]
100. Bimpisidis, Z.; De Luca, M.A.; Pisanu, A.; Di Chiara, G. Lesion of medial prefrontal dopamine terminals abolishes habituation of accumbens shell dopamine responsiveness to taste stimuli. *Eur. J. Neurosci.* **2013**, *37*, 613–622. [CrossRef]
101. Beyer, C.E.; Steketee, J.D. Dopamine depletion in the medial prefrontal cortex induces sensitized- like behavioral and neurochemical responses to cocaine. *Brain Res.* **1999**, *833*, 133–141. [CrossRef]
102. Bimpisidis, Z.; König, N.; Stagkourakis, S.; Zell, V.; Vlcek, B.; Dumas, S.; Giros, B.; Broberger, C.; Hnasko, T.S.; Wallén-Mackenzie, Å. The NeuroD6 subtype of VTA neurons contributes to psychostimulant sensitization and behavioral reinforcement. *eNeuro* **2019**, *6*. [CrossRef] [PubMed]
103. Chung, C.Y.; Seo, H.; Sonntag, K.C.; Brooks, A.; Lin, L.; Isacson, O. Cell type-specific gene expression of midbrain dopaminergic neurons reveals molecules involved in their vulnerability and protection. *Hum. Mol. Genet.* **2005**, *14*, 1709–1725. [CrossRef] [PubMed]
104. Greene, J.G.; Dingledine, R.; Greenamyre, J.T. Gene expression profiling of rat midbrain dopamine neurons: Implications for selective vulnerability in parkinsonism. *Neurobiol. Dis.* **2005**, *18*, 19–31. [CrossRef]
105. La Manno, G.; Gyllborg, D.; Codeluppi, S.; Nishimura, K.; Salto, C.; Zeisel, A.; Borm, L.E.; Stott, S.R.W.; Toledo, E.M.; Villaescusa, J.C.; et al. Molecular Diversity of Midbrain Development in Mouse, Human, and Stem Cells. *Cell* **2016**, *167*, 566.e19–580.e19. [CrossRef]
106. Poulin, J.F.; Zou, J.; Drouin-Ouellet, J.; Kim, K.Y.A.; Cicchetti, F.; Awatramani, R.B. Defining midbrain dopaminergic neuron diversity by single-cell gene expression profiling. *Cell Rep.* **2014**, *9*, 930–943. [CrossRef]

107. Kramer, D.J.; Risso, D.; Kosillo, P.; Ngai, J.; Bateup, H.S. Combinatorial Expression of Grp and Neurod6 Defines Dopamine Neuron Populations with Distinct Projection Patterns and Disease Vulnerability Combinatorial expression of Grp and Neurod6 defines dopamine neuron populations with distinct projection patterns and disease vulnerability. *eNeuro* **2018**, *5*. [CrossRef]
108. Khan, S.; Stott, S.R.W.; Chabrat, A.; Truckenbrodt, A.M.; Spencer-Dene, B.; Nave, K.-A.; Guillemot, F.; Levesque, M.; Ang, S.-L. Survival of a Novel Subset of Midbrain Dopaminergic Neurons Projecting to the Lateral Septum Is Dependent on NeuroD Proteins. *J. Neurosci.* **2017**, *37*, 2305–2316. [CrossRef]

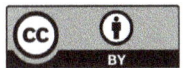

© 2019 by the authors. Licensee MDPI, Basel, Switzerland. This article is an open access article distributed under the terms and conditions of the Creative Commons Attribution (CC BY) license (http://creativecommons.org/licenses/by/4.0/).

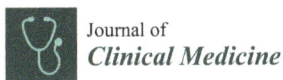

Review

Addiction as Learned Behavior Patterns

Andreas Heinz [1], Anne Beck [1], Melissa Gül Halil [1], Maximilian Pilhatsch [2], Michael N. Smolka [2,3] and Shuyan Liu [1,*]

[1] Department of Psychiatry and Psychotherapy, Charité–Universitätsmedizin Berlin (Campus Charité Mitte), 10117 Berlin, Germany
[2] Department of Psychiatry and Psychotherapy, Technische Universität Dresden, 01187 Dresden, Germany
[3] Neuroimaging Center, Technische Universität Dresden, 01187 Dresden, Germany
* Correspondence: siyan908@hotmail.com

Received: 24 June 2019; Accepted: 19 July 2019; Published: 24 July 2019

Abstract: Individuals with substance use disorders (SUDs) have to cope with drug-related cues and contexts which can affect instrumental drug seeking, as shown with Pavlovian-to-instrumental transfer (PIT) tasks among humans and animals. Our review addresses two potential mechanisms that may contribute to habitual or even compulsive drug seeking and taking. One mechanism is represented by Pavlovian and PIT effects on drug intake. The other is a shift from goal-directed to habitual drug intake, which can be accessed via model-based versus model-free decision-making in respective learning tasks. We discuss the impact of these learning mechanisms on drug consumption. First, we describe how Pavlovian and instrumental learning mechanisms interact in drug addiction. Secondly, we address the effects of acute and chronic stress exposure on behavioral and neural PIT effects in alcohol use disorder (AUD). Thirdly, we discuss how these learning mechanisms and their respective neurobiological correlates can contribute to losing versus regaining control over drug intake. Utilizing mobile technology (mobile applications on smartphones including games that measure learning mechanisms, activity bracelets), computational models, and real-world data may help to better identify patients with a high relapse risk and to offer targeted behavioral and pharmacotherapeutic interventions for vulnerable patients.

Keywords: substance use disorders; alternative reward; cue exposure; animal and computational models; behavioral control; craving and relapse; habit formation

1. Introduction

Drugs of abuse stimulate dopamine release and thus reinforce drug intake [1]. Wise originally suggested that dopamine release is tied to pleasure and hedonic changes that strongly reinforce the behavior of repetitive drug use [2]. Robinson and Berridge later suggested that dopamine release is more associated with reward motivation rather than mediating hedonic pleasure, contributing to "wanting" or "craving" instead of "liking" drugs of abuse [3]. This hypothesis was based on studies by Schulz and co-workers [4]. They found that phasic dopamine release is modulated by an unexpected reward and a conditioned stimulus, which in turn reliably predict reward. They suggested dopamine signals code reward prediction errors (i.e., the difference between received and predicted rewards) which drive reward-motivated behaviors. Accordingly, dopamine D2-receptor blockade in humans was associated with motivational deficits, but not anhedonia [5]. Based on the observations above, dopamine is not only associated with the encoding of unexpected rewards, but also the attribution of incentive salience to reward-related cues [3]. Further research is required to better understand how such learning mechanisms may shed light on drug seeking and intake. Specifically, recreational drug use elicits a rather strong dopamine release, thus reinforcing drug consumption [6]. Habitual drug use is characterized by a shift from ventral to dorsal striatal processing, including the dopaminergic modulation in fronto-striatal brain circuitries [6]. Ultimately, drug consumption was independent of rewarding or aversive outcomes [6,7]. The pathways from the orbitofrontal cortex to the dorsal striatum play a key role in compulsive drug use, in spite of aversive consequences [8]. Obsessions and compulsions in obsessive compulsive disorder (OCD) differ from drug craving and intake [9]. However, drug addiction is characterized by compulsive drug intake and has substantial similarities with other disorders of compulsions, including OCD, on phenomenological and neurobiological levels [10,11]. In this review, we discuss two potential mechanisms that may contribute to habitual drug intake and, ultimately, drug seeking and taking. One mechanism is the stimulus response associations as represented by Pavlovian effects on drug intake and the other is a shift from goal-directed to habitual drug intake, which can be accessed via model-based versus model-free decision-making in respective learning tasks [11,12].

2. Pavlovian Mechanisms in Addictive Behavior

Drug-associated cues can elicit drug craving and promote drug seeking [3,13]. From a theoretical point of view, Pavlovian unconditioned cues, such as food, elicit unconditioned responses, including increased salivation and food craving. Conditioned cues, such as pictures of alcoholic beverages, may elicit drug craving as a conditioned response [14]. However, most drugs of abuse do not often come accidentally to an addicted person. Instead, patients with drug dependence actively search for available drugs. One of our patients described the situation with the following words: "When the evening comes and the sky turns grey, I pass by these bars with their warm yellow light and hear the clinging of glasses. I'm lost." In this context, conditioned cues include the clinging of glasses, certain colors of light in a bar, and the kind of loneliness while looking at the dark gloomy sky. These conditioned cues have been previously paired with positive/pleasant activities/evenings. Such conditioned contextual cues elicit drug craving and have an impact on goal-directed behavior; the afflicted person changes his or her direction, enters the bar, orders a drink, and consumes it. The implicated mechanism has been called Pavlovian-to-instrumental transfer (PIT) [15]. During PIT, a Pavlovian conditioned cue (e.g., the clinging of glasses) can have an impact on a series of obviously unrelated approach behavioral sequences, including entering a certain place, talking to bartenders, and ordering a drink. Regarding cue reactivity, imaging studies show that functional activation elicited by drug-associated cues, particularly in the medial prefrontal cortex, was correlated with a high risk of relapse for detoxified patients with alcohol use disorder (AUD) [16,17]. Moreover, naltrexone, which blocks µ-opioid receptors that have been reported to be elevated in AUD, also reduces cue-induced functional activation in the ventral striatum in AUD patients [18,19]. Another neurotransmitter system implicated in cue-induced brain activation in addictive disorders is the dopamine system. A low availability of dopamine D2-receptors in the ventral striatum is associated with increased functional activation elicited by alcohol cues in the medial prefrontal cortex [20]. Low dopamine D2-receptor availability following detoxification may represent a counter-regulatory new adaptation following excessive dopamine release due to the consumption of drugs of abuse and delayed recovery of dopamine D2-receptor sensitivity following detoxification was associated with poor treatment outcomes [21].

So how can alcohol cues trigger not only drug craving and functional activation in the ventral striatum, amygdala, and medial prefrontal cortex [17,22], but also bias complex goal-directed behavior toward drug seeking and intake? A subclass of environmental cues is called Pavlovian conditioned stimuli due to the ability to elicit a conditioned response, which is usually inborn (such as the production of saliva in a hungry dog or avoidance of malodors) and hence hard-wired in the central nervous system [23]. As suggested above, such Pavlovian conditioned stimuli can also impact ongoing instrumental behavior, even if the instrumental behavior was acquired independently of Pavlovian conditioning, a process called Pavlovian-to-instrumental transfer (PIT) [24]. In PIT, positively valued Pavlovian cues promote instrumental responses and approach behaviors (e.g., enhance the frequency of pressing a button) [24], while negatively valued Pavlovian cues promote inhibition or withdrawal actions (e.g., lower the frequency of pressing a button for instrumental approach or enhance the frequency of pressing a button for instrumental withdrawal [25] (Figure 1)). Thus, in drug addiction, Pavlovian conditioned cues can bias instrumental behavior toward drug seeking and intake [26–28].

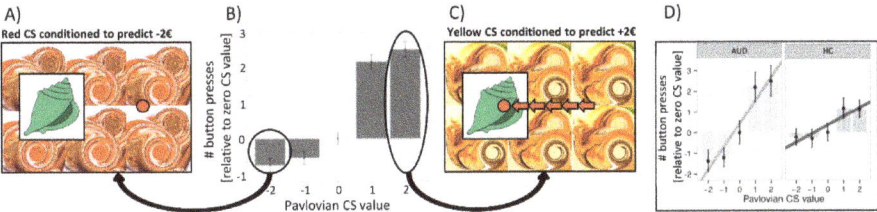

Figure 1. The Pavlovian-to-instrumental (PIT) effect. (**A**) The unrelated Pavlovian stimulus (conditioned stimulus (CS)) presented in the background is negatively valued because it has previously been paired with passive monetary loss. (**B**) The PIT effect is indicated by the number of button presses (instrumental response) as a function of the value of the respective Pavlovian background stimulus (−€2, −€1, €0, +€1, +€2). (**C**) Combining the shell with a positive Pavlovian cue in the background of the screen increases approach behavior (number of button presses) in the unrelated instrumental task. (**D**) The PIT effect was significantly stronger in subjects with alcohol use disorder (AUD) compared to healthy controls (HC).

In outcome-specific PIT, presenting a particular reward-predicting cue can selectively elevate instrumental responses that are associated with the same unique reward, while in general PIT, a reward- or loss-predicting cue can generally modify instrumental responses toward any outcome [24]. So-called single-lever PIT tasks (see Figure 1) usually reflect general PIT, while a full transfer task enables the disentanglement between general and outcome-specific PIT [24]. Like habits, PIT effects may help to prune a complex "decision tree" by biasing an individual to instrumental approaches or withdrawal behaviors in the presence of certain background stimuli [29]. Indeed, a general tendency to rely on habitual rather than complex goal-directed decision-making was associated with increased PIT effects in healthy volunteers [30]. Moreover, we observed PIT effects being modulated by personality traits, such as impulsive decision making, with the strongest PIT effects observed in high impulsive alcohol-dependent patients compared to low impulsive patients [31].

PIT effects may be specifically strong in stressful situations, when decisions have to be fast, and profit from an overall "atmospheric" evaluation of the dangerousness or safety of the current situation [32]. Various forms of stress promote substance use and relapse, as evidenced by a broad range of literature [33,34]. In this context, Quail and co-workers suggested that stress exposure modifies the influence of Pavlovian cues on behavior [35]. They observed that subjects reporting high stress were impaired to suppress instrumental responding under no-reward Pavlovian cues [35]. Moreover, acute stress selectively increased cue-triggered wanting independently of hedonic properties of the reward [36]. Stress exposure and long-term endocrine stress measures (e.g., hair cortisol) in addicts have so far not been studied with respect to PIT and its association with losing versus regaining control over drug intake. Moreover, we did not find gender and age effects [31,37,38], which would require further research.

With respect to neurobiological correlates, animal experiments and human studies suggest that activation of the basolateral amygdala, the nucleus accumbens shell, and the ventrolateral putamen contribute to an outcome-specific form of PIT [15,39,40]. The central nucleus of the amygdala and the nucleus accumbens core are involved in the general form of PIT [15,39,40]. These neurobiological differences are in line with a goal-directed aspect of specific PIT compared to an arousing effect of general PIT. In the outcome-specific form of PIT, the Pavlovian cue has been conditioned with the same rewarding outcome that can also be gained when performing the instrumental response. For example, the smell of wine promotes ordering and consuming a glass of wine instead of lemonade. In the general form of PIT, the Pavlovian cue has been conditioned to a positive outcome that is not associated with the outcome available by the instrumental action. For example, upbeat music played in a shopping mall motivates customers to spent more money. Thus, general PIT appears to promote instrumental actions by modulating arousal, while outcome-specific PIT may facilitate the retrieval of particular actions based on their outcomes [26].

In line with this, stronger general PIT effects elicited by positive non-drug cues and functional PIT-related brain activation in the nucleus accumbens were observed in prospective AUD relapsers [37,41]. This phenomenon of increased PIT effects was also observed in studies when animals were pretreated with drugs of abuse [24].

In smokers, tobacco-related PIT effects have been demonstrated in several studies in satiated and deprived smokers [42,43], but contrary to our findings in AUD patients, studies in smokers did not see stronger PIT effects in more dependent subjects or compared to non-dependent controls. In cocaine addicts, cocaine-paired cues can provoke the pursuit of cocaine through a Pavlovian motivational process [27]. In general, there are a limited numbers of studies examining whether different types of drug abuse, such as opioids and amphetamine, can support PIT [24]. Establishing these effects may deepen our understanding of the behavioral and neural processes underlying cue-motivated drug-seeking behavior.

The PIT effects of drug-related cues were also studied in subjects with AUD. Regarding alcohol versus water cues, we expected that alcohol cues would promote approach behaviors and predict poor treatment outcomes, as was the case with general PIT effects. The appetitive and aversive Pavlovian cues were passively conditioned with monetary reward or loss. Surprisingly, however, patients with poor treatment outcomes behaved similar to the healthy controls. Patients with good treatment outcomes who did not relapse in the follow-up period of three months showed a significant difference both in behavior and in functional brain responses to alcohol cues in a general PIT task [38]. They showed both an increased functional activation of the ventral striatum when confronted with these Pavlovian-conditioned alcohol cues, as well as an inhibition of approached behavior and increased withdrawal behavior in the presence of such alcohol cues [38]. Interestingly, alcohol-dependent patients with good treatment outcomes appeared to learn a specific inhibitory reaction to alcohol cues. At least, they significantly differed both from healthy controls and patients who later relapsed during the follow-up period. Increased activation of the ventral striatum may be due to salience attribution to alcohol cues, which apparently did not simply trigger approach behaviors, but instead enabled subjects to inhibit unrelated goal-directed behaviors. Thus, patients with good treatment outcomes could use alcohol cues as warning signs and—unlike the patient in the example explained above—resist drug-approach tendencies. For example, they may not enter the bar with the warm yellow light or avoid going to the supermarket where they used to buy their alcoholic beverages.

Patients may learn to use environmental cues as warning-signs and thus train to avoid rather than approach situations in which drugs are available. One training program targeting such drug-approach tendencies is the so-called Zooming Joystick Task. Patients with addictive disorders learn to push pictures of alcohol beverages away instead of pulling them toward themselves. Four training sessions appear to be sufficient to successfully reduce the relapse-risk during an one year follow-up period, with the number needed to treat (NNT) being around 10, suggesting that 10% of all patients would benefit from this intervention [44]. From a neurobiological perspective, such alcohol cues activate the medial prefrontal cortex and further brain areas, including the amygdala, implicated in PIT mechanisms; successfully learning to push alcohol cues away was associated with reduced amygdala activation in AUD patients [45,46]. The success of such training programs encourages studies to better understand the neurobiological correlates and to identify patients who may respond particularly well to such training programs.

In line with the key role of the amygdala and nucleus accumbens, behavioral PIT effects are understood as driven by bottom-up processes. Nevertheless, a conflict—like in a Stroop task—should be elicited in situations in which Pavlovian and instrumental cues are incongruent (i.e., collecting "good" shells when negatively valued context stimuli are shown, or leaving "bad" shells during presentation of positively valued contexts) and this conflict should trigger the allocation of top-down control. Indeed, the results of Sommer and co-workers [31] revealed that instrumental behavior during PIT is more error-prone when instrumental and Pavlovian cues are incongruent, in line with the assumption of such a conflict between Pavlovian and instrumental control (Figure 2). Importantly, the incongruence effect was more pronounced in AUD subjects than in controls, indicating that reduced interference control may impair goal-directed behavior, especially in AUD subjects.

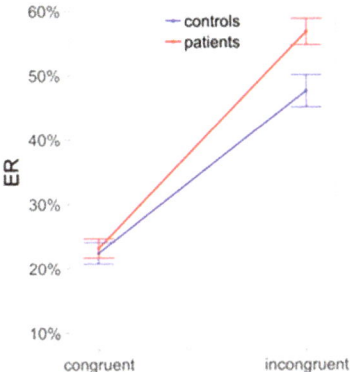

Figure 2. Conflict between Pavlovian and instrumental control: Subjects with alcohol use disorder (AUD) compared to controls. ER = error rates.

3. From Goal-Directed to Habitual Drug Seeking—The Importance of Contextual Cues

Dual-process theories of learning and addiction propose that the development of drug addiction involves a shift from goal-directed to habitual control of action [6,7]. Animal models of drug addiction suggest that occasional drug use becomes habitual and ultimately compulsive (i.e., it is maintained in spite of aversive consequences) [7]. In humans, complex model-based behavior is reduced in patients with different substance use disorders (SUDs) as well as with OCD [11]. This may help to explain why aversive outcomes associated with drug consumption do not affect the respective behavior and enforce modification. Regarding patients with AUD, the results of the recent studies were inconsistent. In a study by Voon and co-workers [11], a shift was not observed from model-based toward model-free behavior in AUD patients, while such a shift was observed by Sebold and co-workers [47]. However, Sebold and co-workers did not replicate their previous findings in a larger independent sample [48]. There was no overall reduction in model-based behavior in patients with AUDs and in patients with poor treatment outcomes compared to patients with good treatment outcomes [48].

Model-based versus model-free behavior and goal-directed versus habitual behavior are assessed by different tasks. Model-based versus model-free behavior is assessed via taking complex decision-making processes into account, while goal-directed versus habitual behavior is operationalized via the impact of reward devaluation. Nevertheless, both tasks are intercorrelated in the sense that individuals who tend to behave in a model-based way also show stronger goal-directed behaviors, while individuals who tend to respond in a habitual way rely more strongly on model-free decision-making [49]. Therefore, failure to observe effects of a reduction in model-based behavior in AUD patients may challenge the assumption that these patients have a general tendency for habit-formation at the expense of goal-directed decision-making. However, Sebold and co-workers also observed that model-based versus model-free behavior can predict treatment outcomes when taking alcohol expectancy into account [48]. Patients with high alcohol expectancies showing low model-based behavior, thus shifting the balance toward model-free behavior, had poor treatment outcomes [48]. These findings suggest that shifts from goal-directed to habitual decision-making depend on contextual stimuli. It may be specifically relevant for a subset of behavior patterns associated with drug seeking and drug consumption. Instead of searching for general tendencies to form habits, specific context-dependent learning mechanisms that may interfere with cognitive control and conscious decisions to remain abstinent must be identified. Cognitive abilities such as working memory have been discovered to interplay between these two behavioral systems [50,51]. Acute [52] or chronic [53] stress are thought to impair executive resources underlying working memory and were found to impair goal-directed decision-making, inducing a relative shift toward habitual behavioral control. Stress is also an important factor in the development and maintenance of AUD and has been shown to increase alcohol intake [54–56]. Human imaging studies revealed that acute stress enhanced stimulus–response learning, which was accompanied by increased amygdala activity during a spatial learning task [57], as well as biased choices for immediately rewarding food stimuli and increased functional connectivity between the ventromedial prefrontal cortex and amygdala and striatal regions encoding tastiness [58]. Therefore, the acute stress experience might promote loss of control over alcohol intake by diminishing goal-directed responses and promoting habitual actions, thus undermining the goal to stay abstinent by promoting habitual substance intake. We also observed that goal-directed decision-making was affected by increased life stressors [59], underlining the strong potential of interventions aimed at altering stress-related effects on losing and regaining control over substance use. In future studies, researchers could model learning and cognitive control systems in interaction with real-life monitoring of stressors, cue responsivity, and ecological momentary assessment of alcohol consumption.

4. Summary and Outlook

Human behavior is more flexible and dependent on context than previously assumed in straight-forward models (i.e., increased PIT effects and habitual decision-making in drug addiction). Researchers should consider contextual cues, such as expectancies and availabilities, mood states, individual stress-levels, and cognitive control processes. Modern technology allows ambulatory assessments, including reports of mood-states, recordings of geolocation, and psychomotor activity in real life [60]. An important future focus should be on the development and establishment of computational models for learning and decision-making in humans. To date, cue exposure in general has limited effects and individual differences in cue effects, including ambulatory assessments of learning mechanisms like PIT, may help to target those patients [61,62]. Thus, utilizing a model's predictions and real-world data may help to better identify patients with a high relapse risk and to offer specific behavioral or pharmacological interventions for vulnerable patients.

Author Contributions: Conceptualization, A.H.; Writing—original draft, A.H., S.L.; Writing—review and editing, A.H., A.B., M.G.H., M.P., M.N.S., and S.L.

Funding: This research was funded by the German Research Foundation (grant number SFB/TRR 265).

Acknowledgments: The authors would like to thank the German Research Foundation for grant.

Conflicts of Interest: The authors declare no conflict of interest.

References

1. Di Chiara, G.; Bassareo, V. Reward system and addiction: What dopamine does and doesn't do. *Curr. Opin. Pharmacol.* **2007**, *7*, 69–76. [CrossRef] [PubMed]
2. Wise, R.A. Neuroleptics and operant behavior: The anhedonia hypothesis. *Behav. Brain Sci.* **1982**, *5*, 39–53. [CrossRef]
3. Robinson, T.E.; Berridge, K.C. The neural basis of drug craving: An incentive-sensitization theory of addiction. *Brain Res. Rev.* **1993**, *18*, 247–291. [CrossRef]
4. Schultz, W.; Dayan, P.; Montague, P.R. A neural substrate of prediction and reward. *Science* **1997**, *275*, 1593–1599. [CrossRef] [PubMed]

5. Heinz, A.; Knable, M.B.; Coppola, R.; Gorey, J.G.; Jones, D.W.; Lee, K.-S.; Weinberger, D.R. Psychomotor slowing, negative symptoms and dopamine receptor availability—An IBZM SPECT study in neuroleptic-treated and drug-free schizophrenic patients. *Schizophr. Res.* **1998**, *31*, 19–26. [CrossRef]
6. Everitt, B.J.; Robbins, T.W. Neural systems of reinforcement for drug addiction: From actions to habits to compulsion. *Nat. Neurosci.* **2005**, *8*, 1481–1489. [CrossRef] [PubMed]
7. Everitt, B.J.; Robbins, T.W. Drug addiction: Updating actions to habits to compulsions ten years on. *Annu Rev. Psychol.* **2016**, *67*, 23–50. [CrossRef] [PubMed]
8. Lüscher, C. Drug-evoked synaptic plasticity causing addictive behavior. *J. Neurosci.* **2013**, *33*, 17641–17646. [CrossRef] [PubMed]
9. Schoofs, N.; Heinz, A. Pathological gambling: Impulse control disorder, addiction or compulsion? *Der Nervenarzt* **2013**, *84*, 629–634. [CrossRef]
10. Ersche, K.D.; Gillan, C.M.; Jones, P.S.; Williams, G.B.; Ward, L.H.; Luijten, M.; de Wit, S.; Sahakian, B.J.; Bullmore, E.T.; Robbins, T.W. Carrots and sticks fail to change behavior in cocaine addiction. *Science* **2016**, *352*, 1468–1471. [CrossRef]
11. Voon, V.; Derbyshire, K.; Ruck, C.; Irvine, M.A.; Worbe, Y.; Enander, J.; Schreiber, L.R.; Gillan, C.; Fineberg, N.A.; Sahakian, B.J.; et al. Disorders of compulsivity: A common bias towards learning habits. *Mol. Psychiatry* **2015**, *20*, 345. [CrossRef]
12. Friedel, E.; Schlagenhauf, F.; Beck, A.; Dolan, R.J.; Huys, Q.J.; Rapp, M.A.; Heinz, A. The effects of life stress and neural learning signals on fluid intelligence. *Eur. Arch. Psychiatry Clin. Neurosci.* **2015**, *265*, 35–43. [CrossRef]
13. Kühn, S.; Gallinat, J. Common biology of craving across legal and illegal drugs—A quantitative meta-analysis of cue-reactivity brain response. *Eur. J. Neurosci.* **2011**, *33*, 1318–1326. [CrossRef]
14. Heinz, A. *A New Understanding of Mental Disorders: Computational Models for Dimensional Psychiatry*; MIT Press: Cambridge, MA, USA, 2017.
15. Prevost, C.; Liljeholm, M.; Tyszka, J.M.; O'Doherty, J.P. Neural correlates of specific and general Pavlovian-to-instrumental transfer within human amygdalar subregions: A high-resolution fMRI study. *J. Neurosci.* **2012**, *32*, 8383–8390. [CrossRef]
16. Grüsser, S.M.; Wrase, J.; Klein, S.; Hermann, D.; Smolka, M.N.; Ruf, M.; Weber-Fahr, W.; Flor, H.; Mann, K.; Braus, D.F.; et al. Cue-induced activation of the striatum and medial prefrontal cortex predicts relapse in abstinent alcoholics. *Psychopharmacology* **2004**, *175*, 296–302. [CrossRef]
17. Beck, A.; Wüstenberg, T.; Genauck, A.; Wrase, J.; Schlagenhauf, F.; Smolka, M.N.; Mann, K.; Heinz, A. Effect of brain structure, brain function, and brain connectivity on relapse in alcohol-dependent patients. *Arch. Gen. Psychiatry* **2012**, *69*, 842–852. [CrossRef]
18. Heinz, A.; Siessmeier, T.; Wrase, J.; Buchholz, H.G.; Grunder, G.; Kumakura, Y.; Cumming, P.; Schreckenberger, M.; Smolka, M.N.; Rosch, F.; et al. Correlation of alcohol craving with striatal dopamine synthesis capacity and D2/3 receptor availability: A combined [18F]DOPA and [18F]DMFP PET study in detoxified alcoholic patients. *Am. J. Psychiatry* **2005**, *162*, 1515–1520. [CrossRef]
19. Myrick, H.; Anton, R.F.; Li, X.; Henderson, S.; Randall, P.K.; Voronin, K. Effect of naltrexone and ondansetron on alcohol cue-induced activation of the ventral striatum in alcohol-dependent people. *Arch. Gen. Psychiatry* **2008**, *65*, 466–475. [CrossRef]
20. Heinz, A.; Siessmeier, T.; Wrase, J.; Hermann, D.; Klein, S.; Grüsser-Sinopoli, S.M.; Flor, H.; Braus, D.F.; Buchholz, H.G.; Gründer, G. Correlation between dopamine D_2 receptors in the ventral striatum and central processing of alcohol cues and craving. *Am. J. Psychiatry* **2004**, *161*, 1783–1789. [CrossRef]
21. Heinz, A.; Dufeu, P.; Kuhn, S.; Dettling, M.; Gräf, K.; Kürten, I.; Rommelspacher, H.; Schmidt, L.G. Psychopathological and behavioral correlates of dopaminergic sensitivity in alcohol-dependent patients. *Arch. Gen. Psychiatry* **1996**, *53*, 1123–1128. [CrossRef]
22. Tiffany, S.T.; Carter, B.L. Is craving the source of compulsive drug use? *J. Psychopharmacol.* **1998**, *12*, 23–30. [CrossRef]
23. Carey, R.J.; Carrera, M.P.; Damianopoulos, E.N. A new proposal for drug conditioning with implications for drug addiction: The Pavlovian two-step from delay to trace conditioning. *Behav. Brain Res.* **2014**, *275*, 150–156. [CrossRef]
24. Cartoni, E.; Balleine, B.; Baldassarre, G. Appetitive pavlovian-instrumental transfer: A review. *Neurosci. Biobehav. Rev.* **2016**, *71*, 829–848. [CrossRef]

25. Huys, Q.J.M.; Cools, R.; Golzer, M.; Friedel, E.; Heinz, A.; Dolan, R.J.; Dayan, P. Disentangling the roles of approach, activation and valence in instrumental and pavlovian responding. *PLoS Comput. Biol.* **2011**, *7*, e1002028. [CrossRef]
26. Corbit, L.H.; Janak, P.H. Ethanol-associated cues produce general pavlovian-instrumental transfer. *Alcohol. Clin. Exp. Res.* **2007**, *31*, 766–774. [CrossRef]
27. LeBlanc, K.H.; Ostlund, S.B.; Maidment, N.T. Pavlovian-to-instrumental transfer in cocaine seeking rats. *Behav. Neurosci.* **2012**, *126*, 681–689. [CrossRef]
28. Ostlund, S.B.; LeBlanc, K.H.; Kosheleff, A.R.; Wassum, K.M.; Maidment, N.T. Phasic mesolimbic dopamine signaling encodes the facilitation of incentive motivation produced by repeated cocaine exposure. *Neuropsychopharmacology* **2014**, *39*, 2441–2449. [CrossRef]
29. Huys, Q.J.M.; Eshel, N.; O'Nions, E.; Sheridan, L.; Dayan, P.; Roiser, J.P. Bonsai trees in your head: How the pavlovian system sculpts goal-directed choices by pruning decision trees. *PLoS Comput. Biol.* **2012**, *8*, e1002410. [CrossRef]
30. Sebold, M.; Schad, D.J.; Nebe, S.; Garbusow, M.; Jünger, E.; Kroemer, N.B.; Kathmann, N.; Zimmermann, U.S.; Smolka, M.N.; Rapp, M.A.; et al. Don't think, just feel the music: Individuals with strong Pavlovian-to-instrumental transfer effects rely less on model-based reinforcement learning. *J. Cognit. Neurosci.* **2016**, *28*, 985–995. [CrossRef]
31. Sommer, C.; Garbusow, M.; Jünger, E.; Pooseh, S.; Bernhardt, N.; Birkenstock, J.; Schad, D.J.; Jabs, B.; Glockler, T.; Huys, Q.M.; et al. Strong seduction: Impulsivity and the impact of contextual cues on instrumental behavior in alcohol dependence. *Transl. Psychiatry* **2017**, *7*, e1183. [CrossRef]
32. Heinz, A.; Deserno, L.; Zimmermann, U.S.; Smolka, M.N.; Beck, A.; Schlagenhauf, F. Targeted intervention: Computational approaches to elucidate and predict relapse in alcoholism. *Neuroimage* **2017**, *151*, 33–44. [CrossRef]
33. Heinz, A.J.; Beck, A.; Meyer-Lindenberg, A.; Sterzer, P.; Heinz, A. Cognitive and neurobiological mechanisms of alcohol-related aggression. *Nat. Rev. Neurosci.* **2011**, *12*, 400–403. [CrossRef]
34. Sinha, R. How does stress lead to risk of alcohol relapse? *Alcohol. Res.* **2012**, *34*, 432–440.
35. Quail, S.L.; Morris, R.W.; Balleine, B.W. Stress associated changes in Pavlovian-instrumental transfer in humans. *Q. J. Exp. Psychol.* **2017**, *70*, 675–685. [CrossRef]
36. Pool, E.; Brosch, T.; Delplanque, S.; Sander, D. Stress increases cue-triggered "wanting" for sweet reward in humans. *J. Exp. Psychol. Anim. Learn. Cognit.* **2015**, *41*, 128–136. [CrossRef]
37. Garbusow, M.; Schad, D.J.; Sebold, M.; Friedel, E.; Bernhardt, N.; Koch, S.P.; Steinacher, B.; Kathmann, N.; Geurts, D.E.; Sommer, C.; et al. Pavlovian-to-instrumental transfer effects in the nucleus accumbens relate to relapse in alcohol dependence. *Addict. Biol.* **2016**, *21*, 719–731. [CrossRef]
38. Schad, D.J.; Garbusow, M.; Friedel, E.; Sommer, C.; Sebold, M.; Hagele, C.; Bernhardt, N.; Nebe, S.; Kuitunen-Paul, S.; Liu, S.; et al. Neural correlates of instrumental responding in the context of alcohol-related cues index disorder severity and relapse risk. *Eur. Arch. Psychiatry Clin. Neurosci.* **2019**, *263*, 295–308. [CrossRef]
39. Corbit, L.H.; Balleine, B.W. Double dissociation of basolateral and central amygdala lesions on the general and outcome-specific forms of pavlovian-instrumental transfer. *J. Neurosci.* **2005**, *25*, 962–970. [CrossRef]
40. Corbit, L.H.; Balleine, B.W. The general and outcome-specific forms of Pavlovian-instrumental transfer are differentially mediated by the nucleus accumbens core and shell. *J. Neurosci.* **2011**, *31*, 11786–11794. [CrossRef]
41. Garbusow, M.; Schad, D.J.; Sommer, C.; Jünger, E.; Sebold, M.; Friedel, E.; Wendt, J.; Kathmann, N.; Schlagenhauf, F.; Zimmermann, U.S. Pavlovian-to-instrumental transfer in alcohol dependence: A pilot study. *Neuropsychobiology* **2014**, *70*, 111–121. [CrossRef]
42. Hogarth, L.; Chase, H.W. Evaluating psychological markers for human nicotine dependence: Tobacco choice, extinction, and Pavlovian-to-instrumental transfer. *Exp. Clin. Psychopharmacol.* **2012**, *20*, 213–224. [CrossRef] [PubMed]
43. Manglani, H.R.; Lewis, A.H.; Wilson, S.J.; Delgado, M.R. Pavlovian-to-instrumental transfer of nicotine and food cues in deprived cigarette smokers. *Nicotine Tob. Res.* **2017**, *19*, 670–676. [CrossRef] [PubMed]
44. Wiers, R.W.; Eberl, C.; Rinck, M.; Becker, E.S.; Lindenmeyer, J. Retraining automatic action tendencies changes alcoholic patients' approach bias for alcohol and improves treatment outcome. *Psychol. Sci.* **2011**, *22*, 490–497. [CrossRef] [PubMed]

45. Wiers, C.E.; Stelzel, C.; Park, S.Q.; Gawron, C.K.; Ludwig, V.U.; Gutwinski, S.; Heinz, A.; Lindenmeyer, J.; Wiers, R.W.; Walter, H.; et al. Neural correlates of alcohol-approach bias in alcohol addiction: The spirit is willing but the flesh is weak for spirits. *Neuropsychopharmacology* **2014**, *39*, 688–697. [CrossRef] [PubMed]
46. Wiers, C.E.; Stelzel, C.; Gladwin, T.E.; Park, S.Q.; Pawelczack, S.; Gawron, C.K.; Stuke, H.; Heinz, A.; Wiers, R.W.; Rinck, M.; et al. Effects of cognitive bias modification training on neural alcohol cue reactivity in alcohol dependence. *Am. J. Psychiatry* **2015**, *172*, 335–343. [CrossRef] [PubMed]
47. Sebold, M.; Deserno, L.; Nebe, S.; Schad, D.J.; Garbusow, M.; Hägele, C.; Keller, J.; Jünger, E.; Kathmann, N.; Smolka, M. Model-based and model-free decisions in alcohol dependence. *Neuropsychobiology* **2014**, *70*, 122–131. [CrossRef] [PubMed]
48. Sebold, M.; Nebe, S.; Garbusow, M.; Guggenmos, M.; Schad, D.J.; Beck, A.; Kuitunen-Paul, S.; Sommer, C.; Frank, R.; Neu, P.; et al. When habits are dangerous: Alcohol expectancies and habitual decision making predict relapse in alcohol dependence. *Biol. Psychiatry* **2017**, *82*, 847–856. [CrossRef] [PubMed]
49. Friedel, E.; Koch, S.P.; Wendt, J.; Heinz, A.; Deserno, L.; Schlagenhauf, F. Devaluation and sequential decisions: Linking goal-directed and model-based behavior. *Front. Hum. Neurosci.* **2014**, *8*, 587. [CrossRef] [PubMed]
50. Dolan, R.J.; Dayan, P. Goals and habits in the brain. *Neuron* **2013**, *80*, 312–325. [CrossRef]
51. Schad, D.J.; Jünger, E.; Sebold, M.; Garbusow, M.; Bernhardt, N.; Javadi, A.-H.; Zimmermann, U.S.; Smolka, M.N.; Heinz, A.; Rapp, M.A.; et al. Processing speed enhances model-based over model-free reinforcement learning in the presence of high working memory functioning. *Front. Psychol.* **2014**, *5*, 1450. [CrossRef]
52. Otto, A.R.; Raio, C.M.; Chiang, A.; Phelps, E.A.; Daw, N.D. Working-memory capacity protects model-based learning from stress. *Proc. Natl. Acad. Sci. USA* **2013**, *110*, 20941–20946. [CrossRef] [PubMed]
53. Radenbach, C.; Reiter, A.M.; Engert, V.; Sjoerds, Z.; Villringer, A.; Heinze, H.-J.; Deserno, L.; Schlagenhauf, F. The interaction of acute and chronic stress impairs model-based behavioral control. *Psychoneuroendocrinology* **2015**, *53*, 268–280. [CrossRef] [PubMed]
54. Brady, K.T.; Back, S.E.; Waldrop, A.E.; McRae, A.L.; Anton, R.F.; Upadhyaya, H.P.; Saladin, M.E.; Randall, P.K. Cold pressor task reactivity: Predictors of alcohol use among alcohol-dependent individuals with and without comorbid posttraumatic stress disorder. *Alcohol. Clin. Exp. Res.* **2006**, *30*, 938–946. [CrossRef] [PubMed]
55. Thomas, S.E.; Bacon, A.K.; Randall, P.K.; Brady, K.T.; See, R.E. An acute psychosocial stressor increases drinking in non-treatment-seeking alcoholics. *Psychopharmacology* **2011**, *218*, 19–28. [CrossRef] [PubMed]
56. McGrath, E.; Jones, A.; Field, M. Acute stress increases ad-libitum alcohol consumption in heavy drinkers, but not through impaired inhibitory control. *Psychopharmacology* **2016**, *233*, 1227–1234. [CrossRef] [PubMed]
57. Vogel, S.; Klumpers, F.; Schroder, T.N.; Oplaat, K.T.; Krugers, H.J.; Oitzl, M.S.; Joels, M.; Doeller, C.F.; Fernandez, G. Stress induces a shift towards striatum-dependent stimulus-response learning via the mineralocorticoid receptor. *Neuropsychopharmacology* **2017**, *42*, 1262–1271. [CrossRef] [PubMed]
58. Maier, S.U.; Makwana, A.B.; Hare, T.A. Acute stress impairs self-control in goal-directed choice by altering multiple functional connections within the brain's decision circuits. *Neuron* **2015**, *87*, 621–631. [CrossRef]
59. Friedel, E.; Sebold, M.; Kuitunen-Paul, S.; Nebe, S.; Veer, I.M.; Zimmermann, U.S.; Schlagenhauf, F.; Smolka, M.N.; Rapp, M.; Walter, H.; et al. How accumulated real life stress experience and cognitive speed interact on decision-making processes. *Front. Hum. Neurosci.* **2017**, *11*, 302. [CrossRef]
60. Wray, T.B.; Merrill, J.E.; Monti, P.M. Using ecological momentary assessment (EMA) to assess situation-level predictors of alcohol use and alcohol-related consequences. *Alcohol. Res. Curr. Rev.* **2014**, *36*, 19–27.
61. Mellentin, A.I.; Skøt, L.; Nielsen, B.; Schippers, G.M.; Nielsen, A.S.; Stenager, E.; Juhl, C. Cue exposure therapy for the treatment of alcohol use disorders: A meta-analytic review. *Clin. Psychol. Rev.* **2017**, *57*, 195–207. [CrossRef]
62. Loeber, S.; Croissant, B.; Heinz, A.; Mann, K.; Flor, H. Cue exposure in the treatment of alcohol dependence: Effects on drinking outcome, craving and self-efficacy. *Br. J. Clin. Psychol.* **2006**, *45*, 515–529. [CrossRef] [PubMed]

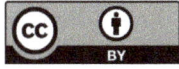 © 2019 by the authors. Licensee MDPI, Basel, Switzerland. This article is an open access article distributed under the terms and conditions of the Creative Commons Attribution (CC BY) license (http://creativecommons.org/licenses/by/4.0/).

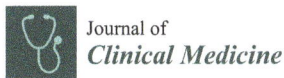

Review

The Potential of Cannabidiol as a Treatment for Psychosis and Addiction: Who Benefits Most? A Systematic Review

Albert Batalla [1,*,†], Hella Janssen [1,†], Shiral S. Gangadin [1,2] and Matthijs G. Bossong [1]

1. Department of Psychiatry, UMC Utrecht Brain Center, University Medical Center Utrecht, 3508 GA Utrecht, The Netherlands
2. Section of Neuropsychiatry, Department of Biomedical Sciences of Cells and Systems, University Medical Center Groningen, 9713 AV Groningen, The Netherlands
* Correspondence: abatallacases@gmail.com; Tel: +31-(0)88-755-8180
† These authors contributed equally to this work.

Received: 24 June 2019; Accepted: 18 July 2019; Published: 19 July 2019

Abstract: The endogenous cannabinoid (eCB) system plays an important role in the pathophysiology of both psychotic disorders and substance use disorders (SUDs). The non-psychoactive cannabinoid compound, cannabidiol (CBD) is a highly promising tool in the treatment of both disorders. Here we review human clinical studies that investigated the efficacy of CBD treatment for schizophrenia, substance use disorders, and their comorbidity. In particular, we examined possible profiles of patients who may benefit the most from CBD treatment. CBD, either as monotherapy or added to regular antipsychotic medication, improved symptoms in patients with schizophrenia, with particularly promising effects in the early stages of illness. A potential biomarker is the level of anandamide in blood. CBD and THC mixtures showed positive effects in reducing short-term withdrawal and craving in cannabis use disorders. Studies on schizophrenia and comorbid substance use are lacking. Future studies should focus on the effects of CBD on psychotic disorders in different stages of illness, together with the effects on comorbid substance use. These studies should use standardized measures to assess cannabis use. In addition, future efforts should be taken to study the relationship between the eCB system, GABA/glutamate, and the immune system to reveal the underlying neurobiology of the effects of CBD.

Keywords: cannabidiol; CBD; cannabis; psychosis; schizophrenia; substance use disorders; addiction

1. Introduction

Schizophrenia is a complex mental disorder, which has a profound impact on patients. The burden of schizophrenia is explained by the early onset, often in early adulthood or late adolescence, its chronic course, and its relatively high prevalence [1]. The symptomatology is highly heterogeneous and often overlaps with comorbid disorders, such as affective or substance use disorders [2,3]. Psychotic symptoms are grouped into three dimensions: Positive symptoms (e.g., delusions, hallucinations), negative symptoms (e.g., blunted affect, anhedonia), and cognitive symptoms (e.g., attention, memory, executive functioning; see for reviews [4–6]). Different combinations of symptoms and comorbidity lead to different clinical profiles and treatment needs. However, the pharmacological treatment of schizophrenia is mainly based on dopamine blockade, the effect of which is limited to the positive symptoms [7]. Moreover, two-thirds of the patients experience a suboptimal response with dopaminergic treatment [8], and these results are even worse when comorbid substance use disorders (SUDs) are present [9]. Therefore, there is an urgent need for alternative and more effective pharmacological interventions aimed to reduce the burden of complex and overlapping symptom profiles.

One of these interventions may involve the endocannabinoid (eCB) system, which is a promising new pharmacological target in this respect. The eCB system consists of at least two types of receptors and their endogenous ligands (i.e., endocannabinoids; [10,11]). The cannabinoid receptors are predominantly present in the central nervous system, in particular, in several limbic and cortical brain structures [12]. The eCB system is a retrograde messenger system that regulates both excitatory glutamate and inhibitory GABA neurotransmission according to an 'on-demand' principle: Endocannabinoids are released when and where they are needed [10,11,13]. This endocannabinoid-mediated regulation of synaptic transmission is a widespread phenomenon in the brain and is thought to play an important role in higher brain functions, such as cognition, motor function, and processing of sensory input, reward, and emotions [14–17]. eCB receptors are also present on immune cells in the central nervous system (i.e., microglia), which suggests their involvement in processes such as cytokine release, immune suppression, and induction of both cell migration and apoptosis [18,19].

The role of the eCB system in the pathophysiology of schizophrenia has been suggested in an accumulating amount of evidence [20,21]. First, epidemiological studies suggest that cannabis use increases the risk for developing schizophrenia [22] and lowers the age of onset of the disorder [23,24]. This risk increases with a higher frequency of cannabis use (e.g., daily use), and with the consumption of more potent cannabis (i.e., a higher amount of Δ9-tetrahydrocannabinol; THC) [22,25–27]. Second, modulation of the eCB system by the administration of THC (i.e., the main psychoactive component in cannabis) to healthy volunteers showed that THC can induce positive psychotic symptoms, effects that resemble negative symptoms (e.g., blunted affect, lack of spontaneity) and deficits in cognition (reviewed in [28]). Importantly, in schizophrenia patients, enhanced levels of endocannabinoids were demonstrated in cerebrospinal fluid and blood [29–31], and increased CB receptor density and availability were shown in the brain [32,33].

In addition to its role in schizophrenia, there is overwhelming evidence that the eCB system is implicated in the pathophysiology of addiction, in particular in processes such as drug-seeking behaviour, reward, withdrawal, and relapse (see for reviews [34–37]). For example, animal studies have shown that addictive properties reflected in behaviours such as self-administration or conditioned place preference of opiates, nicotine, and alcohol are absent or attenuated in cannabinoid CB1-receptor knockout mice and after administration of CB1 antagonists [35]. In addition, whereas the drug seeking behaviour of drugs of abuse was blocked with CB1 antagonists, it was reinstated after the administration of CB1 agonists [34,36]. Finally, endocannabinoid concentrations are affected by active drug seeking behaviour and eCB signalling seems to modulate the rewarding effects of addictive drugs [38].

SUDs and psychotic disorders such as schizophrenia co-occur frequently. Prevalence rates of any SUD (excluding nicotine and caffeine) in patients with schizophrenia are up to 45% [39,40], with the most frequently used substances being cannabis and alcohol. Considering nicotine use disorders, the prevalence rates rise up to 60%–90% [40]. Persistent use of licit or illicit drugs has been associated with adverse consequences in the overall course of psychotic disorders, and increased morbidity and mortality [40]. In addition, SUDs are also related to poor medication adherence, increasing the risk of relapse [39]. For example, in patients with schizophrenia, cannabis use has been related to higher relapse rates, increased severity of symptoms, and poor outcome [41–45]. Despite the high co-occurring rates, patients with comorbid SUDs and psychotic disorders are often excluded from clinical trials, which limits the generalization of results and ignores the potential (positive or negative) effects of the intervention on substance use.

While THC can trigger both schizophrenia and SUD and worsen the course of both disorders, the non-psychoactive cannabinoid compound cannabidiol (CBD) may have opposite or even beneficial effects. For example, CBD may have the ability to counteract psychotic symptoms and cognitive impairment associated with cannabis use as well as with acute THC administration [46,47]. In addition, CBD may lower the risk for developing psychosis that is related to cannabis use [48]. These effects are possibly mediated by the opposite effects of CBD and THC on brain activity patterns in key regions implicated in the pathophysiology of schizophrenia, such as the striatum, hippocampus, and prefrontal cortex [28]. Therefore, CBD displays a highly favourable profile for development as a new antipsychotic agent [48]. Similarly, CBD may serve as a treatment for SUDs, since evidence from preclinical studies suggests that CBD reduces negative withdrawal effects, motivation for self-administration, and reinstatement of drug use [37]. As a result, CBD-containing compounds are increasingly being investigated in the context of substance abuse in humans as well.

The eCB system appears an interesting target for schizophrenia, SUDs, and their comorbidity, due to the implication of the eCB system in their pathophysiology and the beneficial effects of CBD in both disorders. However, one may expect that CBD treatment may be most effective in a subgroup of patients, for example patients who show alterations in the eCB system or have a specific symptom profile. CBD may restore an imbalance in the eCB system, which may result in clinical improvement. Although previous excellent reviews (e.g., [37,48,49]) described the potential of CBD as a treatment for psychosis and SUD, this review provides a detailed and up-to-date systematic literature overview of clinical studies that investigated the efficacy of CBD treatment for schizophrenia and/or SUD. In addition, this review examined whether there are specific subgroup of patients with schizophrenia, SUD, or both that may benefit the most from CBD treatment.

2. Experimental Section

Clinical trials and case reports published up to February 2019, which described the effects of CBD on the symptomatology of psychotic disorders (i.e., schizophrenia and related disorders), SUD, or both were included. Reviews, non-English articles, pre-clinical or animal studies, studies that investigate CBD tolerability and pharmacokinetics or compare the acute effects of CBD with THC, and articles describing psychiatric or neurologic disorders other than psychotic disorders and SUD were excluded.

A literature search was conducted in the PubMed database. The following two searches were used: (1) "((((cannabidiol [MeSH Terms]) OR CBD[Text Word])) AND ((((((Substance-Related Disorders[MeSH Terms]) OR addiction[Text Word]) OR addictive behavior[Text Word]) OR drug abuse[Text Word])) OR drug dependence[Text Word])", (2) "(((((((Schizophrenia Spectrum and Other Psychotic Disorders[MeSH Terms])) OR schizophrenia[Text Word]) OR schizophrenic[Text Word]) OR psychosis[Text Word]) OR psychotic[Text Word])) AND ((cannabidiol[MeSH Terms]) OR CBD[Text Word])".

3. Results

The searches resulted in 214 articles, which included one duplicate (Figure 1). The articles were screened by two authors independently, according to the PRISMA guidelines [50]. After full-text screening, ten articles from the systematic search were included and six additional papers were selected through references in other papers. Of these 16 included articles, seven studies were related to CBD treatment for schizophrenia and eight studies described the treatment of SUD with CBD-containing compounds. Only one study assessed the effects of the treatment with medicinal cannabis for patients with a psychotic disorder and a comorbid cannabis use disorder.

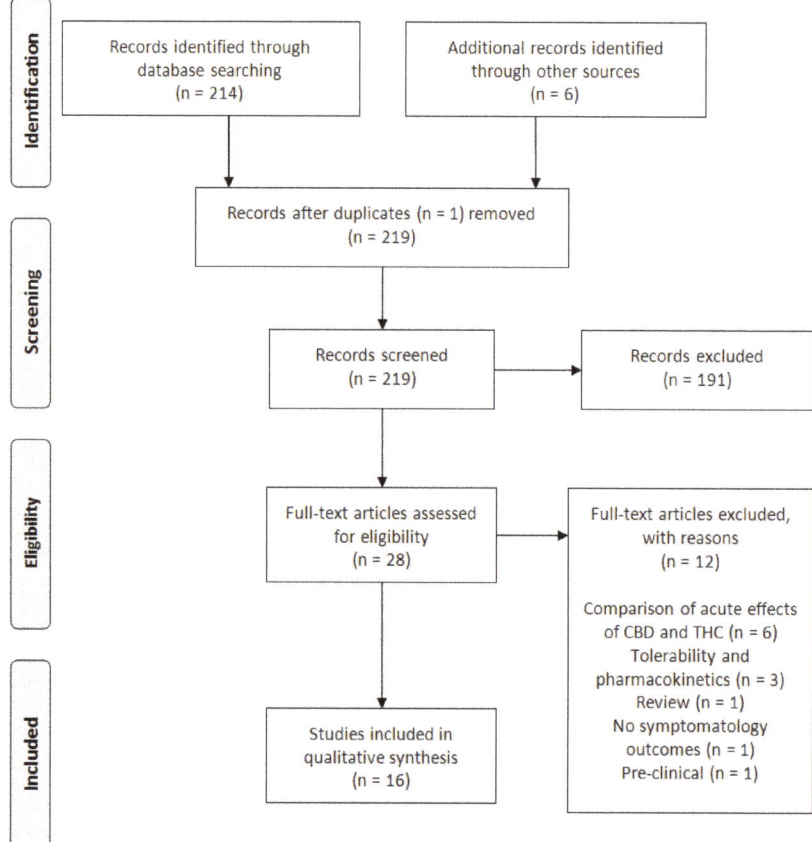

Figure 1. Study inclusion process. CBD: Cannabidiol; THC: Δ9-Tetrahydrocannabinol.

3.1. CBD—Psychosis

Four randomized controlled trials (RCTs) and three case reports assessed the efficacy of CBD as a treatment for psychotic disorders (Table 1).

Zuardi et al. (1995) described a 19-year-old woman with schizophrenia who received progressive increase of CBD monotherapy for 26 days (maximum of 1500 mg/day) [51]. CBD treatment was associated with the improvement of symptomatology as measured with the Brief Psychiatric Rating Scale (BPRS). This improvement did not further increase on haloperidol treatment [51]. In a second case report of the same group, three treatment-resistant schizophrenia male patients were treated with CBD monotherapy for four weeks. The authors reported mild improvement of positive and negative symptoms of one patient after CBD treatment (BPRS score decreased from 29 to 22). Moreover, CBD was well tolerated and no side effects were reported [52]. Makiol and Klunge (2019 described a case of a 57-year-old woman with treatment-resistant schizophrenia, which persisted for 21 years [53]. On admission she had a total PANSS (Positive and Negative Syndrome Scale) score of 117 and a negative symptom score of 41. Adjunctive to treatment with clozapine (275 mg/day) and lamotrigine (225 mg/day), the patient received CBD 500 mg twice daily, which was increased to 750 mg twice daily after seven weeks. On discharge, the PANSS total score decreased to 68 and negative symptom score to 21, which the authors indicated as accomplishment of remission criteria with only mild negative symptoms. CBD did not affect clozapine levels and was well tolerated apart from a mild hand tremor [53]. Leweke et al. (2012) performed a double-blind randomized controlled trial in which 39 acutely psychotic inpatients were treated with either CBD ($N = 20$) or amisulpride 800 mg ($N = 19$) for four weeks [54]. The authors did not provide information about illness duration before hospitalization. Both treatments were associated with clinical improvement, considering a decrease of positive and negative symptoms (change from baseline to 28-day assessment in positive PANSS score -9.0 ± 6.1 and -8.4 ± 7.5, and in negative PANSS score -9.1 ± 4.9 and -6.4 ± 6.0 after CBD and amisulpride, respectively; all comparisons $p < 0.001$). However, CBD treatment had a superior side-effect profile in terms of less severe changes in weight gain, extrapyramidal symptoms, prolactin levels, and sexual functioning. In addition, Leweke et al. (2012) measured anandamide levels in serum before and after treatment with CBD or amisulpride and the relationship with psychotic symptoms [54]. As compared to treatment with amisulpride, CBD showed a significant increase in anandamide levels and this was associated with the improvement of psychotic symptoms (i.e., decrease of total PANSS score). These findings suggest that anandamide levels could serve as a possible biomarker for the efficacy of CBD treatment [54]. In the largest randomized placebo-controlled trial to date, McGuire et al. (2018) assessed the effect of six-week treatment with CBD (1000 mg/day) added to antipsychotic medication in 88 moderately ill (total PANSS score >60) outpatients with schizophrenia [55]. After six weeks, positive symptoms (change from baseline -3.2 after CBD and -1.7 after placebo, treatment difference $= -1.4$, 95% CI $= -2.5, -0.2$) and global clinical impression significantly improved in the CBD group compared with placebo (treatment difference $= -0.5$, 95% CI $= -0.8, -0.1$ for improvement rates and $= -0.3$, 95% CI $= -0.5, 0.0$ for change in severity of illness) [55]. These case studies and RCTs suggest that CBD treatment for psychosis is beneficial and could possibly be as effective as antipsychotic medication.

Two RCTs showed less conclusive results of CBD treatment on positive, negative, and cognitive symptomatology. The randomized placebo-controlled trial by Hallak et al. (2010) presented the effect of acute treatment with single doses of CBD on selective attention as measured with the Stroop Colour and Word Test in a heterogeneous group of 28 schizophrenia patients (illness duration <5 years ($N = 11$), >5 years ($N = 17$)) [56]. These patients performed the Stroop test twice: The first time without the administration of any drug and the second time after oral administration of either placebo, 300 mg, or 600 mg CBD. After the two sessions, all groups showed improvement in cognitive performance (i.e., reduced number of errors during the Stroop test). Improvement was greater in the placebo and CBD 300 mg groups, compared with the patients who received CBD 600 mg. There was no effect of CBD treatment on both positive and negative symptoms [56]. Second, the most recent double-blind, randomized placebo-controlled trial by Boggs et al. (2018) examined treatment with oral CBD (600 mg/day) or placebo adjunctive to a stable dose of antipsychotic medication in 36 chronic schizophrenia patients (mean illness duration >25 years) [57]. Although positive, negative, general, and total PANSS decreased and cognitive performance increased over time in both groups, there were no significant differences between groups. Thus, in this trial, symptomatology and cognitive performance did not improve after adjunctive CBD treatment in schizophrenia outpatients who were receiving long-term polypharmacy for a myriad of psychiatric symptoms (Boggs et al., 2018) [57]. One possibility is that these results may be explained by the significant difference in the use of multiple antipsychotics between the placebo (38.9%) and CBD groups (11%) [57].

In summary, most of abovementioned studies provided evidence for the potential of CBD as an antipsychotic treatment, which could alleviate both cognitive and psychotic symptoms in patients with psychotic disorders. The studies that showed negative results provided either a single dose of CBD [56] or included chronic schizophrenia patients who received multiple types of antipsychotic medication [57].

Table 1. Case reports and clinical trials on the efficacy of cannabidiol (CBD) as a treatment for psychotic disorders.

Study	Study Design	Participants	Substance Use	Intervention	CBD Administration	Primary Outcomes
Zuardi et al. (1995) [51]	Case report	19-year-old female schizophrenia inpatient (two years after first hospitalization)	Not reported	Progressive increase of CBD monotherapy over four weeks, followed by haloperidol treatment	Oral; up to 1500 mg/day	Improvement of symptomatology. Improvement did not continue on haloperidol. No side effects.
Zuardi et al. (2006) [52]	Case series	Three male inpatients with treatment-resistant schizophrenia	Not reported	Progressive increase of CBD monotherapy over four weeks, followed by olanzapine treatment	Oral; up to 1280 mg/day	Mild improvement of symptomatology of one patient after CBD treatment. No side effects.
Makiol and Klunge (2019) [53]	Case report	57-year old-female treatment-resistant schizophrenia inpatient	Not reported	Treatment with CBD adjunctive to clozapine and lamotrigine	Oral; up to 1500 mg/day	Improvement of symptomatology and the patient fulfilled remission criteria with only mild negative symptoms.
Leweke et al. (2012) [54]	Double-blind CBD vs. amisulpride RCT	39 acutely psychotic inpatients	Not reported, exclusion criteria were SUD or positive urine drug screening for illicit drugs in general and cannabis in particular.	Hospitalization and four-week treatment with CBD or amisulpride	Oral; up to 800 mg/day	Treatment with either CBD or amisulpride is associated with improvement of symptomatology, but CBD has a superior side-effect profile.
McGuire et al. (2018) [55]	Double-blind placebo RCT	88 outpatients with schizophrenia	Not reported, substance use was not an exclusion and not prohibited during the study.	A six-week treatment with CBD adjunctive to antipsychotic medication.	Oral solution; 1000 mg/day	Improvement of symptomatology, no side effects.
Hallak et al. (2010) [56]	Single dose double-blind placebo RCT	28 schizophrenia outpatients	Not reported	Acute treatment with a single dose of CBD	Oral; 300 or 600 mg	CBD 300 mg and placebo both improved cognitive performance as compared to CBD 600 mg. No effects on symptomatology.
Boggs et al. (2018) [57]	Double-blind placebo RCT	36 outpatients with chronic schizophrenia	Not reported, patients with substance abuse in the past three months or dependence in the past six months were excluded.	Six-week treatment with CBD added to a stable dose of antipsychotic medication	Oral; 600 mg/day	Cognitive performance improved after placebo, symptomatology improved in both groups, no differences between groups.

CBD: Cannabidiol; RCT: Randomized clinical trial.

3.2. CBD—Substance Use Disorders

To date, eight studies assessed the potential effect of CBD as treatment for SUD (Table 2). Six studies focussed on cannabis dependence and two on tobacco dependence.

3.2.1. Cannabis Dependence

The treatment of cannabis dependence with a cannabis-extracted CBD/THC mixture (Sativex) was assessed in three clinical trials. In the first double-blind randomized controlled trial by Allsop et al. (2014), 51 inpatients with cannabis dependence received Sativex or placebo for six days along with cognitive behavioural therapy [58]. Immediately after treatment, Sativex significantly decreased cannabis withdrawal and craving symptoms and improved treatment retention rates. At 28 days, both groups showed a decrease in cannabis use, in the amount of cannabis-related problems, and in the severity of cannabis dependence from baseline to follow-up, but the differences between groups were no longer significant [58]. A second double-blind randomized placebo-controlled trial assessed the effects of an eight-week treatment with self-titrated or fixed doses of Sativex in nine subjects with cannabis dependence [59]. During treatment sessions, when cannabis use was not allowed, both fixed and self-titrated doses of Sativex reduced cannabis withdrawal symptoms, however, the high fixed dose seemed the most effective. Sativex did not influence cannabis craving. The same research group performed a larger double-blind randomized placebo-controlled trial in which 27 cannabis-dependent subjects were treated with self-titrated dosages of Sativex in combination with cognitive behavioural therapy over 12 weeks [60]. The abstinence rate did not change significantly between baseline and follow-up. Cannabis use, withdrawal, and craving symptoms reduced over time in both groups. Sativex was associated with a greater reduction in cannabis craving symptoms when compared with placebo.

While the previous studies used CBD/THC mixtures, the following three studies described treatments of cannabis dependence with pure CBD. The first study by Crippa et al. (2013), reported a 19-year-old female with cannabis dependence who was treated with oral CBD over 11 days [61]. The dose was 300 mg on day 1, 600 mg on days 2–10 and 300 mg on day 11. During treatment, cannabis withdrawal, anxiety, and dissociative symptoms progressively decreased. A six-month follow-up period revealed a relapse of cannabis use, however at a lower frequency than on admission [61]. In a second case report, Shannon and Opila-Lehman (2015) described the treatment with 24–18 mg CBD oil adjunctive to citalopram and lamotrigine for a 27-year-old male with cannabis disorder and bipolar disorder. During the use of CBD oil, the patient did not use cannabis, showed a decrease in anxiety, and demonstrated improved sleep quality [62]. Third, the open-label clinical trial by Solowij et al. (2018) assessed the effects of ten-week treatment with CBD (200 mg/day) on psychological symptoms, cognition, and plasma concentrations [63]. Twenty frequent and ongoing cannabis users, of which twelve were dependent users (severity dependence scale score ≥3) and ten were nondependent users (severity dependence scale score <3), participated in this trial. Between baseline and post treatment sessions, cannabis use and withdrawal did not change, but cannabis-related experiences (i.e., euphoria and feeling high) decreased. Anxiety, depressive, and psychotic-like symptoms showed greater reductions in dependent than nondependent users. Attentional switching, verbal learning, and memory improved in all participants. Remarkably, higher CBD plasma concentrations were associated with lower psychotic-like symptoms (total and negative), distress, anxiety, and severity of cannabis dependence [63]. These results suggest greater effects of CBD in dependent users which can possibly be detected through CBD plasma concentrations.

Taken collectively, CBD shows some promise in the treatment of cannabis dependence as it reduces behaviour relevant to addiction such as craving and withdrawal in almost all studies. Because double-blind placebo-controlled RCTs with pure CBD are lacking, the evidence for the efficacy of products containing a combination of CBD and THC in the treatment of cannabis dependence is more convincing.

Table 2. Case reports and clinical trials on the efficacy of CBD as a treatment for substance use disorders.

Study	Study Design	Participants	Intervention	CBD Administration	Primary Outcomes
Cannabis Dependence					
Allsop et al. (2014) [58]	Double-blind placebo RCT	51 inpatients with cannabis dependence	A six-day treatment with Sativex in combination with CBT	Intranasal; maximum daily: 86.4 mg THC and 80 mg CBD	Sativex reduced cannabis withdrawal and cravings, and improved treatment retention rates.
Trigo et al. (2016) [59]	Double-blind placebo RCT	Nine individuals with cannabis dependence	Eight-week treatment with self-titrated or fixed doses of Sativex or placebo.	Intranasal; up to 108 mg THC and 100 mg CBD	During interruption of cannabis use both fixed and titrated doses of Sativex reduced cannabis withdrawal symptoms (but not craving), however the high fixed dose seemed the most effective.
Trigo et al. (2018) [60]	Double-blind placebo RCT	27 individuals with cannabis dependence	Twelve-week treatment with self-titrated dosages of Sativex next to weekly CBT sessions.	Intranasal; up to 113.4 mg THC and 105 mg CBD/day	Cannabis use, cravings, and withdrawal decreased in both groups over time. Sativex reduced cannabis cravings.
Crippa et al. (2013) [61]	Case report	19-year-old female diagnosed with cannabis dependence	Hospitalization and progressive increase of CBD	Oral; 300 to 600 mg	A progressive reduction of cannabis withdrawal, anxiety, and dissociative symptoms.
Shannon and Opila-Lehman (2015) [62]	Case report	27-year-old male diagnosed with bipolar disorder and cannabis dependence	Treatment with CBD oil added to citalopram and lamotrigine	Intranasal; decreasing from 24 to 18 mg	Abstinence from cannabis, better sleep quality, and decrease in anxiety during the use of CBD oil.
Solowij et al. (2018) [63]	Open-label clinical trial	20 ongoing cannabis users	Ten-week treatment with CBD	Oral; 200 mg daily	CBD improved psychological and cognitive symptomatology. Greater benefits were observed in dependent than in nondependent cannabis users.
Tobacco Dependence					
Morgan et al. (2013) [64]	Double-blind placebo RCT	24 individuals who smoked >10 cigarettes per day and intended to quit	Optional CBD treatment during one week	Inhalation; 400 µg CBD per dose	CBD reduced the total number of cigarettes smoked. Reduction of craving in both groups after one week of treatment, but this did not maintain at follow-up.
Hindocha et al. (2018) [65]	Single dose double-blind placebo RCT	30 individuals with tobacco dependence	Treatment with a single dose of CBD after an overnight of cigarette abstinence	Oral; 800 mg CBD	CBD reduced the salience and peasantness of cigarette cues but had no effect on craving and withdrawal.

CBD: Cannabidiol; CBT: Cognitive behavioural therapy; RCT: Randomized clinical trial; THC: Δ9-Tetrahydrocannabinol.

3.2.2. Tobacco Dependence

Morgan et al. (2013) assessed the effects of the optional use of an inhaler containing CBD (400 µg/dose) during one week in 24 individuals who smoked >10 cigarettes/day and intended to quit [64]. Results showed that CBD reduced the total number of cigarettes smoked during the treatment period. However, CBD did not have an effect on craving symptoms. In addition, craving was reduced in both groups at the end of treatment, but this did not maintain at follow-up [64]. Additionally, a second clinical trial into the efficacy of CBD treatment for tobacco dependence provided information about treatment outcomes related to motivation and evaluation. Hindocha et al. (2018) treated 30 tobacco-dependent individuals with a single dose of CBD 800 mg [65]. Attentional bias to pictorial cigarette cues was measured using a visual probe and an explicit rating task. In addition, craving, withdrawal, and side effects were assessed. After overnight cigarette abstinence, CBD reduced attentional bias to cigarette cues and pleasantness of cigarette cues, which could suggest that CBD has a potential effect on the motivational aspects of addiction. In this trial, CBD did not have an effect on craving and withdrawal. Moreover, no significant differences were found between CBD and placebo on side effects [65].

3.3. CBD—Psychosis and SUD

Schipper and colleagues (2018) were the first who described the efficacy of CBD treatment for patients with a psychotic disorder and a comorbid treatment-resistant cannabis use disorder (Table 3) [66]. Seven hospitalized patients received eight weeks of treatment with Bedrolite, medicinal cannabis that contains 0.4% THC and 9% CBD, as add-on therapy to conventional antipsychotic medication. The medicinal cannabis was supposed to substitute street cannabis used by the patients but was only provided at fixed moments during the day. Doses ranged from 0.125 to 0.5 g daily (11–45 mg CBD), depending on dose and frequency of the use of street cannabis before admission. Treatment with CBD-rich medicinal cannabis did not affect psychosis- or dependence-related symptomatology. Patients preferred street cannabis over the medicinal cannabis and started to use additional street cannabis during the treatment program [66]. The most likely explanation for these negative results was the low THC concentration in Bedrolite as compared to street cannabis. As a result, the substitution of THC-rich street cannabis by medicinal cannabis with mainly CBD may have been too abrupt for most patients.

Table 3. Studies on CBD treatment for patients with a psychotic disorder and a comorbid cannabis use disorder.

Study	Study Design	Participants	Intervention	CBD Administration	Primary Outcomes
Schipper et al. (2018) [66]	Case report	Seven inpatients with a psychotic disorder and a comorbid treatment-resistant cannabis use disorder	Eight-week treatment with medicinal cannabis (Bedrolite: 0.4% THC and 9% CBD) adjunctive to antipsychotic medication.	Inhalation: 11–45 mg/day	No effect on symptomatology or craving.

CBD: Cannabidiol; THC: Δ 9-tetrahydrocannabinol.

4. Discussion and Conclusions

The current review aimed to provide a detailed and up-to-date systematic literature overview of studies that investigated the efficacy of CBD treatment for schizophrenia and/or SUD. Based on this overview, a second aim was to examine whether there is a specific subgroup of patients with schizophrenia, SUD, or both that may benefit most from CBD treatment. In some but not all studies, CBD seemed effective as a treatment for psychosis and SUD. CBD may have the capacity to alleviate positive, negative, and cognitive symptoms in schizophrenia, as well as craving and withdrawal in SUD. Although most of the studies showed promising results, differences in study design, patient population, and use of concomitant medication make it difficult to define specific subgroups to whom CBD should be administered. In addition, CBD doses and administration were different between studies and most of the reviewed studies did not describe the source of CBD (i.e., synthetic or cannabis extracted), which may have different efficacy. However, the results of the reviewed studies suggested some features that may contribute to the identification of patients who may benefit most from CBD treatment.

Research into CBD treatment for psychosis provided evidence for a few possible clinical and biological characteristics of the subgroup. The effects of CBD were studied in patients in both early and later stages of psychotic disorders. Overall, acutely psychotic and early onset patients demonstrated reductions of positive and negative symptoms [51,54], while treatment resistant and chronic patients showed less promising improvement [56,57]. Even though Makiol and Kluge (2019) described a chronic schizophrenia patient who exhibited great clinical improvement (i.e., change of total PANSS score: 49) [53], the majority of the results suggest that CBD may be more effective in the early stage of psychotic disorders. This is in line with previous studies suggesting that immune dysregulation (i.e., microglial activation) is mainly involved in the early stage of psychotic disorders [67,68]. As cannabinoid receptors are also present on microglia, it is possible that CBD exerts its effects by decreasing microglial activity [69]. Furthermore, anandamide levels in serum could serve as a possible biomarker for the efficacy of CBD treatment. For instance, Leweke et al. (2012) reported a significant increase in anandamide levels after CBD treatment, which was associated with the improvement of psychotic symptoms (i.e., decrease of total PANSS score) [54]. This is in concurrence with a previously reported inverse association between elevated anandamide levels in cerebrospinal fluid and psychotic symptoms in antipsychotic-naïve patients [29–31].

Research into CBD treatment for SUD primarily focussed on cannabis dependence. Taken collectively, CBD shows promise in the treatment of cannabis dependence as it reduces craving and withdrawal in almost all studies. However, these studies have heterogeneous study designs and administration methods. The differences in administration and dosages may provide a possible explanation for the different results observed in the included studies. For instance, THC/CBD mixtures might be more effective in reducing some features of cannabis dependence (i.e., craving, use and withdrawal) than pure CBD. Moreover, the level of cannabis dependence and intrinsic motivation for treatment, may help to define a possible subgroup of patients in which CBD is more effective. Dependent users (i.e., those with a severity dependence scale score ≥3), showed reduced anxiety, depression, and psychotic-like symptoms after a 10-week treatment with CBD, compared with nondependent users [63]. However, studies that include individuals with more symptoms at baseline can show greater reductions after treatment. Therefore, it is difficult to determine whether symptom severity is truly a patient characteristic that could predict better outcomes after CBD treatment. Solowij et al. (2018) also found that cannabis-related experiences decreased after treatment [63], which is in accordance with previous studies that indicate that CBD counteracts the effects induced by THC [46,47]. Intrinsic motivation for treatment seems an important aspect as well, as it may increase medication adherence [65]. Conversely, patients that do not seek treatment are less inclined to follow strict study protocols [66]. The majority of the discussed studies recruited individuals with cannabis dependence from the community, which suggests that these individuals were at least open for treatment. To a certain extent, this may explain why the study by Schipper et al. (2018) found that CBD administration was not effective [66], as they included individuals that did not seek treatment.

Considering the efficacy of CBD in both psychotic disorders and SUD, one can speculate that CBD should also be effective in the treatment of the comorbidity. However, only Schipper et al. (2018) studied this population, with negative results [66]. As discussed previously, these patients were treatment resistant for SUD and showed lack of motivation for treatment. An additional limitation of this study was the good baseline functioning in five out of seven patients. Moreover, this study administered CBD in a formulation that contained very little THC, which possibly explains why the participants preferred street cannabis.

Future studies could take these limitations into account and should focus on examining the effects of CBD in the different stages of psychotic disorders, considering the high prevalence of comorbid SUD. Studies into psychotic disorders could use CBD (i.e., either as monotherapy or add-on) to treat psychotic symptoms and to prevent relapse in early stages, while exploring the effects on comorbid substance use (e.g., cannabis). These studies should use standardized measures to assess cannabis use. In later stages and comorbid treatment-resistant SUD, CBD studies may aim to reduce cannabis use, using harm-reduction strategies (e.g., gradually shift the THC/CBD ratio in medicinal cannabis in favour of CBD) [70]. Currently, nine ongoing clinical trials that study the effects of CBD on psychotic disorders or SUD (including alcohol and cocaine misuse) are registered in clinicaltrials.gov, of which one (NCT03883360) includes patients with recent-onset psychotic disorder and cannabis use. Therefore, more results on this topic are expected in the near future.

It remains unclear if the efficacy of CBD in schizophrenia, addiction, and their comorbidity could be explained by shared or different biological mechanisms. To elucidate this, future efforts should be taken to study the relationship between the eCB system, GABA/glutamate, and the immune system. For example, neuroimaging studies (e.g., positron-emission tomography, PET and magnetic resonance spectroscopy, MRS) could measure CB1 receptor densities and markers for glia in patients with schizophrenia and/or SUD who were treated with CBD.

In conclusion, CBD treatment is a promising and novel tool with several potential applications in the treatment of psychotic disorders, substance use disorders, and their comorbidity. Large-scale trials are needed to establish its clinical utility.

Author Contributions: Conceptualization, A.B. and M.G.B.; methodology, H.J. and S.S.G.; investigation, H.J.; data curation, H.J. and S.S.G.; Writing—Original draft preparation, A.B., H.J. and S.S.G.; Writing—Review and editing, A.B. and M.G.B.; visualization, H.J. and S.S.G.; supervision, A.B. and M.G.B.

Funding: M. Bossong was supported by a Veni fellowship from the Netherlands Organization for Scientific Research (grant number 016.166.038).

Conflicts of Interest: The authors declare no conflict of interest.

References

1. Rössler, W.; Joachim Salize, H.; van Os, J.; Riecher-Rössler, A. Size of burden of schizophrenia and psychotic disorders. *Eur. Neuropsychopharmacol.* **2005**, *15*, 399–409. [CrossRef] [PubMed]
2. Buckley, P.F.; Miller, B.J.; Lehrer, D.S.; Castle, D.J. Psychiatric Comorbidities and Schizophrenia. *Schizophr. Bull.* **2009**, *35*, 383–402. [CrossRef] [PubMed]
3. Volkow, N.D. Substance Use Disorders in Schizophrenia—Clinical Implications of Comorbidity. *Schizophr. Bull.* **2009**, *35*, 469–472. [CrossRef] [PubMed]
4. Fioravanti, M.; Carlone, O.; Vitale, B.; Cinti, M.E.; Clare, L. A Meta-Analysis of Cognitive Deficits in Adults with a Diagnosis of Schizophrenia. *Neuropsychol. Rev.* **2005**, *15*, 73–95. [CrossRef] [PubMed]
5. Tandon, R.; Nasrallah, H.A.; Keshavan, M.S. Schizophrenia, "just the facts" 4. Clinical features and conceptualization. *Schizophr. Res.* **2009**, *110*, 1–23. [CrossRef] [PubMed]
6. Van Os, J.; Kenis, G.; Rutten, B.P.F. The environment and schizophrenia. *Nature* **2010**, *468*, 203–212. [CrossRef] [PubMed]
7. Tandon, R. Antipsychotics in the Treatment of Schizophrenia. *J. Clin. Psychiatry* **2011**, *72*. [CrossRef]
8. Samara, M.T.; Nikolakopoulou, A.; Salanti, G.; Leucht, S. How Many Patients with Schizophrenia Do Not Respond to Antipsychotic Drugs in the Short Term? An Analysis Based on Individual Patient Data from Randomized Controlled Trials. *Schizophr. Bull.* **2019**, *45*, 639–646. [CrossRef]
9. Green, A.I. Schizophrenia and comorbid substance use disorder: Effects of antipsychotics. *J. Clin. Psychiatry* **2005**, *66* (Suppl. 6), 21–26.
10. Kano, M.; Ohno-Shosaku, T.; Hashimotodani, Y.; Uchigashima, M.; Watanabe, M. Endocannabinoid-Mediated Control of Synaptic Transmission. *Physiol. Rev.* **2009**, *89*, 309–380. [CrossRef]
11. Katona, I.; Freund, T.F. Multiple Functions of Endocannabinoid Signaling in the Brain. *Annu. Rev. Neurosci.* **2012**, *35*, 529–558. [CrossRef]
12. Wong, D.F.; Kuwabara, H.; Horti, A.G.; Raymont, V.; Brasic, J.; Guevara, M.; Ye, W.; Dannals, R.F.; Ravert, H.T.; Nandi, A.; et al. Quantification of cerebral cannabinoid receptors subtype 1 (CB1) in healthy subjects and schizophrenia by the novel PET radioligand [^{11}C]OMAR. *Neuroimage* **2010**, *52*, 1505–1513. [CrossRef]

13. Heifets, B.D.; Castillo, P.E. Endocannabinoid Signaling and Long-Term Synaptic Plasticity. *Annu. Rev. Physiol.* **2009**, *71*, 283–306. [CrossRef]
14. Hill, M.N.; Hillard, C.J.; Bambico, F.R.; Patel, S.; Gorzalka, B.B.; Gobbi, G. The Therapeutic Potential of the Endocannabinoid System for the Development of a Novel Class of Antidepressants. *Trends Pharmacol. Sci.* **2009**, *30*, 484–493. [CrossRef]
15. Zanettini, C. Effects of endocannabinoid system modulation on cognitive and emotional behavior. *Front. Behav. Neurosci.* **2011**, *5*. [CrossRef]
16. Bossong, M.G.; Jager, G.; Bhattacharyya, S.; Allen, P. Acute and non-acute effects of cannabis on human memory function: A critical review of neuroimaging studies. *Curr. Pharm. Des.* **2014**, *20*, 2114–2125. [CrossRef]
17. Bossong, M.G.; Jansma, J.M.; Bhattacharyya, S.; Ramsey, N.F. Role of the endocannabinoid system in brain functions relevant for schizophrenia: An overview of human challenge studies with cannabis or ∆9-tetrahydrocannabinol (THC). *Prog. Neuro-Psychopharmacol. Biol. Psychiatry* **2014**, *52*, 53–69. [CrossRef]
18. Pertwee, R.G. Ligands that target cannabinoid receptors in the brain: From THC to anandamide and beyond. *Addict. Biol.* **2008**, *13*, 147–159. [CrossRef]
19. Cabral, G.A.; Griffin-Thomas, L. Emerging role of the cannabinoid receptor CB2 in immune regulation: Therapeutic prospects for neuroinflammation. *Expert Rev. Mol. Med.* **2009**, *11*, e3. [CrossRef]
20. Leweke, F.M.; Koethe, D. Cannabis and psychiatric disorders: It is not only addiction. *Addict. Biol.* **2008**, *13*, 264–275. [CrossRef]
21. Bossong, M.G.; Niesink, R.J.M. Adolescent brain maturation, the endogenous cannabinoid system and the neurobiology of cannabis-induced schizophrenia. *Prog. Neurobiol.* **2010**, *92*, 370–385. [CrossRef]
22. Marconi, A.; Di Forti, M.; Lewis, C.M.; Murray, R.M.; Vassos, E. Meta-analysis of the Association Between the Level of Cannabis Use and Risk of Psychosis. *Schizophr. Bull.* **2016**, *42*, 1262–1269. [CrossRef]
23. Large, M.; Sharma, S.; Compton, M.T.; Slade, T.; Nielssen, O. Cannabis Use and Earlier Onset of Psychosis. *Arch. Gen. Psychiatry* **2011**, *68*, 555. [CrossRef]
24. Di Forti, M.; Sallis, H.; Allegri, F.; Trotta, A.; Ferraro, L.; Stilo, S.A.; Marconi, A.; La Cascia, C.; Reis Marques, T.; Pariante, C.; et al. Daily Use, Especially of High-Potency Cannabis, Drives the Earlier Onset of Psychosis in Cannabis Users. *Schizophr. Bull.* **2014**, *40*, 1509–1517. [CrossRef]
25. Schubart, C.D.; van Gastel, W.A.; Breetvelt, E.J.; Beetz, S.L.; Ophoff, R.A.; Sommer, I.E.C.; Kahn, R.S.; Boks, M.P.M. Cannabis use at a young age is associated with psychotic experiences. *Psychol. Med.* **2011**, *41*, 1301–1310. [CrossRef]
26. Di Forti, M.; Marconi, A.; Carra, E.; Fraietta, S.; Trotta, A.; Bonomo, M.; Bianconi, F.; Gardner-Sood, P.; O'Connor, J.; Russo, M.; et al. Proportion of patients in south London with first-episode psychosis attributable to use of high potency cannabis: A case-control study. *Lancet Psychiatry* **2015**, *2*, 233–238. [CrossRef]
27. Di Forti, M.; Quattrone, D.; Freeman, T.P.; Tripoli, G.; Gayer-Anderson, C.; Quigley, H.; Rodriguez, V.; Jongsma, H.E.; Ferraro, L.; La Cascia, C.; et al. The contribution of cannabis use to variation in the incidence of psychotic disorder across Europe (EU-GEI): A multicentre case-control study. *Lancet Psychiatry* **2019**, *6*, 427–436. [CrossRef]
28. Murray, R.M.; Englund, A.; Abi-Dargham, A.; Lewis, D.A.; Di Forti, M.; Davies, C.; Sherif, M.; McGuire, P.; D'Souza, D.C. Cannabis-associated psychosis: Neural substrate and clinical impact. *Neuropharmacology* **2017**, *124*, 89–104. [CrossRef]
29. Leweke, F.; Giuffrida, A.; Wurster, U.; Emrich, H.M.; Piomelli, D. Elevated endogenous cannabinoids in schizophrenia. *Neuroreport* **1999**, *10*, 1665–1669. [CrossRef]
30. Giuffrida, A.; Leweke, F.M.; Gerth, C.W.; Schreiber, D.; Koethe, D.; Faulhaber, J.; Klosterkötter, J.; Piomelli, D. Cerebrospinal Anandamide Levels are Elevated in Acute Schizophrenia and are Inversely Correlated with Psychotic Symptoms. *Neuropsychopharmacology* **2004**, *29*, 2108–2114. [CrossRef]
31. Leweke, F.M.; Giuffrida, A.; Koethe, D.; Schreiber, D.; Nolden, B.M.; Kranaster, L.; Neatby, M.A.; Schneider, M.; Gerth, C.W.; Hellmich, M.; et al. Anandamide levels in cerebrospinal fluid of first-episode schizophrenic patients: Impact of cannabis use. *Schizophr. Res.* **2007**, *94*, 29–36. [CrossRef]
32. Ceccarini, J.; De Hert, M.; Van Winkel, R.; Peuskens, J.; Bormans, G.; Kranaster, L.; Enning, F.; Koethe, D.; Leweke, F.M.; Van Laere, K. Increased ventral striatal CB1 receptor binding is related to negative symptoms in drug-free patients with schizophrenia. *Neuroimage* **2013**, *79*, 304–312. [CrossRef]

33. Ranganathan, M.; Cortes-Briones, J.; Radhakrishnan, R.; Thurnauer, H.; Planeta, B.; Skosnik, P.; Gao, H.; Labaree, D.; Neumeister, A.; Pittman, B.; et al. Reduced Brain Cannabinoid Receptor Availability in Schizophrenia. *Biol. Psychiatry* **2016**, *79*, 997–1005. [CrossRef]
34. De Vries, T.J.; Schoffelmeer, A.N.M. Cannabinoid CB1 receptors control conditioned drug seeking. *Trends Pharmacol. Sci.* **2005**, *26*, 420–426. [CrossRef]
35. Maldonado, R.; Valverde, O.; Berrendero, F. Involvement of the endocannabinoid system in drug addiction. *Trends Neurosci.* **2006**, *29*, 225–232. [CrossRef]
36. Fattore, L.; Fadda, P.; Spano, M.S.; Pistis, M.; Fratta, W. Neurobiological mechanisms of cannabinoid addiction. *Mol. Cell. Endocrinol.* **2008**, *286*, S97–S107. [CrossRef]
37. Chye, Y.; Christensen, E.; Solowij, N.; Yücel, M. The Endocannabinoid System and Cannabidiol's Promise for the Treatment of Substance Use Disorder. *Front. Psychiatry* **2019**, *10*. [CrossRef]
38. Parsons, L.H.; Hurd, Y.L. Endocannabinoid signalling in reward and addiction. *Nat. Rev. Neurosci.* **2015**, *16*, 579–594. [CrossRef]
39. Hunt, G. Medication compliance and comorbid substance abuse in schizophrenia: Impact on community survival 4 years after a relapse. *Schizophr. Res.* **2002**, *54*, 253–264. [CrossRef]
40. Crockford, D.; Addington, D. Canadian Schizophrenia Guidelines: Schizophrenia and Other Psychotic Disorders with Coexisting Substance Use Disorders. *Can. J. Psychiatry* **2017**, *62*, 624–634. [CrossRef]
41. Schoeler, T.; Petros, N.; Di Forti, M.; Klamerus, E.; Foglia, E.; Murray, R.; Bhattacharyya, S. Poor medication adherence and risk of relapse associated with continued cannabis use in patients with first-episode psychosis: A prospective analysis. *Lancet Psychiatry* **2017**, *4*, 627–633. [CrossRef]
42. D'Souza, D.C.; Abi-Saab, W.M.; Madonick, S.; Forselius-Bielen, K.; Doersch, A.; Braley, G.; Gueorguieva, R.; Cooper, T.B.; Krystal, J.H. Delta-9-tetrahydrocannabinol effects in schizophrenia: Implications for cognition, psychosis, and addiction. *Biol. Psychiatry* **2005**, *57*, 594–608. [CrossRef]
43. Foti, D.J.; Kotov, R.; Guey, L.T.; Bromet, E.J. Cannabis use and the course of schizophrenia: 10-year follow-up after first hospitalization. *Am. J. Psychiatry* **2010**, *167*, 987–993. [CrossRef]
44. Batalla, A.; Bhattacharyya, S.; Yücel, M.; Fusar-Poli, P.; Crippa, J.A.; Nogué, S.; Torrens, M.; Pujol, J.; Farré, M.; Martin-Santos, R. Structural and Functional Imaging Studies in Chronic Cannabis Users: A Systematic Review of Adolescent and Adult Findings. *PLoS ONE* **2013**, *8*, e55821. [CrossRef]
45. Foglia, E.; Schoeler, T.; Klamerus, E.; Morgan, K.; Bhattacharyya, S. Cannabis use and adherence to antipsychotic medication: A systematic review and meta-analysis. *Psychol. Med.* **2017**, *47*, 1691–1705. [CrossRef]
46. Zuardi, A.W.; Shirakawa, I.; Finkelfarb, E.; Karniol, I.G. Action of cannabidiol on the anxiety and other effects produced by δ^9-THC in normal subjects. *Psychopharmacology (Berl.)* **1982**, *76*, 245–250. [CrossRef]
47. Englund, A.; Morrison, P.D.; Nottage, J.; Hague, D.; Kane, F.; Bonaccorso, S.; Stone, J.M.; Reichenberg, A.; Brenneisen, R.; Holt, D.; et al. Cannabidiol inhibits THC-elicited paranoid symptoms and hippocampal-dependent memory impairment. *J. Psychopharmacol.* **2013**, *27*, 19–27. [CrossRef]
48. Iseger, T.A.; Bossong, M.G. A systematic review of the antipsychotic properties of cannabidiol in humans. *Schizophr. Res.* **2015**, *162*, 153–161. [CrossRef]
49. Leweke, F.M.; Mueller, J.K.; Lange, B.; Rohleder, C. Therapeutic Potential of Cannabinoids in Psychosis. *Biol. Psychiatry* **2016**, *79*, 604–612. [CrossRef]
50. Moher, D.; Liberati, A.; Tetzlaff, J.; Altman, D.G. Preferred Reporting Items for Systematic Reviews and Meta-Analyses: The PRISMA Statement. *PLoS Med.* **2009**, *6*, e1000097. [CrossRef]
51. Zuardi, A.W.; Morais, S.L.; Guimarães, F.S.; Mechoulam, R. Antipsychotic effect of cannabidiol. *J. Clin. Psychiatry* **1995**, *56*, 485–486.
52. Zuardi, A.W.; Hallak, J.E.C.; Dursun, S.M.; Morais, S.L.; Sanches, R.F.; Musty, R.E.; Crippa, J.A.S. Cannabidiol monotherapy for treatment-resistant schizophrenia. *J. Psychopharmacol.* **2006**, *20*, 683–686. [CrossRef]
53. Makiol, C.; Kluge, M. Remission of severe, treatment-resistant schizophrenia following adjunctive cannabidiol. *Aust. New Zeal. J. Psychiatry* **2019**, *53*, 262. [CrossRef]
54. Leweke, F.M.; Piomelli, D.; Pahlisch, F.; Muhl, D.; Gerth, C.W.; Hoyer, C.; Klosterkötter, J.; Hellmich, M.; Koethe, D. Cannabidiol enhances anandamide signaling and alleviates psychotic symptoms of schizophrenia. *Transl. Psychiatry* **2012**, *2*, e94. [CrossRef]

55. McGuire, P.; Robson, P.; Cubala, W.J.; Vasile, D.; Morrison, P.D.; Barron, R.; Taylor, A.; Wright, S. Cannabidiol (CBD) as an adjunctive therapy in schizophrenia: A multicenter randomized controlled trial. *Am. J. Psychiatry* **2018**, *175*, 225–231. [CrossRef]
56. Hallak, J.E.C.; Machado-de-Sousa, J.P.; Crippa, J.A.S.; Sanches, R.F.; Trzesniak, C.; Chaves, C.; Bernardo, S.A.; Regalo, S.C.; Zuardi, A.W. Performance of schizophrenic patients in the Stroop Color Word Test and electrodermal responsiveness after acute administration of cannabidiol (CBD). *Rev. Bras. Psiquiatr.* **2010**, *32*, 56–61. [CrossRef] [PubMed]
57. Boggs, D.L.; Surti, T.; Gupta, A.; Gupta, S.; Niciu, M.; Pittman, B.; Schnakenberg Martin, A.M.; Thurnauer, H.; Davies, A.; D'Souza, D.C.; et al. The effects of cannabidiol (CBD) on cognition and symptoms in outpatients with chronic schizophrenia a randomized placebo controlled trial. *Psychopharmacology (Berl.)* **2018**, *235*, 1923–1932. [CrossRef] [PubMed]
58. Allsop, D.J.; Copeland, J.; Lintzeris, N.; Dunlop, A.J.; Montebello, M.; Sadler, C.; Rivas, G.R.; Holland, R.M.; Muhleisen, P.; Norberg, M.M.; et al. Nabiximols as an agonist replacement therapy during cannabis withdrawal: A randomized clinical trial. *JAMA Psychiatry* **2014**, *71*, 281–291. [CrossRef] [PubMed]
59. Trigo, J.M.; Soliman, A.; Staios, G.; Quilty, L.; Fischer, B.; George, T.P.; Rehm, J.; Selby, P.; Barnes, A.J.; Huestis, M.A.; et al. Sativex associated with behavioral-relapse prevention strategy as treatment for cannabis dependence: A case series. *J. Addict. Med.* **2016**, *10*, 274–279. [CrossRef] [PubMed]
60. Trigo, J.M.; Soliman, A.; Quilty, L.C.; Fischer, B.; Rehm, J.; Selby, P.; Barnes, A.J.; Huestis, M.A.; George, T.P.; Streiner, D.L.; et al. Nabiximols combined with motivational enhancement/cognitive behavioral therapy for the treatment of cannabis dependence: A pilot randomized clinical trial. *PLoS ONE* **2018**, *13*, 1–21. [CrossRef] [PubMed]
61. Crippa, J.A.S.; Hallak, J.E.C.; Machado-De-Sousa, J.P.; Queiroz, R.H.C.; Bergamaschi, M.; Chagas, M.H.N.; Zuardi, A.W. Cannabidiol for the treatment of cannabis withdrawal syndrome: A case report. *J. Clin. Pharm. Ther.* **2013**, *38*, 162–164. [CrossRef]
62. Shannon, S.; Opila-Lehman, J. Cannabidiol Oil for Decreasing Addictive Use of Marijuana: A Case Report. *Integr. Med. (Encinitas)* **2015**, *14*, 31–35.
63. Solowij, N.; Broyd, S.J.; Beale, C.; Prick, J.-A.; Greenwood, L.; van Hell, H.; Suo, C.; Galettis, P.; Pai, N.; Fu, S.; et al. Therapeutic Effects of Prolonged Cannabidiol Treatment on Psychological Symptoms and Cognitive Function in Regular Cannabis Users: A Pragmatic Open-Label Clinical Trial. *Cannabis Cannabinoid Res.* **2018**, *3*, 21–34. [CrossRef]
64. Morgan, C.J.A.; Das, R.K.; Joye, A.; Curran, H.V.; Kamboj, S.K. Cannabidiol reduces cigarette consumption in tobacco smokers: Preliminary findings. *Addict. Behav.* **2013**, *38*, 2433–2436. [CrossRef]
65. Hindocha, C.; Freeman, T.P.; Grabski, M.; Stroud, J.B.; Crudgington, H.; Davies, A.C.; Das, R.K.; Lawn, W.; Morgan, C.J.A.; Curran, H.V. Cannabidiol reverses attentional bias to cigarette cues in a human experimental model of tobacco withdrawal. *Addiction* **2018**, *113*, 1696–1705. [CrossRef]
66. Schipper, R.; Dekker, M.; de Haan, L.; van den Brink, W. Medicinal cannabis (Bedrolite) substitution therapy in inpatients with a psychotic disorder and a comorbid cannabis use disorder: A case series. *J. Psychopharmacol.* **2018**, *32*, 353–356. [CrossRef]
67. Monji, A.; Kato, T.; Kanba, S. Cytokines and schizophrenia: Microglia hypothesis of schizophrenia. *Psychiatry Clin. Neurosci.* **2009**, *63*, 257–265. [CrossRef]
68. Gangadin, S.S.; Nasib, L.G.; Sommer, I.E.C.; Mandl, R.C.W. MRI investigation of immune dysregulation in schizophrenia. *Curr. Opin. Psychiatry* **2019**, *32*, 164–169. [CrossRef]
69. Gomes, F.V.; Llorente, R.; Del Bel, E.A.; Viveros, M.-P.; López-Gallardo, M.; Guimarães, F.S. Decreased glial reactivity could be involved in the antipsychotic-like effect of cannabidiol. *Schizophr. Res.* **2015**, *164*, 155–163. [CrossRef]
70. Englund, A.; Freeman, T.P.; Murray, R.M.; McGuire, P. Can we make cannabis safer? *Lancet Psychiatry* **2017**, *4*, 643–648. [CrossRef]

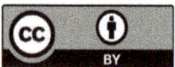

© 2019 by the authors. Licensee MDPI, Basel, Switzerland. This article is an open access article distributed under the terms and conditions of the Creative Commons Attribution (CC BY) license (http://creativecommons.org/licenses/by/4.0/).

MDPI
St. Alban-Anlage 66
4052 Basel
Switzerland
Tel. +41 61 683 77 34
Fax +41 61 302 89 18
www.mdpi.com

Journal of Clinical Medicine Editorial Office
E-mail: jcm@mdpi.com
www.mdpi.com/journal/jcm

www.ingramcontent.com/pod-product-compliance
Lightning Source LLC
LaVergne TN
LVHW070627100526
838202LV00012B/747